SHIPWRECK

OF THE

SINGULAR

HEALTHCARE'S CASTAWAYS

Crusoe,
We say was 'Rescued'.
So we have chosen.

Obsessed, bewildered
By the shipwreck
Of the singular
We have chosen the meaning
Of being numerous.

George Oppen
Of Being Numerous

Cover Design/Illustration: Billiam James

First Printing, 2021

Title: Shipwreck of the Singular: Healthcare's Castaways

ISBN: 978-1-989963-16-6

Publisher: Samizdat Health Writer's Co-operative Inc.

www.samizdathealth.org
www.davidhealy.org
www.study329.org

SHIPWRECK
OF THE
SINGULAR

HEALTHCARE'S CASTAWAYS

DAVID HEALY

Samizdat Health

Samizdat Health Writer's Co-operative Inc.

CONTENTS

Sources and References: Author's Note

Serious books come festooned with references. If checked these often do not support the author. There are no references in *Shipwreck*. This will annoy some and please others.

Shipwreck notes the source of quotes and little else. Dates of birth and death, Sigmund Freud (1856–1939), can be googled. Googling every drug, theme or person mentioned will throw up fascinating material, much of it at odds with what is here.

Online however, at www.samizdathealth.org/shipwreck/, there is more reference material than most books have—what I've been reading while writing *Shipwreck*, and all interviews undertaken as background material, much of it downloadable.

Part 1, The Early Years, was shaped by research on the history of medicine, that included creating historical epidemiology, and a fate that roped me into translating the work of Philippe Pinel.

Part 2, The Intervening Years, was shaped by a decade spent in early neuroscience, which put me in a position to interview the makers of psychopharmacology. Seen at close quarters, the neuroscience adopted by pharmaceutical marketing looks like a biobabble, closer to hucksterism, than science. These are all downloadable from Samizdat.

Part 3, Castaways, was shaped by a series of treatment scandals that gave me a passport into the bowels of the corporations at the heart of this story. Samizdat has many documents on how they manage the risks we pose them. Other documents are bound by confidentiality clauses but I've been saying these things regularly for years without being sued, despite companies scrutinizing everything I write and placing people in lectures I give with a view to suing me if they can. You will have to make your own mind up about these points.

The entire book is shaped by something else. In 2008 *Pharmageddon* took a first stab at outlining forces tearing healthcare apart. It focused on America but was as much about the threat posed to Britain's National Health System, and an inevitable drop in life expectancy. It took four years to find a publisher. In 2008 I worked clinically in a rural part of Britain unaffected by these forces. The local mental health services were the safest and most cost-efficient in the UK. Colleagues said they would work for free if they won the lottery. Since 2012 staff have left or been fired, stress leave has rocketed, the service hemorrhages money, and suicide rates have risen. Clinicians have been replaced by managers and the culture is now one of bullying and harassment. This catastrophic collapse in care has shaped *Shipwreck*.

When she saw the first draft of *Shipwreck* my agent said it would never get published. This led to a parting of our ways and to Samizdat, a writer's co-operative dedicated to books that see the world through a health lens —books that other publishers appear nervous about taking.

Samizdat enables me to change mistakes or add details and useful sources at will. I hope every reader will think about contributing, by pointing out where details are wrong, adding references that might help other readers, and engaging in debates.

Even if annoyed by some positions, I hope you will focus on the big picture and critique or comment on issues that bother you. A lot more could be said about Trauma or Conflicts of Interest, for instance, and my approach may seem to downplay the importance of these and other topics. Samizdat will publish anything sent this way and help spread any discussions that take off. Send all comments to david.healy@rxisk.org.

Shipwreck offers a HealthCare platform. It has been sent to several political parties, and we welcome input from anyone who has an interest in these issues or connections to someone who has.

Introduction

Life expectancy in the United States had been falling since 2014. In 2019 Britain's Office of National Statistics estimated babies born there today will live 3 years less than had been expected 5 years before. In France and Germany, countries that along with America and Britain made modern medicine, and other European countries, life expectancy has stalled.

Some view the pre-Covid increased US death rates as stemming from America's opioid crisis and lack of access to healthcare. Deaths of despair. Britain, France, and Germany, however, have good access to healthcare and no opioid crises. Poverty kills in all these countries, but a greater intensity of health services also kills and disables, regardless of social class. Questions as to why more health services might harm us emerged in 1990s America. They were shot down as 'rationing'. US politicians who tried to re-open the issue in 2010 faced claims they were creating 'death panels'

The response to a fall in life expectancy has been silence. Mental illness, often the canary in the medical mine, offers a cautionary tale. Reports of falling life expectancy in schizophrenia appeared in 2000. By 2006 there was agreement people with schizophrenia lose up to 20 years of life compared to the rest of us. The greatest risk of death lies in the first 5 years of the illness. A century ago, people with schizophrenia lived as long as the rest of us. These data, so at odds with medicine's vision of itself, have met silence.

Faced with horrific birth defects caused by a sleeping pill, thalidomide, in 1962 the US Food and Drug Administration (FDA) adopted a set of regulations that today are the greatest influence on healthcare in every country on earth. These regulations are key to the fall in life expectancy. They have led to an increase in drug wrecks (treatment-related adverse events) that regulations were supposed to solve or at least manage.

Treatment related deaths are now the third leading cause of hospital deaths, even though the contribution of drugs is written out of the script in, for instance, cancer or cardiovascular deaths, when our treatments often kill us. Our medicines must be an even commoner cause of death and disability in our homes and workplaces where the conditions treated are less severe though the treatments are just as toxic. But this has not been looked at.

In 1980 comparatively few of us were taking more than 1 drug per day and then only in short courses. As of 2020, over 50% of us of all ages are on at least one drug every day, 40% over 45 are on at least 3 drugs, and 40% over 65 are on 5 drugs or more. For a decade, an increasing amount of evidence shows that reducing drug burdens to 5 or less drugs per day increases life expectancy, reduces hospitalizations, and improves quality of life. Yet even though we can do something to solve the problem, the evidence that our treatments may be shortening our lives is met with silence.

Tobacco's contribution to cancers and heart attacks led to a wobble in (male) life expectancies in 1962. This adds to the point, especially if we add in alcohol and opioids, that the substances we consume can harm us. Medicines are on prescription because they are thought to be more dangerous than alcohol and tobacco. An ever-increasing number of us, however, blithely take 5 or more of these substances every day.

There are fates worse than death. Over 15% of us take antidepressants, 80% taking them indefinitely, primarily because we can't stop. Every drug has a hundred effects. For antidepressants, sexual dysfunction is one of the 99 other things every drug does that pharmaceutical companies don't want us to know about. These drugs compromise the sex life of everyone who takes them, and thousands remain permanently sexually dysfunctional for decades after stopping.

All other best-selling treatments, the statins for cholesterol, drugs for osteoporosis, reflux, asthma, or Type II diabetes, can also cripple us. These treatments may not offer a clear enough benefit to warrant being included among the 5 or less drugs whose disabling effects we might have to put up with as part of a life-saving trade-off. But our health systems now force these drugs on us.

We have forgotten the lesson of thalidomide, that modern medicines are dangerous miracles. As a result of thalidomide, pregnant women avoid soft cheeses, uncooked meats, hot showers, tobacco, and alcohol. But because of thalidomide, with every drug we take we swallow an invisible set of techniques that all but force 15% of pregnant women to take antidepressants, despite evidence these drugs double birth defects, miscarriages, and Autistic Spectrum Disorder rates, about which there is silence.

Every time a solider with Post-Traumatic Stress Disorder (PTSD), obeying orders, swallows an antidepressant, unaware it won't help, he increases the pressure on women to take antidepressants and other medicines, while pregnant. This book grapples with this extraordinary situation and the silence in which it is shrouded.

Shipwreck looks at medical techniques through the window of our falling life expectancies and increasing disabilities and beyond that at the role of technique in driving history. It looks at one set of techniques in particular, as invisible as carbon dioxide, that have changed the climate of medicine in a manner that is a real and present danger to each of us.

Techniques include technologies like guns and the behavioral techniques built into social media platforms aimed at nudging us one way or the other. All techniques are one-dimensional, but our lives are not. Whether techniques enhance or diminish us depends on our willingness to take responsibility for their use. There is no better place to see this than with the combination of physical and behavioral techniques that is a medicine. When we control medical techniques, we have healthcare; when they control us, health becomes a service industry.

The Changing Climate

The change in the global climate is not yet something we clearly experience. But there has been a climate change in our health services that you can experience when you visit a doctor and is now a daily experience for staff working in these systems.

In response to a person being injured by a prescribed drug, most doctors now sign up to the claim that the plural of anecdote is not data. If hundreds of people are harmed that is still anecdotal. This claim upends traditional medicine, which regarded reports of something new on a drug as serious science and accumulating reports as strengthening evidence. The claim also inverts the original—the plural of anecdote is data. If the plural of anecdote is not data, medicine and Google are heading toward each other on the same piece of track. How did this happen? What will happen when they meet?

If we paid heed to them, drug wrecks remain the best way to discover new drugs. Between keeping us safe and discovering new drugs, there is money to be made from drug wrecks. Instead, we now go to extraordinary lengths to avoid acknowledging the possibility of wrecks. The claim that drug wrecks are anecdotes is at the heart of these efforts, leaving us marooned where we have been drug-wrecked.

Many doctors notionally accept the 'known' side effects of a treatment. For anyone on a cocktail of drugs they may figure some interaction could cause difficulties. Faced with us raising something not in the drug's label, however, they go blank. No doctors today are trained in how to establish if a drug is causing an adverse event. We are often better placed than our doctor to decide if things are going wrong. If privately they accept our treatment is causing issues, few will support us publicly. Many become nasty if pushed.

Medical arrogance might be something to live with if doctors were doing something without which we would die. Today, however, they are as likely to disable as save us. In 1962 we who knew little about medicine were up against medical expertise. Today, we are up against an expert ability to ignore or deny what is in front of everyone's nose. This denial is more profound than the denial experienced by those who have been sexually abused.

The adverse effects of psychotropic drugs—suicidality, homicidality, agitation, loss of libido, brain fog, and others—overlap with the symptoms of the disorders for which they are prescribed. If we claim our drugs are causing difficulties, at best this will lead to entries in our medical record about our lack of insight. If we insist, we risk detention and compulsory treatment with the cause of our 'illness'. Across the Western world more people are now detained and treated by mental health services than were detained in the 1980s.

At present, conflicts of interest are the favorite explanation for this situation. Doctors aren't supposed to have interests other than their patients, but they supposedly get money from drug companies. Conflict of interest is important. Unless doctors recognize drug-wrecks they risk going out of business. If that's not an incentive to recognize treatment hazards, it's hard to know what is. But doctors are paying ever less heed.

Anne-Marie offers a paradigmatic case of the issues drug wrecks pose. A nervous 33-year-old, she choked on food at her father's funeral. A few weeks later, having difficulties swallowing, she went to a doctor who put her on liquid paroxetine, a selective serotonin reuptake inhibiting (SSRI) antidepressant. Her choking cleared like magic. She was less nervous driving and more confident socially.

A year later a friend cautioned her that her drinking was getting out of control. She began hearing stories of what she had done the night before of which she had no memory.

When she was arrested for being drunk and disorderly, she wondered about paroxetine. She contacted GlaxoSmithKline, the makers of paroxetine, who told her it wouldn't cause anyone to drink but they would contact her doctor. Her doctor put her questions about paroxetine down to alcoholic denial. This was easily done—she had dropped out of school at 16 and had no background in healthcare. At her insistence, months afterwards he switched her to citalopram. Her drinking got worse. She didn't realize she had been switched from one SSRI to another. Suggesting a link between her drinking and her medication at AA meetings, she was told her thinking proved she was an alcoholic.

Several arrests, a crashed car, and lost job later, she began researching the serotonin system on which SSRIs work. After months of interneting, she asked her doctor to switch her to mirtazapine. This acts in the opposite way to SSRIs. Either she was more insistent than most patients, or he was less nasty than many doctors, but he did so. Her drinking stopped. This research, however, was not enough to prevent a conviction for disorderly behavior that made her unemployable and shredded her belief in justice.

As Anne-Marie's story unfolded, the Western world's largest selling newspaper, a guardian of conservative values, Britain's *Daily Mail*, ran an increasing number of stories about women killing pedestrians while driving drunk, being divorced by high profile partners because of their drinking, or having their children removed because of their inability to control their drinking. Antidepressants lurk at the heart of many of these cases.

Meanwhile, as signs proliferated in restaurants warning pregnant women not to drink, a study reported that pregnant women taking SSRIs were ten times more likely to have a baby born with Fetal Alcohol Spectrum Disorder (FASD). The researchers put this striking finding in a footnote; they had no idea SSRIs can compel people to drink.

Even without alcohol, SSRIs are more likely to cause birth defects and disturbed behaviors in children born to women taking them in pregnancy than modest alcohol intake is. Far from warnings against the use of antidepressants in pregnancy, many women are browbeaten into taking them when pregnant.

Anne-Marie had no studies of SSRIs and alcoholism to appeal to. Apart from anecdotes, the only source of evidence was drug development pipelines. Working with anecdotes like Anne-Marie's, industry had also concluded that SSRIs can cause alcoholism and mirtazapine like drugs can reduce cravings for alcohol. Should industry bring a drug that suppresses cravings to market, doctors will very quickly slip into making a connection between the serotonin system and alcoholism. They will likely never remember they regarded a series of Anne-Maries as flawed, almost depraved, women.

This case struck me because I have a doctorate in the serotonin system. Here was a school drop-out educating me about this system. Over 80% of observations made in this way turn out to be correct. While the authority of a doctor might help transform the observation into a medical fact, it is the Anne-Maries of this world who make the observations. With internet access, they often do a lot more. Motivation is worth more than expertise. Both however are up against power.

Becoming Invisible

September 20 1991 is a key date in this history. We had survived 1984. The Berlin Wall had come down. There was talk of the End of History. We were being told we now lived in Risk Societies. Through to August, unexpected clinical events like Anne-Marie's were welcomed as an important way to advance medical science. By October, we could become alcoholic on an SSRI, and our doctors would miss it.

On this day, Eli Lilly, defending their blockbuster antidepressant, Prozac, against compelling reports it could cause suicidality, ran a which are you going to believe defense—the anecdotes or the data? The company did this with the blessing of the FDA. It had help of the *BMJ*, the medical journal most 'anti' the pharmaceutical industry. The brave new evidence-based world ushered in that day has descended into medical fascism now. There is fake news on all sides. Truth is a discredited commodity. And health care has been transformed into a service industry.

When things go this badly wrong, our need for an account of what is happening puts us at risk of succumbing to a fiction. Two hundred years ago, we could turn to Providence as a repository for questions that don't have answers. The fiction we are now offered is some version of: "We're making progress. If something went wrong, it was an accident." Whatever the ultimate answers to life might be, the answer this book offers to what happens when something goes wrong on treatment is: "*There are no accidents.*"

Mentioning drug-induced difficulties to your doctor offers a glimpse on the inner structure of our world. Tiananmen-Square like, you will find yourself staring down the barrel of a tank facing someone whose options are to shoot you or get shot. If you dare say drug wreck while he is deciding whether to blow you away, he will demur and say side effect, or adverse event, which suggest something accidental that could not be foreseen. But there is nothing accidental about drug wrecks, or about efforts to write off such events as accidental. These events that might wreck your life are intrinsic to the nature of a drug.

Economics is from Mars, Medicine from Venus

In terms of making sense of what you might glimpse down the barrel of a tank, the narratives that have dominated our thinking from 1800 to 2020 stemmed from a set of signature events linked to the Industrial and French Revolutions. Efforts to grapple with these issues around 1848 gave rise to conservatism, liberalism, socialism, communism, anarchism, and religious fundamentalism. We were all forced to wear a new set of tribal badges.

In 1848 this new world's issues stared every urban dweller or factory owner and worker in the face. A new beast, the economy, was replacing religion as the thing we had to get right. Today's key issues stare us and our doctors in the face when we meet.

Modern medicine and modern economics were born at the same time. In 1848 there was little to choose between Rudolph Virchow, a Berlin physician, who claimed politics was nothing more than medicine on a grand scale and Karl Marx writing *The Communist Manifesto*. Doctors did more to shape this manifesto than economists.

Since then, economics has taken a lead in shaping the rules (*nomos*) of our common house (*oikos*) to the disadvantage of many, especially women. The *oikos-nomos* books that shave shaped our lives since 1848 were written by people who likely found the medical world as impenetrable as many of us find economics. Almost all of them, Marx repetitively, attended doctors.

None of them thought that medical offices rather than factories then or banks now might be a place to interrogate the modern world.

The split has been of 'Economics is from Mars and Medicine is from Venus' proportions. Viewed through a health lens, the most primitive divide is between fortunate and unfortunate rather than rich and poor, black and white, male and female.

In 1848 factory owners had to manage industrial 'accidents', aware some workers viewed them as industrial 'murder'. These 'events', to pick a neutral word, were comparatively rare, but they shaped medicine and briefly made doctors a revolutionary force. Drug wreck 'events' now happen on an industrial scale. Doctors are at the forefront in suppressing information about them.

The medical world is not a world of self-made men. It is or should be a world of relationships. Economics centers on the impersonal—money. Healing is interpersonal. Medicine might seem to many even more dependent on expertise than economics but at least the way the story is told here the motivation of an Anne-Marie counts for more than expertise.

Calls for sustainable economic growth in response to climate change sound like rationing, a settling for second best. Falling life expectancies and the changing climate in healthcare call on us to sustain what we cherish rather than ask us to give things up.

This said, Marx and others faced an irruption into daily life of new techniques and commodities. Their efforts aimed at understanding the transformations in what it meant to be human triggered by these changes rather than just the economics of a marketplace. It has only been since the emergence of a new kind of pharmaceutical in 1935 that medicine has had to grapple with commodification. Given a century to prepare, we should have been better able to predict and manage the impact of pharmaceuticals.

We face challenges in health from the growing costs of drugs to a degradation of care. Top-downs solutions for these issues look to health policies, incentives, patents, and barriers to access to medicines, and propose changes which often make things worse.

Shipwreck calls on your experience of healthcare. Drug wrecks bring the difficulties of our time into focus more clearly than anything else. They are, and so long as we use medicines, will continue to be, an Achilles Heel for technique. An answer to drug wrecks cannot be imposed from above.

Robinson Crusoe

Shipwreck maps onto *Robinson Crusoe* for a few reasons. His journey and ours began around 1660, the year in which the first shoots of modern economics and medicine appeared and the birth of what was then openly called political medicine, a combination of words both medicine and politics now try to avoid.

Crusoe was an Adventurer, an 'entrepreneur,' as the French termed it, facing a New World. Rather than settle down as his father advised, risks were there to be taken. The politics of his day hinged on religion but would soon center on property ownership. The invisible hand of Providence, then the main driver of events, was about to be replaced by the invisible hand of the Market. Crusoe prefigures this.

We too face a new world, where progress in health is the lodestar of politics. Beneath the skin, however, this progress is beginning to look like a morally neutral advance of technique. Techniques that might once have enhanced us now risk diminishing us. The arc of this moral universe does not bend toward justice as Martin Luther King—whom we can imagine as a descendant of slaves Crusoe planned to transport from Africa to the Americas on his fateful voyage—hoped. Technique is amoral. Any bending must come from us.

When Crusoe set sail, a pendulum in European society had swung toward individuals and risk taking and away from solidarity and tradition. Away from accidents and toward crashes and disasters. His adventurism led him to the Americas and his shipwreck. The pendulum is swinging again. Our singular experiences when drug-wrecked are now weighed in a balance against a statistical collective and declared accidents rather than crashes.

If a mine collapses now or a ship sinks, while not admitting responsibility, we search for survivors. But no-one will search for you if you are marooned by a drug wreck, even though we know where you are. Regulators and politicians would prefer you dead than discovered. Marooned, you will face questions Crusoe asked: Why Me, Why Now?

The Early Years

Both *Shipwreck* and *Robinson Crusoe* involve a break with the past (Early Years), a period of consolidation and voyages of hope (Intervening Years), interrupted by a wreck, leading to a period as a castaway threatened by savagery (Castaway). *Crusoe* ends with an escape. *Shipwreck* doesn't.

Everyone knows where Crusoe ends up. Few read his account of the elements of his character and moral ambiguities of his time that led him to leave his family and later sail in search of slaves to transport from Africa to his Brazilian plantation. When marooned, he wonders if these traits and ambiguities 'caused' his shipwreck.

A good account of the journey to the place we are now marooned should shed light on socialism, conservatism, communism, neoliberalism, identity politics, and climate change. *Shipwreck* also juxtaposes JFK and Louis XVI, sheds light on the roots of our current opioid epidemic, touches on Brexit, and names the originator of thalidomide, a drug of which it could be said it's still too early to judge the consequences.

Getting history to make sense is a tall order, when even watching a single relationship break up can leave us uncertain about what has just happened. There is no option but to eliminate 99.99% of the pain and rage of the last 220 years, voices silenced by age, sex, race, and class. But this story of a silencing happening now might shed light on past silencings.

At the risk of demonstrating a tin ear for American, German, or other 'realities', I have used versions of France, Britain, Germany and America to bring out the origins of the medical model (France), political medicine (Britain), pharmaceutical technique (Germany), and Big Medicine (America).

Wars emerge from this narrative as perhaps the greatest factor shaping the trajectory of medicine, nicely symbolized by the term Magic Bullet. War has been a grisly medical experiment, in which through to 1904 disease killed more than weapons did. To win a War the best medical techniques were as important as the best military techniques.

The Intervening Years

The years between 1929 and 1989 saw Britain turn to single payer healthcare as America went private. The 1962 Food and Drugs Act cut across all else, even these diametrically opposite systems. We now have increasingly similar systems in both countries, neither public nor private, more health service than healthcare.

Well-intentioned initiatives now seem to make things worse. Randomized Controlled Trials (RCTs), the Holy Grail of Evidence Based Medicine (EBM), have become the key generator of misinformation about drug wrecks. Campaigns for access to high-cost medicines now drive polypharmacy. Efforts to ensure a degree of consistency between doctors has produced a service industry that brings illnesses to us to induce us to consume drugs. Pharmaceutical companies, meanwhile, no longer see cures for the diseases we want remedied as a viable business model.

Key sections of this story are told through the careers of Louis Lasagna and William Haddad. Lasagna was responsible for introducing RCTs into medicine, a move he later regretted. RCTs laid the basis for what is now called EBM. Haddad was the driving force behind the emergence of a generic pharmaceutical industry and access to medicine campaigns.

Using anyone to tell a story risks turning a real person into a cipher. Lasagna's early work gave rise to a famous article, "The Powerful Placebo". Thirty years later he tracked what had become of the placebo concept in a piece called "The Powerful Cipher". All celebrity and most concepts become ciphers.

Knowing where individual stories end up, the temptation is to draw a line through selected points to make events seem inevitable. The twists and turns in the Haddad and Lasagna stories defy straight lines. Mark

Twain said Truth is stranger than Fiction because Fiction has to make sense. Those convinced of their claim on truth invariably tell a simple story. *Shipwreck* is neither simple nor comforting.

The cost of medicines was an issue that tied Lasagna and Haddad together. Since 1960, escalating drug costs have alarmed and bewildered everyone. Every apparently foolproof initiative to contain these costs has seen them rise even faster. The costs of health services now risk toppling entire economies.

Despite drug costs rising faster than anything else in health for over 60 years, companies claim drug expenditures have remained a constant fraction of health budgets. The simple three-card trick behind this claim stumps politicians and policy wonks.

While taking opposite sides on many of these issues, Lasagna and Haddad both fought to increase access to medicines for patients with AIDS (Acquired Immune Deficiency Syndrome). Their efforts helped shape one of the greatest triumphs of modern medicine, the discovery of and access to Triple Therapy for AIDS.

In any decent romance, Triple Therapy would have led us to a new sunny medical upland. Instead, Triple Therapy was a sideshow to a replacement of healthcare by health services, characterized by a focus on risk, an emphasis on individual responsibility rather than collective action, and increased managerialism.

These changes in medicine paralleled a turn by politicians and economists to neoliberalism, a vague term used indiscriminately to account for the ills of the modern world. It is invoked to explain everything that has gone wrong since 1980. But neoliberalism is a slogan not an explanation. We are facing a neo-something and desperately need to work out neo-what.

While tackling AIDS, Lasagna and Haddad were unaware of CIDS, also born in 1980. CIDS (Clinical Immune Deficiency Syndrome) like AIDS is caused by a new kind of virus, a Clinical Immunodeficiency Virus (CIV). This is transmitted by doctors, as surely as they once killed patients by not washing their hands. CIV causes CIDS (drug wrecks).

By 1980 pharmaceutical companies had begun to sequester the data from trials of their drugs, ghostwrite the articles reporting these trials, and put in place a hands-off public relations operation the National Rifle Association would die for. These are aimed at disabling the clinical immune system we need functioning properly if we are to gamble on taking a poison or submit to a mutilation. The greatest concentration of Fake News on the planet now centers on the drugs your doctor gives you, as it has done for 3 decades.

These changes have made it easy to cast Big Pharma as a pantomime villain. Big Risk (health insurance and government) were once seen as having opposing market interests to Pharma, but they now comfortably share a bed with Pharma. Are we up against a mindless totalitarianism, or is there an engineer of human souls at the controls?

We could now offer good healthcare for free but instead every effort to make the system add to the wealth of nations, from Lasagna's RCTs and Haddad's generic pharmaceuticals to Evidence Based Medicine, increases costs, reduces access, and compromises care. Can anything be done to make our systems work for us rather than against us?

This is not a dry economic issue. Healthcare was there for us when we had medical difficulties. Health services now invade us, giving us disorders not just with our cholesterol levels but with our 'identity'. The tremendous pressure these services exert on each of us force us to establish and maintain an identity, fueling identity-based epidemics based on gender, or neurodiversity. More epidemics spread by Health Apps are coming our way. We once had religion to cope with an indifferent universe. It is not clear what if any shelter there is in a health universe, indifferent to us other than as consumers.

Castaways

Most people know that Crusoe ends up facing off against savages and few want to spend time on moral ambiguity. You can cut straight to the shipwreck and savagery in Castaways which is a stand-alone horror story. Afterwards, you can look back and see how the savagery became inevitable.

For over a century, the stories told about the events covered in *Shipwreck* were a set of paeans of praise to medical progress. Written by medical people, they featured in introductions to medical books, and now embarrass everyone. They have been replaced since 1960 by accounts of a more problematic medicine, but in these it is difficult to pick out a story beneath the bristling academic asides and counters. More recently again, history has become silent. Its leading practitioners claim it's difficult to write history in an age of biomedicine. These historians have never engaged with those marooned by drugs and health services even though the critical step in determining whether treatment has caused a wreck lies in establishing a history. The history leading up to Castaways will take you beyond academic jargon and make you queasy. Castaways will shock you.

Upton Sinclair in 1906 changed the food industry by dropping into *The Jungle*, an account of Chicago's meatpacking industry, the fact that there might be human in your hamburger. Eric Schlosser, a century later, electrified us by dropping into *Fast Food Nation* an image of feces in our hamburgers.

The Jungle revealed rotten apples in the barrel. It worked because it pointed to something that could be put right. Castaways reveals a rotten barrel. No politician is going to brandish *Shipwreck* the way Roosevelt brandished *The Jungle* as a call to change. They are going to respond like Pius XII, the Pope who failed to intervene in the Holocaust.

If you rarely visit doctors and have never become a castaway, the terrain on which I claim we are now stranded will seem incredible. Recent medical travel tales or an experience of modern health services might have left some wary of savages linked to Big Risk or Big Pharma, but no one expects the 'savages' who visit your island to be doctors. If marooned, these are the people likely to stew you in a pot and eat you.

You may spot one of them trussed up, waiting to be eaten. Should you try to rescue her? I don't mean, can you see a way to undertake a risky maneuver; I mean, is there any point?

Castaways doesn't offer an escape plan. It nails itself to a Cathedral Door, setting up a what's next moment. Five hundred years ago, what was next was a century of bloodshed.

The pharmaceutical industry and the rapidly developing service industry, we used to call medicine, are now handling rather than helping us. This handling, and the question of what Google and Facebook are up, require an engagement with the issue of who has power over us, what the basis of that power is, and how it is likely to be deployed.

Our Singular Times

There is an art to history as there is, or was, to medicine. Beyond knowing what to include and what to omit, there is a need to make a diagnosis rather than just amass detail. This was caught in a famous parable, *On Rigor in Science*, by Jorge Luis Borges that runs through this book.

> *In that Empire, the Art of Cartography attained such perfection that the map of a single province occupied the entirety of a city, and the map of the Empire, the entirety of a province. In time, those Unconscionable Maps no longer satisfied, and the College of Cartographers set up a Map of the Empire whose size was that of the Empire, and which coincided point for point with it. Following generations, who were not as addicted to Cartography as their forebears, saw the vast map as useless, and unceremoniously delivered it up to the inclemency of the seasons. In the deserts of the West, there are still some tattered remnants of the Map… but in the rest of the country geography has ceased to exist.*

Traditionally the word accident refers to something unintended and unforeseeable—an Act of God. It can also refer to something incidental—having arms is incidental to being human, as the thalidomiders born without them have demonstrated. Unwelcome consequences are a foreseeable part of taking a drug. But if your child is born now without arms after you took a drug while pregnant, you will be told it was an accident.

Increasingly incapable of seeing the role of systems in what happens to us, we accept it when told the system is not to blame.

What's singular about our times is that whether we view ourselves as individuals or as members of a community, we are increasingly incidental to a story that was once the human story. When told to, we take our drugs.

We get on the train rather than take to the woods. But as we found out in the 1940s, process-based technocracies can stop working. We thought a cancerous element had been excised in 1945. Faced now with a rising tide of drug wrecks, and plastic laden water, and the perils of a complete one-dimensionality that Full Artificial Intelligence (AI) poses, we need to re-examine the diagnosis.

More than any other diagnoses, drug wrecks point to the most primitive of divisions between us, between the fortunate and the unfortunate. They call on us to frame rules (nomos) for our common house (oikos) to manage this divide. The drug wrecked, the stone the builders currently reject, more than anyone else are forced to be entrepreneurial (risk takers). Their experience offers the best basis for a house we might call home.

We need to move beyond Descartes *Cogito ergo Sum*, I think therefore I am, and Luther's *Credo ergo Sum*, I believe therefore I am, to something like *Decernimus ergo Summus*—it is in grappling together with the effects of bumping into things and into each other that we are. It is in Caring that we are.

Our singular times are not an island from which there is an escape. Talk of 'rescue' is where the myths begin.

THE EARLY YEARS

The steel worker on the girder
Learned not to look down, and does his work
And there are words we have learned
Not to look at.
Not to look for substance,
Below them. But we are on the verge
Of vertigo

There are words that mean nothing
But there is something to mean
Not a declaration which is truth
But a thing
Which is.

O the tree, growing from the sidewalk –
It has a little life, sprouting
Little green buds
Into the culture of the streets
We look back
Three hundred years and see bare land
And suffer vertigo.

George Oppen
Building the Skyscraper

1: THE REVOLUTION

The trip had some similarities with the average trip to a doctor. It took longer to get there than the medical procedure took. There was trepidation beforehand, and an abrupt ending. Who knows what the patient thought just before, or even just after the encounter? The trip was for a medically sanctioned procedure that has gone down in history as an encounter whose implications we may still not fully understand.

On Jan 21, 1793, Louis XVI, King of France, travelled from the former headquarters of the Knights Templar to the Place Louis XV, the biggest square in Paris. A priest with him in the carriage described the king as calm, remarking that they must be there when the carriage stopped. Louis was nervous on getting out and in need of support from the priest, rallying before mounting the steps to a platform.

He tried to tell the crowd he forgave them and hoped his blood would not curse them but was manhandled onto an apparatus. The blade of the guillotine dropped. His head was picked up and held out to the crowd who, after a pause, shouted *Vive la République*!

After the opening events of the Revolution in August 1789, Louis had appointed Joseph-Ignace Guillotin, a physician, to the medical brief in the new constitutional monarchy. Guillotin proposed that among available execution techniques, the 'guillotine' was the quickest and least painful, and that it should apply to everybody.

The swift and clean action led to speculation that the severed head might be able to sense and think. The *tricoteuses* knitting at the foot of the guillotine were sure of this. A few months after Louis, Antoine Lavoisier, France's most famous scientist, supposedly told his assistant he would try to communicate by blinking after the blade fell. He blinked twenty times. Medical observations since indicate the facial muscles go into spasm, but afterwards people may be able to make eye movements in response to questions before fading away.

Guillotin had played an earlier part in the build up to the revolution. In February 1778, Franz Anton Mesmer, an Austrian, came to Paris with word of animal magnetism, or mesmerism, as it came to be called. This new healing technique seemed to cure everything from chronic ailments to nervousness. Parisians flocked to Mesmer.

The leading lights of the Enlightenment, Voltaire and Jean-Jacques Rousseau died in 1778, followed by Robert Jacques Turgot in 1781. Their signature ideas, the idea of Progress, the importance of a Social Contract, the harms of inequality and the power of governments to manage poverty, reached a limited audience. Mesmer, and the Montgolfier Brothers with the first successful balloon flight in 1783, changed this. The French were gripped with the idea of progress through science. Balloon flight became a craze. Up to a hundred thousand people turned out to watch flights. While the possibility of disaster was a draw, the mastery of nature's laws caught the imagination. There was enthusiasm on the scale of that for the Wright Brothers in 1903 and space travel in the 1960s.

The enthusiasm for Mesmer had the characteristics of later religious revivals. He set up a Society of Harmony that stressed the need to achieve balance (harmony) within the individual and between the individual and the environment. The Society of Harmony embraced Rousseau's suggestion that the entire social order was held in place by customs that stunt human growth and health. If the chains of custom could be thrown off, society would be restored to a state of Harmony.

These unsettling ideas prompted Louis in 1784 to set up a commission drawn from the Faculty of Medicine, the Academy of Sciences, and the newly created *Sociéte Royale de Médecine* to investigate magnetism. The commission, which included Guillotin, Benjamin Franklin, Antoine

Lavoisier, and six others, reported there was no physical reality to magnetic claims. The patients precipitated into convulsions or cured from paralysis, they said, were affected by suggestion.

Despite circulating 12,000 copies of its report, the Commission failed to chop the head off Mesmerism. Many people didn't believe that all that was involved was suggestion. If suggestion was what was involved, it proved the power of the mind to influence the body for the better. We needed to find a way to harness these forces.

Mesmerists brought ideas about progress, equality and opportunity to people Voltaire and Rousseau could never reach. Many of the Revolutionaries in 1789 were members of the Society of Harmony. They hoped to make a mark in society, but found society only worked if you had the right connections.

One of these aspiring young men, one of the Revolution's early leaders, then a Mesmerist, Nicolas Bergasse, castigated established medicine:

> *It is important to maintain among the common people, as a constant civilizing influence, all the prejudices that can make medicine respectable... The corps of doctors is a political body, whose destiny is linked with that of the state... Thus, within the social order, we absolutely must have diseases, drugs and laws, and the distributors of drugs and diseases influence the habits of a nation perhaps as much as do the guardians of its laws.[1]*

The Revolution began with a vote among an elite to implement what seemed like the most enlightened ideas of the day. 'Progressives' across Europe cheered. Others like Edmund Burke recoiled. In *Reflections on the Revolution in France*, Burke raised alarm at the disintegration of a moral universe, and the replacement of chivalry and honor by economics and technicians. He predicted a descent into chaos. As more and more people were drawn in, the Revolution plunged into a Reign of Terror. This has

---

1   Darnton R, *Mesmerism and end of the Enlightenment in France* (Harvard University Press, 2009), 84.

left a marker for over two hundred years of the molten passions that lie beneath a thin crust of civilization, passions mesmerism seemed to release.

Guillotin was imprisoned in 1794 but later pardoned. He retreated from politics to medicine, becoming, with Philippe Pinel, an advocate for a new public health measure, vaccination. When efforts to rename the guillotine failed, he changed his name.

The Revolution replaced both mesmerism and balloon flights as a spectacle. Those who remained interested in the healing function of mesmerism began to exploit the possibilities that their cures hinged on manipulating attention. Magnetism became hypnosis. Seventy years later this change in emphasis gave birth to our ideas about psychodynamics, and later placebos, brainwashing and behavior modification.

In 1971 when Richard Nixon visited China and asked the Chinese Premier Chou En-Lai what he made of the French Revolution, Chou's response that it was too early to tell became an historical moment in its own right. It was cited as a symbol of the long view Chinese leaders take. Others suggest Chou was referring to the revolts in France in 1968, which looked more revolutionary outside America than within.

Whatever happened politically in the 1790s and 1960s in France and elsewhere, there were medical revolutions in the 1790s and 1960s that connect directly to the experience each of us has going to a doctor today, and whose consequences are still working themselves out.

A Medical Revolution

In the American and French Revolutions, subjects became citizens. The French Revolution created patients—the citizens of a new medical domain.

Louis XVI succeeded to the throne in 1774 at the age of 19. His brother-in-law, Joseph II, the Holy Roman Emperor, based in Vienna, seen as an Enlightened Monarch, had set about emancipating the serfs in the Empire and liberalizing trade. When Louis appointed Robert Turgot as his Comptroller-General, it looked like he was moving in the same direction.

While Voltaire and Rousseau are now more celebrated, in 1750 Turgot helped create modernity by crystalizing the Idea of Progress. Rather than viewing the human situation fatalistically, he insisted on the possibility of progress through risk taking and a turn to a market economy. This Idea of Progress, through markets and science, came to replace Providence as the lodestone of human affairs. Along with Francois Quesnay and Samuel du Pont, Turgot was part of a group of moral philosophers called *Les Économistes*, those who would make the house (*oikos*) rules (*nomos*). Later castigated by Burke as sabotaging moral philosophy, they were committed to Free Trade before Adam Smith. Gournay, coined the term *laissez-faire, laissez passer* to capture a new spirit of economic and social liberalism in which people rather governments would shape the country. Jean-Baptiste Say coined the term *entrepreneur* to connote an adventurer, one who takes risks in a marketplace.

Turgot set about liberalizing trade, abolishing monopolies, reforming taxes, and eliminating the vestiges of serfdom in France. He also set about reforming medicine, which like economics had been a branch of moral philosophy. He drew up a Bill to abolish Guilds, but lost office before it could be brought into law.

European medicine was dominated by Guilds (corporations), which were thought to eliminate inefficiencies and maintain quality standards. They laid down the guidelines and protocols which regulated practice. The Parisian Faculty of Medicine was the center of medicine's Guild power in France. It controlled a medical education that as a branch of moral philosophy aimed at producing an individual learned in Latin, Greek, logic, and philosophy. Entry to the guild hinged on handing over money and attending a certain number of meals. Science had not penetrated this domain.

Forty years before the Revolution, Denis Diderot, Rousseau, and other Enlightenment figures envisaged a medicine driven by science, central to which was the idea that man was the product of his environment. Diderot's *Encyclopedia*, to which Turgot contributed, and Rousseau's *Social Contract* advocated self-help, a way of a life not injurious to health, and hygienic measures imposed at a social level. This project was a first stab at public health and behavioral economics.

The project did not need democracy. An Enlightened Monarch could promote the right changes. While self-interest might lead some citizens to look after their health, the elite largely thought the people, sunk in ignorance, would need their environment changed from above.

Turgot persuaded Louis to establish the Sociéte Royale de Médecine to supplant Paris' medical guild and to appoint as its head a doctor committed to science, Felix Vicq d'Azyr. D'Azyr and the Sociéte Royale survived Turgot's dismissal.

In 1789 there was little medicine could do to help anyone. Conditions regarded as medical today, congenital and obstetric disorders, fractures, trauma, joint problems, fevers and a handful of disorders, now seen as metabolic or endocrine, were managed by bonesetters, barber-surgeons, apothecaries and midwives. Guild medicine regarded these as artisans, empirics, or charlatans, who operated on the basis of what seemed to work rather than by keeping to medical theory. 'Empiric' was a term of abuse.

Medical theory centered on the 4 humors. Real doctors bled their patients or used herbs or other methods to purge them, cause them to sweat, vomit or pass water, reproducing what appeared to be the body's own methods to handle disorders. Medical recommendations on foods to eat or activities to manage melancholia for instance made sense as remedies for blood that was dark, thick, and sluggish. They embodied knowledge about what herbs or foods can do in terms of purging us or raising or lowering body temperature. Physicians also employed biologicals, such as opium and foxglove, and chemicals such as antinomy, arsenic and mercury that certainly did things to the human body. This medical knowledge aimed at achieving a balance between our environments and our constitutions. It shaped not just the potions we took but the food we grew and global trade. But like the Ptolemaic framework of the Heavens, theoretical elegance stood in the way of progress.

In 1800 heart attacks, strokes, and cancers were largely non-existent. Occurring after 50, they lay beyond the average life expectancy. They also, unlike infections, happened within the body making them invisible except for tumors such as breast cancer. Mental illness was invisible because the realm of the mental was then vanishingly small.

The Sociéte Royale was tasked with bringing science into medicine and looking after the health of the nation. Science was seen as universal and disruptive, where guilds were hostile to competition and innovation. D'Azyr's blueprint for a new medicine foresaw an education in anatomy, physiology, pathology, hygiene, and obstetrics. This would be delivered by a College that would promote science, do research, and combat prejudice. Some of the doctors it produced would work for health councils to ensure the health of regions rather than treat private patients. This was anathema to the Faculty of Medicine.

D'Azyr also envisaged treatment at home free of charge, an emphasis on inoculation for smallpox, and good maternity care to reduce maternal and infant mortality. Medical officers would keep statistics on births, deaths and marriages, track epidemics, the changing climate, the state of the soil, swamps, and drainage.

The Revolution abolished Feudalism in August 1789, and the Aristocracy in June 1790. The initial plan was to keep the monarchy but to sweep away the *ancien regime* of which guild medicine and aristocratic privilege were part. Turgot's Bill banishing Guilds became law in 1791. This abolished the Faculty of Medicine and medical licensing. In Assembly debates, Guillotin proposed that it was the task of the state to establish proper cures.

The Revolution proclaimed a Right to Equality. Some petitions for equality argued that ill-health was one reason for poverty and inequality. When a person broke an arm or leg and couldn't work, they were at risk of destitution. So, reducing the occasions for injury was important. If epidemics or even birth left people disabled, these disorders would cause poverty. Unchangeable though a loss of sight or hearing might appear, something could still be done to enable these citizens to more productive lives. The later development of Montessori teaching methods, Braille, and

Sign languages demonstrated this. There was a new Can-Do spirit when it came to social well-being.

D'Azyr's blueprint was adopted. Everybody, it was decreed, had a right to free healthcare. Not only could the nation afford this, but it would make the nation wealthier, especially if science, rather than politicians or the clergy, shaped what happened.

The emphasis on treatment at home may seem remarkable. But this was prudence rather than an early form of boutique medicine. Paris had a set of enormous insanitary hospices, where the destitute and frail had come to die since 1650. Some of these were vagabonds, or beggars. Most were medically indigent. They were crippled, insane, blind or with chronic respiratory, arthritic, or gut conditions or paralyses that made it impossible to work. And they had no-one to look after them. The medically indigent, who were mostly elderly (over the age of 45), outnumbered the medically ill, those with acute disorders like typhoid, tuberculosis, or dysentery, by 2 to 1. Both were looked after by nuns more concerned for their souls rather than doctors concerned for their bodies

The biggest of these hospices was the 2,500 bed Hôtel Dieu. Following a fire that destroyed part of this, plans were drawn up to locate hospitals in each of Paris' main quarters, making a system that would be, as Jacques Tenon, a surgeon, in a 1788 report put it, a *Machine à guérir*. In the chaos of the revolution, this idea of a hospital system was adopted and led to the idea that hospitals might specialize. The Hôtel Dieu was infamous for puerperal fever. Up to 25% of the women giving birth died.

Women were given a maternity hospital instead and the mentally ill were given asylums. There was a drop in puerperal infections and peri-natal mortality, and new talk of curing lunacy. These were the first medical hospitals—institutions dedicated to exploring and treating conditions in a manner quite different to traditional medical practice. The hospices had been run by religious orders who provided person centered care. The new emphasis on curing that emerged with hospitals sat uneasily alongside this traditional duty of care.

In return for free healthcare, patients had to play a part in advancing medical science. They faced an assessment at the entrance aimed at restricting admissions to the medically ill. Once admitted, they had to follow medical dictates on hygiene and inoculations. In death, they had to accept postmortems. Medical training moved out of lecture theatres and into hospitals. Previously never examined hospice inmates now encountered daily ward rounds. They had to accept physical examinations and be prepared to give their history to trainees.

The new doctors were oriented to science. When licensing was re-introduced in 1799, it mandated training in anatomy, physiology and pathology, as well as hygiene and obstetrics instead of the works of Hippocrates, Aristotle and Galen. The training was in French rather than Latin. A new Academy of Medicine, combining physicians and surgeons where the old system had kept them apart, was dedicated to science and research. No longer would doctors be expected simply to do something to amuse us while Nature cured us.

In 1802 a Public Health Council was established with a brief to get to grips with matters of temperance, prostitution, sanitation, the adulteration of food, water, and wine and the imposition of quarantine during epidemics. Tackling these issues involved 'police' powers. Police is a loaded word now. Rather than images of men in blue, toting guns, then it meant a set of civil servants to implement the rules (policy) laid down by the city or the municipality (the *polis*). Medical police would keep a social body functioning the way transport or harbor police do now. Their brief included placing foundling children, monitoring wet-nursing, or coordinating midwives. Having health policies and police to operate them was the difference between civilization and barbarism.

Policymakers faced a new question. What to pay doctors? Medical Guilds controlled prices through a monopoly on the supply of a service. In a market economy, Adam Smith argued, the 'market' should set a price for goods and services, with consumers able to take their custom elsewhere if they were not satisfied. Guilds had guaranteed quality of a sort.

Markets could too over the longer run, after injuries and lawsuits. But we need to be able to trust doctors. This is less likely to happen if they are competing to make money out of us, or worried about being sued. Smith's answer was that there are some processes the public can assess and some it can't. In the case of physicians, we can't assess their skills and have to pay to get good men who have a status in society. This gave rise to the idea of a liberal professional, someone trained and certified in a specific field, distinct from learned gentlemen on one hand and tradesmen on the other.

This professional image was something of an ideal before 1880. In France, Britain, Germany and America, family doctors visited people at home doing a little bit of surgery, bloodletting, setting fractures, lancing the gums of teething infants, along with dispensing purgatives or emetics. It was easy to become a doctor and competition pushed down what little there was to be earned from attending the poor or medically indigent. Medical practitioners were better off than tradesmen but lower down the pecking order than lawyers. Their professional politics aimed at improving their status.

The needs of the military were another driver of change. Napoleon's armies embarked on campaigns in Egypt, Russia, and the Caribbean that exposed troops to new disorders like Yellow Fever. These environments were often more threatening than any human enemies. Military campaigns traditionally had medical input, but Napoleon put more store on nutrition, morale, and constitutions than on balancing humors. He wanted bonesetters and surgeons. His surgeon, Jean Larrey, introduced ambulant hospitals to remove the injured from the field of battle as quickly as possible or even treat them on the ground.

Napoleon was a Systematizer. The Code Napoleon standardized the legal system, giving France one legal system rather than a multiplicity of codes based on local custom, making it a national organization. In the same way, ambulances and developments in army provisioning laid the basis for a new medical system. This military medicine marks the emergence of a trajectory that leads through the Crimean War, the American Civil War, two World Wars, Vietnam and beyond.

The French Revolution spawned another development that took nearly two centuries to impinge on clinical medicine, with effects Chou-en-Lai might say are still too early to judge. In 1793, the Revolutionary government adopted a new system of measures, supposedly based on science, which gave us the meter, the liter, and the kilogram. These were an exercise in practical democracy, limiting the discretion of the aristocracy in matters like determining exactly how much wheat constituted a bushel and accordingly how much money should change hands. Standard measures like this are critical to market exchanges. This push to standardize, to limit discretion, and to a certain kind of objectivity, often begins from the bottom up. In 1947 as part of their revolution, Chou and Mao Tse-Tung standardized measurements across China. But those with the most resources are always best placed to exploit new systems and techniques.

THE REVOLUTION
WITHIN THE REVOLUTION

Vicq d'Azyr was not guided by a medical model. His changes to medical education and provision hinged on a belief in the power of people approaching things scientifically to come up with new answers to age-old problems. He did not build on a medical tradition. He overturned it.

There is a balance between authority and observation in any branch of science. Within medicine, the Roman physician, Galen, tipped the balance toward authority. The postmortems of Andreas Vesalius in 1540, and William Harvey in 1620 demonstrating the heart is a pump, began to tip it back. These transformed our understanding of how the body works but had no effect on medicine. The idea an organ or a tissue might be the seat of a disease had not been born. Before 1800 any disturbances noted on postmortem were incidental.

A disorder that killed us was in us rather than our organs. When doctors intervened to rebalance our humors, they were rebalancing us. They were not treating a disorder that might be put right by a magic bullet. Humors affected the entire body. In purging, blistering, and bleeding, doctors copied the ways in which the body seemed to manage disorders. The diuresis, diarrhea, and skin rashes we now regard as treatment side effects were seen then as evidence a treatment was working.

If we rather than our organs were disordered, it was natural to ask what we might have done that led God to strike us down. When cholera or plague struck, communities questioned how they had been behaving before God and repented.

The French Revolution did not make anyone more empirical, rational, observant, or even scientific than they had been. Physicians since Hippocrates had distinguished between disorders like epilepsy and hysteria and linked disorders to observables like the blackening of blood or stools on exposure to air, the bile that can appear in vomit or feces, or the clear fluids within the body that sometimes drown a patient lying in their own bed or spill out of a skull cracked open.

Everyone agreed that charlatans and quacks, who treated patients with things that might seem to work but whose workings couldn't be explained by the theories of the day, were part of the problem not part of the solution. To specialize in an area of medicine, or in a particular cure, rather than treat the whole person was frowned upon.

Who could possibly pick out germs as a cause of disease? Any number of deadly contagious disorders had overlapping symptoms, and there was no way to see germs, or to differentiate one germ from another. Even now, 99% of our germs don't cause disorders. It made sense to think climate, soil, water, and air contributed to the outbreak of a pestilence. It wasn't clear we were dealing with anything wrong within an individual any more than it is now clear that anorexia nervosa or gender identity disorders are better located within individuals.

While some tumors distinguish themselves by obvious swellings on the surface of the body, all diseases, even cancer, provoke a general adaptation syndrome, or stress reaction, that ensures all diseases have features in common.

In 1761 toward the end of his life, Giovanni Morgagni published a thesis on diseases and postmortems *Of the Seats and Causes of Diseases.* This proposed that organs like the liver or kidney could be diseased and give rise to specific disorders. His ideas were wrapped in philosophizing, and while he was on to something, like Mendel a century later, he was ignored.

Even with the Morgagni precedent, it was not inevitable that post-mortems in Paris in 1800 would lead anywhere. The more high-tech our instruments, the more likely postmortems will show what someone can live with rather than what they have died from. But in Paris, postmortems gave rise to what is now called the Medical Model. The new orientation to bedside examinations triggered a recognition that the features a patient displayed while living had correlates after death. This was especially true for tuberculosis (TB), which became the basis for the medical model.

In 1800 Xavier Bichat noted that some corpses at postmortem showed not just diseased organs but evidence of inflammation in specific tissues. Bichat died from TB the following year at the age of 31. Sixty years later Rudolph Virchow pushed this insight further and claimed the cells within tissues were the seat of disorders. The die of specificity had been cast. Our original sin was no longer the issue. Diseases would be linked to discrete malfunctions in the machinery of our bodies.

When René Laennec developed the stethoscope in 1816, before dying from TB, he made it possible to link different breath sounds or cardiac murmurs with postmortem lung or heart abnormalities. This kind of analysis penetrated mental medicine in 1822, when Auguste Bayle discovered postmortem brain changes in patients with tertiary syphilis.

There was no suggestion that all dis-ease would stem from diseases. Just the opposite. Medical diseases were on their way to being shipwrecks that were not linked to flaws of character, the moral ambiguities of an employment or the whims of Providence. The challenge to a clinician was one of pattern recognition. From what this patient tells me, or what I can see, smell, or feel, is it likely there will be an underlying disorder of their biology?

The medical model involved a new set of techniques and practices. A technique is more than an intellectual construct or paradigm. It is a way of doing things within which paradigms can rise and fall. Techniques ground systems that support livelihoods. Like the guillotine or guns, they universalize, unless replaced by something more efficient.

The luck that gave rise to techniques like the stethoscope played a part in this revolution. From stethoscopes to microscopes shortly afterwards, and neuroimaging and genetics since, techniques have enabled us to advance beyond cherished ideas. We never get cleverer, but those who are around when a new technique gives rise to a new observation become famous and, since 1900, win Nobel Prizes.

Technique has increasingly driven history since 1800. Looking back, perhaps because of a bias toward seeing history as arcing toward progress, we see a force for liberation. Looking forward, we are often alarmed. Are we heading toward a utopia or a dystopia? New medical techniques have offered a lot but the medical model has also meant that doctors may show more interest in a disease they are meeting again, in a slightly different form, than they do in us. Our values can take second place to their wish to re-engage with an old foe—tuberculosis in 1820, cancer now.

If it is difficult to pinpoint just why the medical model emerged, it is important to recognize it had a beginning. It may have been important the hospitals did not close. Treating everyone at home would have made it more difficult to recognize commonalities across patients. The continuity in Parisian hospital buildings masked the radical change. This new medicine was as much at odds with the medicine that had gone before it as the Copernican was to the Ptolemaic universe.

The Revolution that decapitated Louis split the elite into progressives and conservatives, with conservatives bemoaning the descent from moral philosophy into technique. Both progressives and conservatives in contrast supported the techniques of the new clinical medicine. Clinical medicine, though, co-existed with a new Public Health model also put in place by Vicq D'Azyr, which has been at the heart of politics since 1790.

A Model Physician

Another way to view what happened is through the career of Philippe Pinel. Born in 1745 into a provincial family, he trained in medicine. Like others, he was drawn to the Parisian Republic of Letters, arriving there in 1778 the same year as Mesmer. His provincial degree was not recognized. Entry to the guild denied, he became as disenchanted as Nicholas Bergasse. But he joined D'Azyr's Sociéte Royale rather than Mesmer's Society of Harmony.

Pinel believed in Rousseau's claim that society alienates people from their true selves. After a stint in a private facility that took mental patients, he developed an interest in madness and lost any wish to treat wealthy hypochondriacs. He frequented salons linked to the Revolution where he met Benjamin Franklin, who tried to persuade him to move to America.

In January 1793, he was present at the execution of Louis XVI. Later that year, given his new connections, he was appointed to look after one of Paris' vast hospices, the Bicêtre, an institution for men. He separated out the destitute from the medically ill and, within the medically ill, defined a new group whom we would now call mad. Madness then was not a distinct entity. It was linked to fevers. The typical mad person was delirious. Treatment involved purging, bloodletting and other efforts to rebalance deranged humors, which may have seemed to help as when the fever passed some patients recovered.

Pinel's attention was drawn to the mad who had no signs of fever and to Jean-Baptiste Pussin. Pussin was a former patient who, as happened in Parisian hospices, after recovering had taken a job looking after the inmates, with Marguerite his wife. His way of handling patients seemed to work. Had he been doing the same thing but selling his services on the street, he would have been dismissed as a charlatan, or an empiric.

Reports around then from England about the management of the madness of King George III supported approaches similar to Pussin's. Getting to know the patient and shaping their behavior by methods that varied from patient to patient might help. The approach came to be called a moral method. In this context moral meant a hygienic method. The patients were to be treated in so far as possible by good nutrition, a regulated day, constructive activities, a firm hand, and the avoidance of vices like drunkenness or prostitution.

Pinel was open to whatever worked. He saw his role as working backwards from an effective treatment to what that meant in terms of how human minds work. In 1795 he moved from the Bicêtre to the even bigger Salpêtrière hospice for women. He brought Pussin with him. He again separated patients into groups, restricted admissions to the medically ill, and distinguished between raving patients with and without fevers.

At this point, the progressive theory of how minds worked came from England's John Locke, who a century before, in *An Essay Concerning Human Understanding*, created psychology. Locke proposed our minds work by making associations—linking impressions. Like the serotonin hypothesis today, this was almost self-evidently wrong. Just as the serotonin hypothesis was a better fit with antidepressants than the more sophisticated psychodynamic theories it replaced however, Locke's ideas were more consistent with the emerging brain sciences of his day than the sophisticated metaphysical theories they replaced.

The immediate practical influence of Locke's theory was on education. If all a child has in its mind are associations laid down by experience, making good associations a matter of habit becomes critically important to the future of society.

This theory faced three conundrums. The first was social. It assumed that people like us with the right education would come to the right kind of judgments, but how to educate the masses who were exposed to so many pernicious impressions? The second involved the role of judgment. For Locke knowledge arises from a distillation of impressions and some correspondence between the distillate and what is out there. This skirt around the question of judgment. How do we know the distillate is right? Before Locke, philosophers were comfortable making judgments. We couldn't survive if we didn't make them. After Locke, they agonized over how judgments arise, and the relation they bear to knowledge.

The third conundrum centered on madness. Why did education not restore the mad to their senses? Before Locke, we had passions. The word stems from the Greek pathos and implies an experience of having one's body acted upon, as in suffering. The body was thought to be porous and open to outside influences. It could be curdled the way wind can sour milk or wine. The rational individual had a duty to civilize outside influences through moderation in diet, activity, sex, and an avoidance of contagion.

Locke helped locate our emotions more clearly in ourselves, helped to privatize our passions. Rousseau didn't agree a rational faculty should subdue all others, or that rationality was the supreme virtue. We needed, he argued, to listen to an inner voice because civilization often alienated us from our true path. In the climate surrounding the Revolution, this alienation looked like it might account for disorders then called mental alienation.

Locke's ideas came to France through Pierre Cabanis, who introduced the term ideology as the science of how ideas link together. Cabanis saw medicine as anthropology, a science of understanding man, but one that needed philosophy to stabilize its facts. He was sure madness was a matter of associations gone wrong.

Pinel turned to the new science of disease entities. As a clinician, he noted the role of puberty, menstruation, the menopause, sex drives, and sensations in the gut and heart when we get emotional. He placed weight on the role of passions such as anger, jealousy, resentment, and joy as triggers to madness. Time and again, the word chagrin crops up in his case descriptions, in which frustration in life and terror leads to collapse. These passions were not metaphysical. They were rooted in the body. Great passion had bodily effects. Where Locke's ideas were based on sensations from without, Pinel figured a mixture of internal and external sensations might compromise the judgment of the mad. Freud later exploited just this nexus.

Following Rousseau, Pinel also noted the extent to which the secondary passions, the desire to gain the esteem of others, honor, or wealth, matters of self-esteem, could be perverted. Mesmerism had shown that imagination was prone to error and that all our associations could be disordered without us realizing it. This way an alienation certainly lies. For Pinel the disturbed associations in mental alienation, however, were more like the disturbances we get with a fever or other toxic state.

An incident catches this new medical world. After emptying out the prisons, a band of Revolutionaries entered the Bicêtre to liberate the people driven mad by the *ancien regime*. Freeing an inmate who seemed entirely sensible, they confronted Pussin demanding at sword point he account for this abuse. Marguerite interposed herself between the marauders and her husband. The band left with their freed prisoner. They returned soon after conceding he was indeed mad. While they may be linked, medical alienation and political alienation are not the same thing.

The question was how to manage the deranged passions of mental illness. Pinel recognized you cannot destroy them. A man of reason only, devoid of feeling, would be a monster who desired nothing, and felt no fear. Passions are necessary to but a problem for judgment.

After Mesmer's departure from Paris, Armand de Puységur emerged as the leading magnetist. Pinel asked him to the Salpêtrière to explore whether magnetism might help his patients. He concluded that Pussin's methods offered a more consistent basis to build on than magnetism. Pussin also engaged patients and shaped their associations. In addition, he had a moral presence, and a street wisdom as to when to approach them and in what way to subdue their unruly passions.

Pinel was lucky in meeting the right empiric. He was also lucky in the Salpêtrière. He would never have seen the full range of mental illnesses in the private institution he worked in previously. Just as in other hospitals, where large collections of patients highlighted the common features of diseases, so having large numbers of the mad together brought differences between disorders into view.

He distinguished between patients with mania, melancholia, dementia, and mental handicap. These distinctions seem extraordinarily simple now. But since Hippocrates it was rare for anyone to categorize patients from the bottom-up rather than the top-down. This was not classification by first principles or logic but by observation of clinical patterns.

In 1802 building on his categories, Pinel was the first to commit medicine to a statistical approach. The typical treatments for the raving included bloodletting, cold baths, being hosed down with water jets, or given purgatives, emetics, diuretics, and other drugs. Although there were elegant rationales for these treatments, and some had been advocated by history's most distinguished physicians, Pinel was skeptical. Patients often improved when the doctor waited before intervening. Learning the typical course of a disorder, he reasoned, would make it possible to predict which patients might recover, and when they might turn a corner on their own or with input from Pussin.

Between April 1802 and December 1805, he followed 1002 admissions to the Salpêtrière to see who recovered and who didn't. Were his new diagnostic labels worthwhile or not?

Pinel laid out his reasons for taking this approach:

In medicine it is difficult to come to any agreement if a precise meaning is not given to the word experiment, since everyone vaunts their own results, and only more or less cites the facts in favor of their point of view. However, to be genuine and conclusive, and serve as a solid basis for any method of treatment, an experiment must be carried out on a large number of patients following the same rules and a set order. It must also be based on a consistent series of observations recorded very carefully and repeated over a certain number of years in a regular manner. Finally it must equally report both events which are favorable and those which are not, quoting their respective numbers, and it must attach as much importance to one set of data as to the other. In a nutshell it must be based on the theory of probabilities, which is already so effectively applied to several questions in civil life and on which from now on methods of treating illnesses must also rely if one wishes to establish these on sound grounds. This was the goal I set myself in 1802 in relation to mental alienation when the treatment of deranged patients was entrusted to my care and transferred to the Salpêtrière.[2]

---

2   Pinel, P, (1809), *Medico-Philosophical Treatise on Mental Alienation, Trans.* Hickish G, Healy D, Charland L (J Wiley & Sons), 153.

Overall, 47% of the patients recovered. Among first admissions treated by watchful waiting or Pussin's methods, up to 85% responded. When left to recover naturally, many more first admissions did so than those with prior admissions. Not only that, soon after admission, based on their clinical features, Pinel could tell who was likely to recover and who was not.

There seemed to be different disorders, and people suffering from some types of disorder would recover if left alone while other types didn't recover regardless of what treatments they were given. Finally, following the patients after discharge brought a new group of periodic disorders into view, laying the basis for the later discovery of manic-depressive illness and other recurrent mental disorders.

Pinel presented his data on February 9, 1807. This was the first time in medicine that results were presented as ratios of patients, rather than accounts of individual cases. It was only through the application of science, he said, that doctors would be able to distinguish among the conditions they were treating and establish the natural history of each, giving them the best chance to discover the anatomical basis of conditions and possible therapies.

In reporting these findings, Pinel was aware personal bias could have colored the results. But, as he noted, while an individual patient in London could not be compared to one in Paris or Munich, the results of complete groups of patients could be, and the registers of Salpêtrière patients were publicly available. He challenged others to contest his findings based on data they could check.

Diagnosis counted. Pinel expected that disordered behavior stemmed from physiological derangements in the gastrointestinal tract or peripheral nerves, as in his hands the patients' brains appeared clear at postmortem. Soon after, Auguste Bayle sealed the triumph of the anatomo–clinical method across medicine when he demonstrated a link between post-mortem brain changes and the clinical picture of General Paralysis of the Insane (tertiary syphilis).

The commitment to data, however, soon drew blood. In 1828 another Parisian physician, Pierre Louis, came to grief when he proposed using numbers to guide treatment:

> *In any epidemic, let us suppose five hundred of the sick, taken indiscriminately, to be subjected to one kind of treatment, and five hundred others, taken in the same manner, to be treated in a different mode; if the mortality is greater among the first than among the second, must we not conclude that the treatment was less appropriate, or less efficacious in the first class than in the second?*[3]

Bleeding works well for heart failure, but it was also used for fevers based on a theory that fever arose from inflamed organs. When Louis compared bleeding to doing nothing in 77 patients with pneumonia, he sparked a crisis. The data stood at odds with the theory:

> *The results of my experiments on the effects of bleeding in inflammatory conditions are so little in accord with common opinion [those who were bled were more likely to die, he found] that it is only with hesitation that I have decided to publish them. The first time I analyzed the relevant facts, I believed I was mistaken, and I repeated my work but the result of this new analysis remains the same.*[4]

These results led outraged physicians to claim it was not possible to practice medicine by numbers. The physicians preferred theories that made sense. They defended themselves with an ethical argument that their duty was to the patient in front of them rather than the population at large. Doctors had to be guided by what they found at the bedside.

> *The practice of medicine according to this [Louis'] view is entirely empirical, it is shorn of all rational induction, and takes a position*

---

3   Louis PCA, cited in Healy D., *The Antidepressant Era* (Harvard University Press) 83

4   Louis PCA, cited in Healy D, *The Antidepressant Era*, 83.

> *among the lower grades of experimental observations and fragmentary facts.*[5]

In contrast to Louis, Pinel offered not just data but a treatment approach, a moral method. This had the potential to support livelihoods rather than undermine them. He was also lucky. He was diffident, but he had a charismatic student, Jean-Etienne Dominique Esquirol. Using Pinel's evidence, Esquirol supervised the building of asylums across France aimed at adopting the new methods. In this way, along with obstetrics, psychiatry became the first branch of medicine to have specialist hospitals, associations, and journals.

Pinel's story contains all the elements that led to breakthroughs across medicine. These had been present before him. Thomas Sydenham in 1690, for example, had argued in principle for classifying diseases from the bottom up, and moral methods had been used in England. But presented with large numbers of lunatics in the one place, Pinel and Esquirol were able to distinguish between patients with delusions, obsessions, or phobias. Some had moods that rose and fell. Others didn't. Some had an early onset and never recovered, others became insidiously deluded in later life.

Recognizing comparable differences among patients led to cardiology, respirology, urology and neurology. The growth in knowledge and techniques seemed to call for specialization. Some argued this would rupture the profession and transform doctors into factory workers. But claiming to be specialists allowed doctors to charge higher fees.

In 1893 the *International Classification of Diseases* (ICD) endorsed classification from the bottom up. The technique born in Paris went global. Data meanwhile had also begun to make its presence felt in public health.

---

5 Lawson L M (1849) cited in Rosenberg C E. *The Therapeutic Revolution: Medicine, Meaning and Social Change in Nineteenth Century America*, in Vogel M J, Rosenberg C E Eds, *The Therapeutic Revolution*. (University of Pennsylvania Press 1979), 20.

PANDAEMONIUM

In 1800 less than 1% of us lived in cities. By 2020 75% of European and over 50% of global populations lived in cities. In 1800 one third of us died by the age of 6. By 2000 death before 6 was rare. In 1800 there was no more than a four-fold difference between the overall wealth of the richest countries on earth and the poorest. By 2020 the gap was several hundred-fold greater and inequality within countries was growing.

Babylon, Jerusalem, Beijing, Athens, and Rome are names with such resonance that we think the city has always been with us. But the cities of antiquity were small. Before 1700 we lived on the land. Economists from Turgot through Marx, a century later, saw wealth as arising from the land with a small elite in the polis extracting value from those who worked the land. Turgot approved. Marx didn't. The growth of cities and a new urban class complicated politics further.

Around 1800, London reached a million people. Just before the Revolution, the population of Paris grew from half a million to three-quarters of a million. Berlin had less than 200,000, and New York only had 60,000 people. Most famous German and Italian cities with thousand-year histories had no more than 40,000 residents. Heading towards 1800, Manchester and Liverpool in England became the first cities to surge on the back of the Industrial Revolution, reaching populations of half a million by 1850.

From antiquity, in the face of ill-health Westerners located the cause in us (Original Sin) or in social settings. Except for Jerusalem, all cities were seen as sick, physically and socially, typified by Pandaemonium (the residence of All Demons). After 1800 we faced an urban future, in which the demons would have to be managed.

The first Public Health Council set up in Paris in 1802 achieved little. By the time the monarchy was restored after Waterloo, though, the public health genie was out of the bottle. One of the first moves of the new government was to create a properly functioning apparatus. A new journal, *Annales d'Hygiène Publique*, provided a focus. Hygienists (sanitarians) began to collect statistics through public health councils to improve society.

When Rousseau had first come to Paris, expecting a gleaming city, he saw it as sick. Air quality was poor, sanitation non-existent, food adulterated. Bad smells, foul and pestilential vapors, as Shakespeare termed them, miasmas as they were more usually called, were regarded as disease carrying. It was thought the smell of putrefaction could kill. Many cities and towns stank, as urine and feces were deposited from houses into drains running down streets.

Just as happened in its hospitals, the concentration of people in Paris' districts brought a new health prospect into view. When people developed diseases in the countryside some died while others didn't, but the deaths did not advance knowledge. The discovery of diseases has been largely an urban thing.

In the 2010s, social inequality became a hot political topic. Growing American inequality was highlighted by winners of the Nobel Prize for Economics, like Joseph Stiglitz and Angus Deaton. Inequality kills, we heard. This is not a new discovery.

In the late 1820s, Louis-René Villermé analyzed Parisian mortality. Conventional thought saw proximity to the river or a city dump as the primary determinant of outcome but Villermé fingered poverty and inequality instead. He argued disease took hold because starvation weakened constitutions and people starved because they were poorly paid. Skeptical these conclusions could be solidly based without using modern statistical techniques, many have analyzed his data since. All agree the data support his claim.

Villermé's inequality findings slipped off the radar until recently. He has been celebrated instead as a founding father of public health for his work on the health of prisoners, and on occupational health. He described respiratory disorders of cotton-workers, illnesses in children from labor in cotton mills, and injuries linked to the use of machinery in factories.

In 1700 Bernardino Ramazzini had noted the difficulties of Venetian mirror workers and other work-related disorders and advised doctors to ask their patients what they worked at. In 1775 Percival Potts noted that chimney sweeps in Manchester linked cancer of the scrotum to exposure to soot in young boys, soot wart. But it was Villermé who put occupational disorders and public health on the map.

In 1832 Alexandre Parent-Duchatelet, mapping a cholera outbreak that killed 18,000 Parisians, showed that those living the closest to the city dump at Montmastre had lower death rates than those living further away. This meant the miasma theories of the disease could not be right. Disproving the miasma theories was one thing but leaving us without an answer as to how we might mitigate the risks was not a comfortable position.

Hygiene now conjures up anodyne images. But in 1832 French hygienists were a new profession, who saw themselves as having a stake in the shape of society. Between them Villermé and Parent-Duchatelet created a medical discipline and a new politics.

In 1840 Villermé described the conditions of cotton, wool, and silk workers centered around Lyons. The workers there were in the vanguard of a militant artisanat (rather than a proletariat). They were very aware that new machines imposed by merchants were designed to break craft-based guilds and the merchants were using the market to do so. In addition to driving down wages, the machines exposed them to new dangers and deskilled them. This was an 1840s version of zero-hours contracts and working conditions we would now link to a precariat. Villermé catalogued the harms these new conditions, allied to a wage depression that led to poor diets, were causing.

English, American and German doctors came to Villermé's lectures. His work triggered a flurry of publications in the 1840s, especially in England, describing the conditions of a new group of factory workers, living in urban settings, a phenomenon found nowhere else in Europe. In England and America, the response was channeled into sanitarian movements, which assumed that filth rather than poverty was the key driver of physical and moral illnesses. Friedrich Engels' 1845 *Condition of the English Working Class* lit a different fuse (chapter 3).

Stimulated by Villermé's work, the early 1840s saw the birth and rapid growth of Etienne Cabet's communist movement, Saint-Simon's socialism, Pierre-Joseph Proudhon's anarchism, syndicalism, and other dreams of refashioning society in an egalitarian direction. Francois-Vincent Raspail, another doctor, was a prominent figurehead. A new urban world was trying to find a political expression. By 1848 there were roughly 100,000 communists in France. At a time when in Paris and Berlin, even doctors were taking to the barricades, communism seemed too pacifist to many.

In response to the 1848 Revolution in Paris, a new French government put a series of public health measures in place. A building program cleared Paris' tenements, widened its streets, created boulevards, installed parks, and produced the Paris people see today. But social unrest erupted again in 1871 in the Paris Commune.

Serendipity and Chance

One of the most famous aphorisms about science is: "In the field of observation, chance favors the prepared mind." Its author, Louis Pasteur, played a key role in the development of both the biosciences, and public health. Like Pinel, Pasteur was not academically top notch, but the new sciences were about problem solving. When it came to puzzles that could be answered by experiments, his skill led to breakthroughs. The first involved demonstrating that some molecules come in mirror image forms, which can have very different properties, a step in the development of biochemistry and pharmacology.

In 1858 he demonstrated that the fermentation of wine and beer was caused by yeast (germs) and that exposure to air led to bacterial molds growing on foods, which caused putrefaction. While fermentation and putrefaction were well known and reproducible in laboratories, nobody had nailed down their causes. It was a short jump from Pasteur's experiments to the idea that germs might colonize blood clots or placentas during childbirth, leading to puerperal fever, or infections in surgery. This led to pasteurization, which made food and drink, especially milk, safer, and improved infant mortality.

When Pasteur noticed that chickens inoculated with out-of-date cholera didn't come down with the full-blown illness, his hunch was that they had developed immunity from a weakened form of the germ. This helped explain the efficacy of inoculation, which had been used to manage smallpox in China and Turkey for centuries, and later vaccination, which produced immunity through an attenuated form of a germ.

There was a growing international dimension to medical science. Pasteur in his work faced competition from Robert Koch in Prussia. Prussia became Germany on the back of an invasion of France and siege of Paris in 1870. After the siege lifted, the Paris Commune saw citizens take controls of the streets. The elimination of tenements and widening the streets after 1848 to control epidemic infections had done nothing to eliminate political infections.

Once this second Reign of Terror had been dealt with, another science took shape. Seventy years after Pinel's meeting with Puységur, the room in which they likely met, later adorned with an iconic picture of Pinel liberating the insane from their chains, was the setting for another scene that became an iconic painting. Holding a limp Blanche de Witt across his arm, the doyen of world neurology, Jean Martin Charcot, is portrayed demonstrating how hypnosis could be used to diagnose hysteria.

Hysteria was the prototype for disorders that fell in between Pinel's mental diseases and the dis-ease in the face of our existential situation that concerned Rousseau. Hysterics often had the trappings of medical disease, convulsions, aphonia, or blindness. It only affected women supposedly. In this hospital, formerly for women only, among the extraordinary ideas Charcot put forward, none was more extraordinary than his claim that men could become hysterical. A claim then as bizarre as the idea that men might have a womb.

The moment, in which Charcot holds Blanche de Witt across his arm, is often seen as a labor pang in the birth of psychodynamics, whose conception can be traced back to Mesmer. Physicians from all over Europe were in the audience at Charcot's presentations, including Pierre Janet from Paris, and Sigmund Freud from Vienna, who became the leading proponents of psychodynamics.

As with all new sciences, this was also a cultural event. We can trace the unconscious back to the Greeks. Shakespeare writing in 1600 produced characters with 'subconscious' motives and depth. Mesmer, however, started something different that came into clearer focus with Janet and Freud, and gave us psyches we never had before.

The 1871 Reign of Terror that was the Paris Commune put the dynamics of crowds on the radar. In the 1880s, General Boulanger looked set to overthrow the new French Republic by mobilizing the crowd. In 1890s America, William Jennings Bryan's Democratic Party created populism. The management of contagious ideas became politically important. In 1895 drawing on Janet's work, Gustav Le Bon's book *The Crowd* analyzed what drove the rabble. In 1890 in *The Laws of Imitation* and in 1895 in *The Social Logic*, Gabriel Tarde offered a sociological view of the crowd that covered not only social movements but made everyone aware of something new—fashions. By 1920 America had become the leader in both the social and psychological sciences, had created public relations and marketing, and was adept at driving fashions.

MEDICAL POLITICS, MEDICAL FASHIONS

Michel Foucault, a French sociologist, published *Madness and Civilization*, ostensibly a history of psychiatry in 1960. This and *The Birth of the Clinic* in 1962 offered a new read on the history of medicine. We had moved, according to Foucault, from a world of bedside medicine before the Revolution to a world of hospital medicine. At the heart of this change lay an objectifying clinical gaze that had produced biomedicine (clinical medicine) and surveillance medicine (public health). This coincided with a great confinement, in which emerging States swept the destitute, the inconvenient, and the mad off our streets. Far from being a liberator, Pinel was part of an apparatus of repression. Any liberation from ancient scourges that medicine brought about came at the cost of accepting a controlling System.

Before Foucault, the introductory chapter of medical texts contained a paean to biomedical progress written by doctors listing the heroes behind breakthroughs on our journey to a medical utopia. A few books by historians based in the United States, Edwin Ackernecht, Oswei Temkin and George Rosen, told a different story. They spoke to the importance of public health. Improved housing and wages and the cleaning up of industrial and urban pollution had improved health and changed culture, not biomedicine. Rudolph Virchow became the patron saint of this medicine.

Foucault's language was impenetrable, especially in translation. Historians examining the details of his claims declared them wrong, especially his claims about madness. But when in 1968 students and workers poured onto the streets of Paris and other cities and Western governments tottered, Foucault's message that something profound had happened to us two centuries previously resonated. It seemed to mesh with both the events and the fiction of the day from *Clockwork Orange* to *One Flew over the Cuckoo's Nest* and later *The Stepford Wives*. The history of medicine became red hot. Was it a system of control or a force for liberation? Social scientists poured into the debate, and many historians saw it as their brief to support a social rather than a bio-medical narrative.

By 2000, some wondered if the critique they embraced with Foucault had become an echo chamber. Others wondered if it was still possible to write history in the era of the Human Genome Project. By 2010, a common future seemed increasingly difficult to imagine.

2: DECAPITATION

As for the people, truly I desire their liberty and freedom as much as anybody… but I must tell you that their liberty and freedom consist in having of government those laws by which their life and their goods may be most their own. It is not for having share in government, sirs: that is nothing pertaining to them; a subject and a sovereign are clear different things. And, therefore, until they do that, I mean that you do put the people in that liberty, as I say, certainly they will never enjoy themselves.

So saying, on January 30, 1649, Charles I, convicted of treason by the English Parliament but given more time to speak than Louis XVI, laid his head on the block, pulled his hair out of the way of the executioner's axe, and was decapitated. Fingers and cloth were dipped in his blood as the blood of Kings was held to cure illnesses.

The French medical model of 1800 was unprecedented, but it had been shaped by scientific, technical, and political changes in England. The anarchy that began with the English Civil War in 1641 led Thomas Hobbes in *Leviathan* (1651) to echo Charles and claim human life in its natural state was nasty, brutal, and short and civilization comes from the top down. A century later, Rousseau argued alienation came from the top down. This issue is key to healthcare and the question of drug wrecks.

Religion was one fault line beneath Charles' execution. The Reformation unsettled Europe leading to the Peasant Wars in the 1530s and the

Thirty Years War in 1618. These brought as much destruction to central Europe as later World Wars. New printing presses allowed many to become their own theologians, lawyers, and scholars. This made governing more difficult. Monarchs, previously seen as standing in for God, could no longer count on the loyalty of dissenters. Some stability was restored with a formula that the religion of a state would be that of its ruler. This solution to the difficulties of governing laid the seeds for the emergence of nation states. The German speaking states became either Protestant or Catholic. England encouraged its dissenters to emigrate to its American colonies.

Health was another fault line. Around 1600, the pace of enclosure of the commons, a privatization of lands formerly held in common, picked up. Private ownership would supposedly maximize the value of holdings. No-one had any incentive to spread dung on common land where it might be stolen for heating purposes in winter. A first welfare system, the Poor Law, was put in place in 1601 to compensate those driven off the land. Many went to London making it by 1640 the most populous city in the world, the center of England's trade, and close to self-governing.

Absolute Monarchs, like Charles, had a brief to ensure the lives and welfare of their subjects, protecting them against corporations, and containing episodes of plague. Facing a plague in 1640, Charles proposed a quarantine. Parliament refused this trade-blocking measure. This led to War in 1641. The monarchy was restored in 1660, but the political struggle continued to 1688, when Parliament won, and Free Trade triumphed over Public Health.

Parliament deployed a New Model Army, drawn from the masses of London's unemployed who formed a literate and politically aware army. This was a first hint of a new role for labor. Seven months after Charles' execution, Oliver Cromwell, the new Lord Protector of England, whose army had not been paid, invaded Ireland promising payment and lands.

The Irish Laboratory

The invasion was financed by monies raised by Adventurers (entrepreneurs). Between executions and deportations, the invasion depopulated

Ireland. In 1652 Royalists and Catholics had their Irish lands confiscated and turned over to Adventurers. One of these was William Petty, who had studied medicine in Oxford. Petty secured a contract to survey Ireland's population, resources, and religious profile.

The survey showed a destitute country. The Catholic Irish lived in smoke-filled, one-room cabins. The potato made it easy to produce enough food to live on, and sheep provided wool for clothes. This was simple living in line with biblical precepts, as Petty noted, but not a recipe for prosperity. The population and wealth data, supplemented by tax and trade data, allowed him to estimate for the first time the Gross Domestic Product of a country.

Petty was struck by Ireland's contrast with Holland, a more crowded country with fewer natural resources, yet wealthier. The Dutch confounded the conventional wisdom that population growth beyond a certain point should reduce wealth and that a country should export more than it imported. Petty concluded that wealth came from productive labor. From hands, not lands. Ireland needed more Irish incentivized to produce and trade.

The standard view claimed competition created by more people would drive wages down and land rents up. Petty argued the more production took place and the more trading of goods surplus to needs the more wealth would increase. More people would lead to more profits and falling taxes. Money would make money the more hands it passed through and the quicker it passed. This was more likely in cities where the lives of others would spur the pursuit of wants in addition to needs. Conspicuous consumption would grow as trade flourished and prices fell. As prices for Irish goods would be better, if free of import duties, he proposed a Free Trade agreement between Ireland and England. A world first.

Following the data flew in the face of Christian thinking. Petty covered his tracks by arguing that Dissenters viewed their labor as a duty to God.

The Monarchy was restored in 1660. One of Charles II's first acts was to create a Royal Society dedicated to science. Petty became one of its eight founders. The guiding principle of the Society was that it would only deal with questions that could be resolved by data and experiment. The Royal Society conjures up images of early physicists and chemists, but it included many physicians, among them Petty, Thomas Willis who transformed our view of the brain, and John Locke the creator of Liberalism. The physicians have been written out of the script. We hear about Copernicus, Galileo, and Newton displacing the earth from the center of the universe, rather than Vesalius' anatomical dissections, and William Harvey displacing the heart from the center of the body. The discovery of the body as a machine was at least as shocking as the idea the earth does not lie at the center of the universe.

By 1660 it was natural to link physics and chemistry with data, but it was not clear human behavior, which involves meaning and values, would yield data. In 1662 Charles II asked the Society to admit John Graunt, a haberdasher. Graunt had analyzed births, deaths, marriages and diseases in London over 50 years. In *Natural and Political Observations on Bills of Mortality Natural and Political Observations on Bills of Mortality*, he contrasted 'epidemical' diseases like the plague or smallpox, here one year and not the next, with a regular rate of injuries, suicides, and homicides from 'chronical' causes of death. Seeming randomness was predictable.

In non-plague years, Graunt could show that on average there were 5 births and 8 deaths a week. The population of the capital therefore depended on immigrants, both commoners and wealthy property owners, with rents supporting consumption and trade. One third of the population died by the age of six. Any country wishing to increase its population and its wealth needed therefore to watch after its births and the conditions of early infancy. This led the later French Revolutionaries to establish Foundling and Maternity Hospitals.

Petty promoted Graunt's work as an example of how to use data in the service of science. He applied the same approach to Dublin and found a similar picture. This work and his earlier survey data led in 1672 to essays on political arithmetic and political anatomy and what he called a political medicine of Ireland.

Petty invited his colleagues to consider: "whether of 100 sick of acute diseases who use physicians, as many die in misery as where no art is used, or only chance." This is a first glimpse of the numerical method later developed by Pinel and Louis in Paris.

Driven by data, Petty embraced a market approach to the national economy, advocated task specialization, put forward a modern theory of money, distinguished between price and value and developed a labor theory of value. These ideas later reappeared in Adam Smith's 1776 *Wealth of Nations* and Karl Marx's 1867 *Kapital*.

In 1665 London was struck with its greatest plague, the most vivid account of which was given by Daniel Defoe in *Journal of a Plague Year*.

The Oxford Laboratory

The English Civil War pitted a society organized from the top down, whose monarch standing in for God squared up to a movement that saw God within each of us and each of us as able to understand the divine plan as the elite. While war raged, the issues played out in the Oxford anatomy laboratory, where Harvey's demonstration that the heart was a pump gave the prospect that the body was a machine real force.

At postmortem, the brain is like a rice pudding. It leaks out of split skulls. It was dismissed as a cold organ. The cavities in this mass, the ventricles, discovered in early dissections were thought to be as key to the brain as they are in the heart. René Descartes proclaimed them as such in *The Passions of the Soul*, published in 1649.

In a set of experiments with preservatives, Thomas Willis revealed a new brain. His *Anatomy of the Brain* in 1664 contained drawings of a solid brain, the most famous of which was of the brain's under surface with its folds and fissures. This had features—a brain stem, the pons, the medulla and a circle of arteries known now as the Circle of Willis. Other views showed the corrugations of the cerebellum and the cerebral cortex.

The brain as an organ of thought came into view. It replaced the fluid containing ventricles. These were thought to be open to outside influence, whether the promptings of God or Satan, or the effects of the seasons, perhaps through the pineal gland. If it was open to influence, the new closed brain must grasp sensory impressions and convert these into thought. The different strata of the brain, the cortex, cerebellum, and midbrain, suggested different systems with different functions. Philosophers began to talk about rational, emotional, and volitional faculties and later up to 40 different faculties.

This brain called for two new sciences. Willis coined the term neurology for the science of nerve fibers and their central controller, the brain, the new governor, or monarch of the body. John Locke coined the term psychology to embrace the functioning of the mind within the brain. In his 1690 *Essay Concerning Human Understanding*, Locke argued that we begin life with a *tabula rasa* and through sensory inputs we lay down associations. These form our personalities and thoughts. A key question for all views of human nature centers on how to guarantee order in society. Locke's psychology reconciled a mechanical man with social order through the shaping of our associations by the correct education.

Willis and Locke made it conceivable we were individuals in a new sense. The motive force that drove us might arise from within rather than from without. Everyone believed there was an order and purpose to the universe. The term atheist at this point meant someone living a godless or immoral life rather than someone who did not believe there was an order in the Universe. Even the scandalous Baruch Spinoza, arguing in the 1660s that man was entirely material, termed himself a Deist, someone who believed in a God-given order from which God stepped back to let the Universe unfold. In 1689 when he became the leading advocate of religious tolerance, Locke also drew a line at tolerating non-belief.

The difficulty lay in understanding how a Godless world would work. What would motivate people to be moral? What would keep them in their place? The people were many and the rulers few. The English Civil War gave a sense of the forces that might be unleashed by too much freedom to do unchecked by fear.

Liberalism & Industry

England through to 1600 had been a minor player on the European stage compared with Austria and France for whom wealth lay in landed Estates. Petty introduced the idea that wealth might come from labor and trade rather than lands. As Defoe put it, *estate's a pond, trade's a spring.*

England and Holland were developing as trading nations. England in 1660 and Holland in 1662 established East India Trading Companies, financed by shares under limited liability laws. The Dutch set up a first ever stock exchange where company shares could be traded and a bank in Amsterdam to finance business. The market for spices, tea and slaves was intense and both companies appreciated in value. It became possible to make money by investing in companies.

In both countries, an emerging middle class argued they needed to be free to speak about different ways to solve problems. Rather than a Divine Right of Kings to rule, we could govern ourselves through a market. Make the right call and there was the pleasure of being right along with wealth. Make the wrong call and there was penury. Science appeared to support this new way. Observations counted whether they came from a scullery maid or a King. The new freedom needed security. Property could offer security, if there was a rule of law, equality before the law, and voting rights.

The emerging order seemed under threat in 1685 when James II, who favored a return to absolute monarchy, succeeded Charles. Locke moved to Holland. In 1688 James was deposed, and Parliament offered a constitutional throne to the Protestant William of Orange. An anonymous book *Two Treatises of Government* appeared. It argued that government requires the consent of the governed, that lawful government does not need a supernatural basis, and that Church and State are separate spheres. Under a social contract, there was a right to liberty of conscience. Individuals might even need protection from government. This marked the birth of Liberalism. The man too nervous to put his name to these subversive ideas was John Locke.

The new climate favored Free Trade. Not all worked out smoothly. In 1700 a Company of Scotland, set up to trade with Africa, failed disastrously taking 25% of Scottish wealth with it. This precipitated political union with England, chronicled by Defoe from his vantage point as an English spy in Edinburgh. In 1711 a South Sea Company formed to trade with South America. Defoe soon after opted to have Crusoe make his fortune in Brazil. Crusoe was published in 1719 and the following year the South Sea Company collapsed. Trading in company shares was banned for a century.

The words liberal and liberalism were rarely used before 1769 when William Robertson, a Scottish historian, used them to cover the combination of religious and political tolerance introduced by Locke and Free Trade. In 1776 Adam Smith's *Wealth of Nations* put an establishment seal on Liberalism. Rather than government from above, if trade were free, an invisible hand would govern our affairs. Unless, when they sought to maximize their own gain, people were irrational, markets should work. A producer might bring something new on the market and charge a high price because of its scarcity. If it sold others would replicate it and the price would fall. If it fell too far people would stop making it. Everything would settle at a reasonable value in a free market.

Dependence on others according to Smith was a source of corruption and ill-health, which would be banished as a rising tide of wealth floated all boats. The discipline of commerce and manufacturing would prevent crimes and ill-health, and so, Smith argued, the role of government should be restricted to national defense and justice. It should not participate in regulation, grant monopolies, or support employers or workers. Not everyone saw it this way. Others found it difficult to distinguish between liberalism and libertinism, freedom from restraint or obligation and illegality. Many agreed with Charles that freedom was only possible within a framework government puts in place.

Markets don't predict concentrations of wealth. They assume innovation goes into increasing the production of goods that people need and not into ways to create artificial scarcity or stimulate a demand in wants rather than needs. Smith did however note: "people from the same trade seldom meet together, even for merriment and diversion, but the conversation ends in a conspiracy against the public, or in some contrivance to raise prices."

Free Traders assumed this conspiracy would wither away in the face of growing trade. The eighteenth and nineteenth centuries however saw a series of booms and busts rather than steady growth. The makers and traders of goods responding with price-fixing and cartels, leading Marx to predict that a system based on competition must collapse.

Even as Smith was writing, techniques were doing an end-run around liberalism. Where he advocated a division of labor to increase productivity, machines, like the Spinning Jenny in 1760, vastly increased productivity and profit. They led to factories, urbanization, and ever more commodities we might want but didn't need.

The machines created new relations between capital and labor. Factories required labor. Previously serfs had been tied to place but had rights linked to local customs. For a labor market to work these had to become legal rights that held regardless of place. Traditional arrangements began to give way to a world of contracts. Workers were now free to go where they wished but the freedom in these contracts was notional as they typically needed the work more than employers needed a job done. Workers took on risks as part of their job, sometimes being paid more but without the safety net of a world in which masters had duties to serfs who were injured or ill. In the new world, an employer owed an injured worker nothing, until negligence was invented.

Accidental Destinies

These changes intersected with another profound shift. As Graunt collected statistics for his Life Tables, Blaise Pascal and Pierre Fermat in France, grappling with how to calculate odds in games of chance, created the mathematics of probability. While the numbers coming up on the next throw of a pair of dice are random, with a large enough set of throws the overall result can be predicted. Until then our understanding of the world came from authority and the use of logic to work down to what was supposedly real. Now it became possible to establish truths about the world starting from what happened in front of us and working up.

Life and death took on a new meaning. In addition to what an individual life and death means, all lives and deaths became beads on a string of lives and deaths that can enable others to pinpoint what leads to health and prosperity or premature death.

Business took on a new meaning. From 1600, English and Dutch clubs pooled money to cover funeral expenses and support a widow and children left behind by a loss at sea. These annuities or tontines appealed as a gamble—the last man standing inherited the pot. Dutch and English ships traveling to China, Indonesia, and the Americas were insured.

In 1762 a marriage between probability and business was consummated, when increasing data on the population of London supported the foundation of an Equitable Life insurance company. Basing its premiums on data, Equitable could charge less than other schemes and still profit. The new insurance business portrayed itself as respectable. There was no appeal to gambling. It would now be a gamble *not* to be insured. This insurance was for the risk averse rather than the risk takers. It was for a middle class anxious not to lose their place in society in the event of mishap. Crusoe could now cover his family, courtesy of a company called Providential or Prudential. Leaving everything to Providence didn't seem prudent.

Unlike cobblers, seamen and healers had to cope with storms and other forces of nature. Theirs was a world of magic and superstition, of reading auguries and runes, a world of fortune and misfortune, governed by Providence. Nothing happened without Gods' knowledge. When misfortune befell an individual or community, it was natural to question what the person or group had done to deserve this fate. Why me? Why now? It was natural to pray in an effort to manage fate. The new numerical orientation, which brought out the predictability of events rather than their singularity, offered some liberation from superstition.

Asking questions about the meaning of events can lead to superstition, but aggregating events can introduce meaninglessness. The regularity of accidents can be used by the owners of factories where accidents happen, or drug companies whose treatments injure, to deny meaning and shuck off responsibility.

Statistics came into play in another way. In 1835 Alphonse Quetelet claimed measures like height and girth distribute normally; they fall inside a Bell-shaped curve. From this, he drew the concept of *l'homme moyenne,* the average or statistical man. Describing variation is one thing. If my differences, especially in terms of behavior, become a deviation from a norm, and someone figures on making money out of fixing the deviation, that's another matter.

Complaints about a loss of individuality in the face of 'biomedicine' are common. This loss is linked to the medical model and leads to a call for a narrative medicine that takes individual stories into account. If medicine is not to lose its soul, we are told, it must answer the questions of Why me? and Why now?

Voices are being silenced, but does this come from the biology in medicine, from collecting data, or from an application of statistics that strips people of their individuality?

Monarch or Bureaucrat?

While it has been difficult to locate the mind in the body, no-one had any difficulty tying our passions to our hearts and viscera. The leading disorder of the passions was hysteria. This was thought to be caused by a wandering uterus which pressing on other organs could cause breathlessness, palpitations, or spasms. In 1662 Willis referred to it as the 'so-called uterine disease," whose true origin lay in the nerves and brain. By means of the nervous system, he wrote, "are revealed the true and genuine reasons for very many actions and passions that take place in our body that would otherwise seem most difficult to explain: and from this fountain, no less than the hidden causes of diseases and symptoms, which are commonly ascribed to the incantations of witches, may be discovered."

When Descartes suggested that the bodies of men and animals might function like machines his idea was that behavior was mediated by an equivalent of ropes and pulleys, or pipes involving fluid and valves. Nerves were the obvious candidates for such threads or pipes. On stimulation by pain, he proposed delicate threads lying in the nerve bundles open valves in the brain that release sensitive substances, which lead to movement—by reflex. Even though some actions seemingly occurred beneath the level of awareness, as in removing one's foot from a flame, these actions were invariably wise. For Descartes, reflexes involved reflection on the part of the ghost in the machine, rather than something automatic.

When François Magendie and Charles Bell described the reflex arc in 1823, ideas about how wisdom got into our behaviors began to fracture. Marshall Hall showed that reflex arcs could operate independently of the brain. Over the next 30 years, Wilhelm Griesinger and Carl Wernicke in Germany, and Thomas Laycock and Hughlings Jackson in Britain claimed increasingly complex behaviors, such as sleepwalking, were automatic and unconscious, tied to higher and higher reflexes.

A new view of man was taking shape. As Laycock put it:

Many will consider it dangerous to concede that apparently pure mental acts are only the results of vital machinery excited into action by physical agencies.[6]

Researches of this kind… whether instituted on the insane, the somnambulist, the dreamer, or the delirious must be considered like researches in analytical chemistry. The reagent is the impression made on the brain; the molecular changes following the application of the reagent are made known to us as ideas.[7]

Reflexes raised the possibility that consciousness might be a spectator of human activity rather than its guiding focus, and no more important, as Thomas Huxley put it, to human functioning than the whistle of a

---

6   Cited in Clark E, Jacyna LS, *Nineteenth Century Origins of Neuroscientific Concepts* (University of California Press, Berkeley, 1987), 143.

7   Laycock T (1844), *On the Reflex Functions of the Brain.* Cited in Dewhurst K *Hughlings Jackson on Psychiatry.* (Sandford Publications, Oxford, 1982).

locomotive to the running of a train, or a mist or steam that hovers over machines while they work.

In 1888 Ramon-y-Cajal radically altered our views of our nervous system when he showed it was not a continuous network but a mass of individual nerve cells—neurons. Freud was ever one to incorporate the latest biology into his theories. In his *Project for a Scientific Psychology* (1895), he proposed that individual memories might reside in these neurons. A splitting of associations previously formed by a reflex linking of these neurons might be the basis for a repression of difficult memories. In this way trauma might cause hysteria as he proposed in his *Studies on Hysteria*, written with Josef Breuer in 1893.

Soon after he decided this was not the way minds fit into brains. He turned to the question of how minds develop. What powers development if it doesn't stem from the unfolding of a divine plan? Fifty years earlier, Alexander Bain, stepping beyond Locke, linked associations to pleasure and pain. Recasting libido as a pleasure principle and pain as a reality principle, Freud argued these principles interacting with how we handle our instincts and impulses as we develop shape our characters.

While Freud was abandoning reflexes in favor of psychoanalysis, Ivan Pavlov married Locke's idea about associations shaping behavior to reflexes and created behaviorism. Thirty years later, linking Pavlov's reflexes with Bain's rewards and punishments, B. F. Skinner created operant conditioning. This behavioral neuroscience now underpins the operations of Google, Facebook and other social media companies and poses fundamental questions for all of us.

As late as 1955, despite reflexes, the dominant view of the brain had an electrical wraith hovering in a mechanical system. The difficulties in investigating the brain were in part responsible for this, but there was also resistance to the idea we are spiritless. We readily swap neurotransmitter biobabble today, but in 1968 students protesting in Paris, Amsterdam and Tokyo laid siege to laboratories engaged in what they saw as new and dehumanizing neuroscience research.

For these students a biochemical brain questioned the continuity of the self, not just after death, but a moment-to-moment continuity. How do we emerge from our chemicals? Does thinking connect with anything? How do we explain to our children why we fall in love, get gripped by causes, or why we should take responsibility for our actions? Are people on psychotropic drugs themselves? These are questions about the link between us and society. Questions about government. Is the brain the monarch of the body, a governor put in place by society, a bureaucrat coordinating bodily functions, or something else?

PROGRESSIVISM

As the body desacralized, society secularized. The Bible became an object of study rather than reverence. The idea of progress based on science became a belief system. We moved from valuing ascetic withdrawal to valuing engagement, from ritual to ethical living, from waiting for Jerusalem to building it and from histories of a few to a history of the many.

While there had been parliamentary government in Britain since 1688, with Liberals (Whigs) facing Conservatives (Tories), political parties only emerged around 1850. By then politics had turned inside out. Health played a key role in the shift. Liberals turned to government intervention for what they termed 'progressive causes', such as universal elementary education and wider suffrage. Where private property had been a liberal weapon against authoritarianism, the Conservatives became the party of private property.

The emergence of nation states catalyzed the new politics. In 1825 the first passenger rail travel triggered a mass laying of tracks in huge construction works that offered fresh investment opportunities. Liberals introduced a Joint Stock Companies Act, which made it possible to invest in business again for the first time since 1720. If the business failed, the investors were only liable to creditors for the amount they invested.

The development of steam-powered rotary presses in 1850 increased the number of copies of newspapers and periodicals. Linked to rail transport, local newspapers became a national press. Journalism, previously seen as an inferior form of life featuring news from the gutter about gambling, divorce and society scandals, along with advertising for food and drugs, became a pulpit. National newspapers like the Times brought a hint that most 'preaching' involves slogans and echo chambers. Like social media now, newspapers confirmed views rather than changed them. Social cohesion, it seemed, owed more to placing views in the hands of as many as possible rather than the accuracy of those views.

Risk Management

In 1820 French ideas about public health were as un-English as Catholicism. Liberal individuals had a duty to look after their own health and that of their family. The growth of industrial cities like Manchester and Liverpool challenged this. After a typhus epidemic in Manchester in 1796 a group of physicians, magistrates, church wardens and businessmen set up a voluntary Board of Health as:

> *The crowded and miserable habitations of the lowest orders… their inattention to cleanliness and ventilation, together with extreme poverty attendant on their dissolute manners of life, had conspired to introduce among them the most fatal and infectious disorders.*[8]

In these cramped quarters, typhus flourished. Was it airborne or spread by contact? The owners of properties near a proposed isolation hospital claimed contamination of their air would be a legal nuisance, and that contagion might be spread by the 'gaddings' of nurses. Any facility should be built on bare land instead. The trustees held firm and were able to show that investment in the new establishment saved money.

The growth of Manchester and other cities soon overwhelmed these voluntary efforts. The numbers of people in new cities linked to factories led to air pollution, a lack of fresh water, sewage disposal issues, increased rates of injuries and street crime especially after dark. Crowded properties

---

8   Harris H. *Manchester's Board of Health in 1796* (Isis 1938), 28, 26-37.

owned by private landlords created vast slums but managing this by providing public housing was anathema.

At just this time, Wordsworth and Coleridge inspired a Romantic Movement in English poetry. Where the order that came with civilization, especially its gardens, had been seen as the height of beauty, now wilderness and an unspoiled nature became the embodiment of beauty, inspiration, and health. By contrast, a string of writers, among them Friedrich Engels in Manchester and Charles Dickens in London, painted vivid pictures of life in industrializing cities, with rat infested buildings, stinking sewers, foul air, dwellings where no light ever penetrated and a sickly population.

Then reports came from India of a new disease—cholera. It began to migrate westwards, arriving in England in October 1831. The initial epidemic was brief but left 23,000 dead. Despite killing more than 100,000 in four visitations over thirty years, cholera killed less than typhoid and typhus. And tuberculosis killed more than smallpox, malaria, typhoid, and cholera combined. But the rapidity with which cholera killed and the gruesome deaths caused panic. It struck down the healthy and working poor as readily as the infirm and old. It threatened all orders of society. It made public health a liberal issue.

Edwin Chadwick was secretary to Jeremy Bentham, Britain's leading liberal. After Bentham's death in 1832, Chadwick lived on bequests from wealthy patrons. He viewed the Irish in England as pests who spread disease. He believed pauperism was gratuitous and preventable. He saw doctors as corrupt, and their education as useless. Most medical men in Britain at this time were apothecaries, who compounded medicines, and undertook some procedures such as setting fractures. They were poorly paid, often Irish or Scots, and had a reputation as political radicals.

In 1832 Chadwick became secretary to a commission to review the workings of the Poor Law. This welfare system put in place in 1601 with the enclosure of common lands was tied to parishes. As the pace of industrialization picked up, growing numbers of people unable to work through injuries or failing health, who could not support themselves, found themselves isolated in cities. These medical indigents ended up in workhouses, which had to be paid for. Chadwick had a horror of giving money to anyone able-bodied. Contrary to liberal principles, which would have trusted to the invisible hand of local relieving officers to get things right, he recommended the creation of a centralized system, which he believed would be more efficient, employ less people and operate to a standard set of procedures.

His report led to an 1834 Welfare Law aimed more at deterring scroungers than providing a safety net. While working on welfare policy, he met Thomas Southwood Smith and William Duncan. Smith was a doctor in the London Fever Hospital, which worked on the French model of postmortems, regular examinations, data collection and research. He persuaded Chadwick of French thinking that disease caused poverty and that the wealth of the nation would be increased if disease were prevented through sanitarian measures.

Duncan worked in Liverpool, then the most rapidly growing city in the world. Its population quadrupled between 1800 and 1840. In 1840 he produced a report, *On the Sanitary State of the Laboring Classes in Liverpool* that laid the basis for Chadwick's 1842 report *The Sanitary Condition of The Laboring Population*. Both sketched grim vistas of the conditions in which people lived, blaming these conditions for diseases, including cholera. The message was that, if people like us wanted to avoid diseases like this, we must clean up the reservoirs from which it came.

Chadwick's Welfare Law recommended appointing medical officers to workhouses. These poorly paid posts had a brief to keep the able-bodied out. Creating the posts linked to medical wards in workhouses, however, unintentionally laid the basis for a state hospital system and state medical care. Chadwick's 1842 Report came peppered with references to sanitary systems and medical police. This was astonishing given that classic liberalism abhorred efforts to regulate public life. In 1842 the British State took 2 pence in every pound in taxes—for defense only. There was no money for public works, unless a case could be made that it would save money. This was the case Chadwick made.

The standard narrative for a century after Chadwick was that the French and Austrian idea of medical police only appeared in England with this Report. The freedom-loving English preferred education and persuasion to controls and resisted his ideas. But there was a divide between English rhetoric for home consumption and English actions in Ireland, and later India and wherever they saw themselves bringing civilization.

In 1833, for instance, the Conservative Prime Minister, Robert Peel, introduced a Bill for a publicly funded police force to support law and order in England. A publicly funded police force had been introduced in Dublin in 1786, which Dubliners did not see as fostering public good but rather as securing English property and suppressing legitimate grievance.

In 1845 fleeing a famine aggravated by English politics, the Irish poured into Liverpool, adding 300,000 to its population of 360,000, bringing typhus with them, it was claimed. Liverpool appointed Duncan as Britain's first Metropolitan Medical Officer with a brief to improve drainage, add sewers, remove refuse, and provide clean drinking water.

The British Parliament passed a Public Health Act in 1848. This was permissive rather than mandatory. It recommended appointing medical policemen around the country, creating sanitation schemes, and inspecting dwellings.

Big Data

The times were also statistical. A Registrar General's Office opened in London in 1836 to collect census and other data. A Royal Statistical Society, a Board of Trade statistical office, and other statistical societies also appeared. John Simon, Chadwick's successor, established an Epidemiological Society in 1850 to "endeavor by the light of modern science to review all those causes which result in the manifestation and spread of epidemic diseases." Statistics meant Big Data, not statistical tests. Data on infant mortality and other deaths were both clamant and value-free. Difficult for governments to ignore.

William Farr was appointed to the Registrar General's Office. A general practitioner who had shown an aptitude for data collection, Farr had authored a chapter on Vital Statistics, set up a journal for population statistics, and attended lectures given by Villermé in Paris. Using census data, his brief was to break mortality out by region and occupation. But how to classify deaths?

Just as with the creation of hospital medicine in 1800 when having enough patients in one place to see commonalities was key, too fine-grained or too broad a classification of deaths risked missing useful commonalities. Farr plumped for 27 causes of deaths divided into 5 groups: deaths by epidemics and contagious diseases, general deaths with no clear cause, diseases by anatomical site, developmental diseases, and violent deaths by external causes, including accidents, suicides, and homicides. With qualifiers like workplace, railroad, domestic, or Acts of God, external cause deaths had the potential to be intensely political. In this way, 180 years after Graunt, medical statistics, or as it is now called epidemiology, was born. It became to social medicine what the laboratory was to biomedicine.

Cholera revisited England in 1849, 1854 and 1866. As in France, it was initially seen as a pestilential vapor, a miasma. The miasma theory supported the development of drainage and sewage systems. When Germany's Justus Liebig, in creating organic chemistry, demonstrated that chemical reactions could produce putrefaction, fermentation and all the smells of disease, science appeared to support miasmatic theories.

Cholera became an epidemiological battleground. Farr's data showed it was less likely on higher ground, leading him to claim it was air-borne rather than water borne. Another London physician, John Snow, produced a map of Battersea cases pointing to contaminated water. Majority opinion sided with Farr. When William Budd in Bristol claimed he had detected a "living organism of distinct species… which could be conveyed in water," in the feces of those affected, no-one paid heed.

When there was another outbreak in London's Soho in 1854, Snow mapped a clustering of cases around Broad Street and argued that water from the Broad Street Pump was the source of infection. His arguments were promoted by the area's abattoir owners and dismissed because abattoirs were notable producers of noisome materials.

Meanwhile, Florence Nightingale came to world attention in the Crimea, where in 1855 English troops were at war with Russia. She distinguished herself by providing nursing care but also by epidemiological maps showing that troops were more likely to die from disease and the management of wounds in insanitary conditions than from battle. Air quality and filth were the issue and cleanliness the answer. She dismissed Filippo Pacini's claim in 1854 to have isolated a vibrio cholera. When London faced the Great Stink in 1858, the worst ever contamination of the River Thames, she dismissed William Budd's data showing a fall in mortality during the period that cast doubt on the miasma theory.

As late as 1860 infection did not imply germs. Basic questions such as whether cholera was contagious remained undecided. Smallpox clearly passed from person to person, but malaria 'infections' were linked to the air from marshy areas, hence the name. It was not contagious. Farr's records were filled with certificates of deaths of people said to have been overcome by sewer or marsh gas.

When Pasteur demonstrated in 1858 that germs also caused putrefaction and fermentation, the tide turned. Budd again categorized typhoid as an intestinal infection transmitted through sewage systems in 1866 and was believed. When the East London Water Company admitted lying to cover up fecal contamination in their water, Farr admitted defeat. In 1867 Joseph Lister promoting the benefits of antiseptic technique in surgery, which he attributed to the management of germs, was celebrated where Ignaz Semmelweis in 1847 was sacked.

Health Systems

The poor who couldn't work and ended up in workhouses brought into view those who were too sick to work and those who were too mad. Opening medical wings in workhouses for the medically indigent sorted the sick but lunacy was more challenging. As of 1800, there were only a handful of publicly funded beds for lunatics in England. Some patients were committed to private madhouses, leading Defoe, a century earlier, to draw attention to the involuntary commitment of people by relatives seeking their money or husbands trying to get rid of wives. His efforts led to Acts aimed at curbing abuses. But now there was another reason to do something about the mad.

In 1845 the Liberal Anthony Ashley-Cooper steered Lunacy and Counties Asylum Acts through Parliament, putting in place an asylum building program across Britain. Where previous Acts had been aimed at curbing abuses, these Acts were based on a belief that clean water and air, good food, a daily routine, the discipline of work, and hygiene, would make recovery from lunacy possible.

This 1845 Act followed Esquirol's 1838 law establishing asylums in France, but, in fact, the Richmond Asylum opened in Dublin in 1815, followed by an asylum building program in Ireland that led to more beds per head of the population than ever seen anywhere else. Double the rates found in Britain or France. Asylums continued to be built even after the Famine halved Ireland's population. These asylums were accompanied by a set of Regional Hospitals on the lines drawn up by French reformers but put in place even earlier in Ireland, Britain's laboratory for testing social programs.

The 1845 Acts mark the start of legislation to manage the new urban environments. An 1848 Public Health Act addressed water and sewage, followed by a Nuisance Removal Act (1855), a Factory Act (1864), a Sanitary Act (1866), and an 1868 Act mandating the improvement of tenement housing. Contagious Disease Acts in 1864, 1866 and 1869 were aimed at prostitutes and garrisons. These were followed by an Artisans Dwelling Act (1875) and a further Public Health Act in 1875 forcing local authorities to appoint Medical Officers.

A General Medical Council was established in 1858 to license doctors. This marks the point at which the French model of clinical medicine was accepted, where apothecaries became doctors, and acceptance of the idea that properly qualified medical practitioners would be self-policing. Similar arrangements, across the Western World at this time, led the excluded hydropaths, homeopaths, and sanitarians, to smell a plot. A division between orthodox and alternative medicine emerged that differed from the older division between learned gentlemen and empirics.

Regulation was an incoming tide. Some saw an effort by a Ruling Class to control the people. But Mass Society was facing all of us for the first time. Medical and social causes could become a matter of national debate within weeks. Invading armies of germs could arrive from nowhere. The choice lay between having a system or anarchy. If it's war and an efficient response is needed, nations systematize (aka militarize).

Safe Food & Drugs

These regulations were designed to make markets work. The Greeks, Romans, and Chinese all produced books on the preparation of medicines (*Materia Medica*). Medicines were modified foodstuffs; herbs sprinkled with eye of newt and toe of frog, and after Paracelsus in 1530 with mercurials, arsenicals and other heavy metals. In Europe, Grocers Guilds were responsible for these compendia. In 1618 the London College of Physicians assumed responsibility for a *Materia Medica*, renamed a *Pharmacopoeia*, and took the apothecaries (family doctors) who compounded medicines into their ranks, leaving grocers to deal in food. The College had the powers to check the quality of medicines and to fine anyone producing false goods. Edinburgh and Dublin followed suit with pharmacopeias. The United States produced a first national pharmacopeia, the USP, in 1820.

The development of chemistry made it possible to detect food adulteration. Potassium, aluminum, and copper sulfates were in use along with chalk to whiten bread. Starch from potatoes, with plaster of Paris and pipe clay, was used to bulk up bread. Almost everything, including medicines, contained lead or other fillers. Tea was cut with used tea leaves or hedgerow clippings 'painted' black or green to look like tea. Beer had strychnine and vitriol (sulfuric acid) added along with wormwood and opium to save on hops. This market was like the street drug market today.

The new chemical capabilities gave Frederik Accum, who arrived in London from Germany in 1793, an opportunity. He set himself up as a Chemist, wrote books, and set up Accum and Garden to sell chemicals and laboratory equipment. The company shipped the equipment and chemicals needed for the first chemical laboratories in Yale and Harvard.

In 1820 Accum published *A Treatise on Adulterations of Food and Culinary Poisons Exhibiting the Fraudulent Sophistications of Bread, Beer, Wine, Spirituous Liquors, Tea, Coffee, Cream, Confectionery, Vinegar, Mustard, Pepper, Cheese, Olive Oil, Pickles and other articles employed in Domestic Economy and Methods of Detecting Them.* It sold out in a month, but it made him enemies and forced him to move back to Germany. The new market was quickly filled with *The Domestic Chemist* and other books.

Confectioners, who wanted to make sweets colorful to entice children, coated them in yellow or orange chromate of lead, vermillion (mercury sulfide) or red lead to make them red, and arsenate of copper, verdigris or copper acetate to make them green. The same compounds were used in lipsticks, rouges, blushers, and mascara.

In 1850 two hundred people were poisoned by food colorings and seventeen deaths were attributed in London to colored lozenges alone, stimulating a debate in Parliament. Several of the businessmen involved were members of Parliament. Foreigners, they argued, were the adulterators; local producers, by contrast, 'sophisticated' foods harmlessly.

The deaths triggered a new form of journalism, medical periodicals. The *Lancet* made its name in the 1830s with articles on food adulteration. In 1850, its editor, Thomas Wakley, set up the Analytical Sanitary Commission with Arthur Hill Hassall as director. Using a new high-powered microscope, Hassall produced an article a week for years covering thousands of substances, naming the companies and individuals responsible for the adulteration. The furor triggered led to a series of Acts in 1860, and 1872, culminating in 1875 with a Safe Food and Drugs Act. The Government had been forced to fetter the God of Free Trade to make the market work.

The opposition of the business community to the new Act was intense. Yet by 1880 food producing companies began supplementing the Act with voluntary self-regulation. The protection of the consumer suddenly coincided with company needs to be protected from unfair trade practices. This was a first hint that regulation can set up market capture.

The second most famous medical journal, the *British Medical Journal,* also tackled market abuses in *Secret Remedies.* This campaign drew attention to continuing failures to label the ingredients of drugs adequately and price mark-ups of a 1,000% or more.

As the *Lancet*'s critiques of food adulteration were unfolding, the world of food and drugs was on the cusp of dramatic change. In 1856 William Henry Perkins isolated a purplish dye from coal tar, he called mauveine. This discovery created a dye industry. New dyes tumbled out of chemical companies offering new ways to color textiles and foods. These dyes were safer than lead. But in the 1890s it became clear that any dyes coloring organic material could potentially bind to human tissues and be a drug or a toxin.

Apart from the poisoning that led to death, food adulteration may have caused many disorders. North West Wales was and is one of the poorest and most rural parts of Britain. Because of geography, its asylum had no patients from out of area. The population was ethnically homogenous and rural, then and now, with no options for private care then or now. Logging all admissions between 1875 and 1924 makes it possible to compare the diagnoses and outcomes then and now.

Between 1875 and 1924, the asylum had 1074 patients admitted with a psychosis, and a striking increase in the incidence of schizophrenia, a disorder not described before 1800. Beginning in the 1860s, English and French physicians reported a new illness, and their concerns that the asylums could not hold a new patient flood. The descriptions paint a picture like the emergence of AIDs in the 1980s. Then, from 2005, there is a marked fall in the incidence of schizophrenia.

There are only a few factors that can explain this pattern. One is lead. A rise in our exposure to lead after 1800 parallels the rise in schizophrenia. The elimination of lead from food and its more recent elimination from paint and gasoline maps onto the decline in the incidence of schizophrenia. A change in obstetrical practices consequent on the discovery of anesthesia might explain a rise in the mid-nineteenth century and fall today but very few other factors can account for both the rise and the fall. Meanwhile of the patients who died in the asylum, 60 cancers were found at postmortem. There were no lung cancers, and one breast cancer. The rest were gastro-intestinal cancers. Was our food killing us?

Saving the People?

In 1905 for French and German politicians managing the Crowd meant containing socialist uprisings. The most significant crowd events in Britain and America involved religion and protests against vaccinations. Against a background of strikes in the largest quarries in the world, and rising deaths from tuberculosis, in 1905 there was a Religious Revival in North Wales. The community was called to temperance and clean living, as the end was nigh. A spike in admissions to the Asylum has made it possible to establish the outcome of what is now called 'Jerusalem Syndrome,' confirming that this socially triggered psychosis, unlike schizophrenia, ordinarily resolves completely.

Vaccination was among the concerns of the religious. In 1798 Edward Jenner demonstrated that vaccination with cowpox was a safe way to confer immunity to smallpox. Smallpox was a feared disease. Up to a quarter of those affected might die, with others left disfigured. It had a major role in the conquest of the Americas by decimating native populations. Vaccination reduced the risks and seemed an obvious benefit to many, but there were ethical, religious, and epidemiological doubters. The vaccine came from cows. The procedure introduced pus from one person into a scarification on another without sterilization. There were convincing claims of syphilis and tuberculosis transmitted in this way. Middle-class mothers had difficulties when their babies were inoculated with pus from a working-class child in public sessions. Others resented the pauperizing stigma of being vaccinated by workhouse medical officers.

When vaccination was made compulsory in 1853, with fines for refusal, resistance grew among those who had previously called for the Abolition of Slavery and supported the Temperance and Co-operative movements. The visible scarification and link to cows were portrayed as the Mark of the Beast as foretold in the Book of Revelation. Vaccinators deployed the new germ theories to justify the procedure. Anti-vaccinators asked for evidence of a smallpox germ and claimed the upper classes didn't get smallpox because of their better food and air. Vaccinators talked about the feckless negligence of the laboring classes for not having their children vaccinated.

An *Anti-Compulsory Vaccination League* (ACVL) was set up in 1866 followed by a National ACVL in 1874, after an 1871 Act made vaccinations compulsory for some employments. Refusing to have a child vaccinated led to a fine, or in the event of being unable to pay, jail. Some vaccination officers went to jail rather than impose the Act. Demonstrations against government policy took place, with 100,000 at a protest in Leicester in 1885 at which an effigy of Edward Jenner was decapitated.

Compulsory vaccination, the protesters claimed, was indistinguishable from compulsory baptism or circumcision. What was needed was tolerance of belief and medical Free Trade rather than medical monopoly. The Liberal Party split between those who held to traditional beliefs that everyone should be able to decide for themselves and those who thought a party prepared to ban child labor could also intervene to protect children with vaccines.

A review commissioned in 1892 branded the anti-vaccine lobby as soft-headed spiritualists, over-influenced by journalism and public opinion. In *The Doctor's Dilemma* George Bernard Shaw, an anti-vaccinationist, portrayed medicine as a conspiracy against the laity. Between the lack of a bug, and apparent establishment lies about the risk of syphilis, there were grounds to doubt medical and government bona fides.

A new Vaccination Act in 1898 allowed for conscientious objection provided parents could 'satisfy' a magistrate they had grounds to opt out. Many magistrates had a conscientious objection to conscientious objectors. The objectors didn't like a law that made them licensed lawbreakers rather than equal citizens. They invoked the 1689 Tolerance Act that brought the

English Civil War to an end by giving Dissenters the right to legally affirm allegiance. A decade later conscientious objectors featured in World War I.

The British Labour Party formed in 1900. One of its founding principles was the abolition of compulsion. When the Liberals returned to power in 1906, they introduced a new act continuing compulsory vaccination, but removed the word 'satisfy' which took discretion out of the hands of magistrates. Within two years, it was estimated that 25% of the children in the country were unvaccinated, with 50% in some regions, and 90% in pockets. Smallpox never returned. With the 1948 National Health Services Act, the Labour Party abolished compulsion. Ironically, the last recorded case in the world happened in Britain when the virus (discovered in 1930) escaped in 1978 from a laboratory in Birmingham.

There are times we prefer to take our chances with what the universe has in store for us rather than run with the herd. This risks reprisals from the herd. Regardless of the name we put on our religion or politics, community beliefs are conservative. They favor civic duty, and loyalty. Having occasional animals stray from the herd is one thing, having the herd split is another, especially if a technical system appears to offer an efficient solution to a significant threat. Splits can almost only be permitted on 'religious' grounds.

Technical systems, in health as elsewhere, do not tolerate pluralism. They reach for guidelines and standards. The vaccination controversies are emblematic of this.

3: THE TWO MEDICINES

I shall not rest and shall not pride myself on having been Lord of the People, unless the farmer is able to have a chicken on his table and is able to restore the forces spent at work with good food.[9]

Johann Peter Frank, the lead physician in the Holy Roman Empire, mentioned these words of Henry of Navarre, King of France, in a graduation day speech for doctors in Milan in 1790. The Empire, begun in France in 800 A.D., was then centered in Vienna. The Emperor Joseph II, the brother of Marie Antoinette, wife of Louis XVI, had just died. Joseph had been the model Enlightened Monarch, but his reforms aroused opposition. Everyone was waiting to see which way the new Emperor, Leopold II, would jump. Be a Henry or a Joseph, was Frank's message, this way a society's wealth lay:

The great majority of all evils from which we suffer derives from man himself... why is it that a vast amount of illness originates in the very society that man of old put in place in order to enjoy a safer life?

The people live in such a slavish condition and are excluded from any property rights as citizens... Those of us who look after the sick

---

9 Frank, J.P. *The People's Misery, Mother of Diseases* (1790). Sigerist, H.E. (Johns Hopkins University Press, Baltimore.) 88-100.

but are healthy do not succumb to contagion which takes away those who been debilitated to begin with...

In these deplorable conditions... women already enfeebled by hard physical labor and poor nutrition are forced to neglect their own children when wealthy women come demanding wet nursing... Abolish servitude and "the mother's fertile womb will produce strong and numerous children, the fields cultivated by sinewy arms will thrive, the diseases will return to the cities that are rotten with debauchery—joy virtue patriotism and the former health of citizens secured by labor will be restored. [10]

Mention Frank and historians say medical police and imply there was something distinctively German about medical police. But Frank's views about enlightened medicine were similar to Diderot's and others. Medical police should avoid being stubborn parents, avoid the iron rod of oppression and use instead the "soft and persuasive advices of friendship".

He advocated land ownership for the peasantry and making all property owners equal before the law. He supported securing the state by developing the lives of individuals. But Louis XVI's decapitation did not encourage Leopold.

In 1805 Napoleon swept across the Rhine bringing liberalism, markets, vaccinations, and ambulances with him. He crushed the 1006-year-old Empire at the Battle of Austerlitz in 1806. Austria-Hungary emerged from its ruins. A year later he defeated Prussia at the Battle of Jena and entered Berlin, a grubby and smelly provincial capital, one third the size of Paris, a sixth the size of London, but triple the size of New York.

In response to defeat, Prussia emancipated its serfs, embraced property owning, restricted Guild control to allow industries to develop, extended the right to vote, gave equality before the law to free peasants, and barred the clergy from government. These reforms aimed at opening government to merit and engaging a peasantry then morphing into a working class. There was talk of a constitutional monarchy. The key change was replacing

---

10 Frank, J.P. ibid.

its aristocracy with a bureaucracy. the place where each of us now encounters government.

Meanwhile science was growing in importance. The exchanges it fostered between universities, along with railroads, the press, and a turn from agriculture to industry, led to talk of unification of the 39 German-speaking states. Many looked to Prussia to take a lead but even Prussia was barely one entity. It had multiple provinces along with Silesia, which was inhabited by Poles. Uncertain if they were Prussians or Germans, many Prussians talked loosely of a Fatherland.

Death of Vitalism

Around 1800, physicians attempting to make diagnoses could look at tumors and areas of discoloration on the body surface. Looking within the body was restricted to evacuations, urine, feces or blood, variations in the color or consistency of which might indicate what was happening within.

Physicians were commonly portrayed holding a urine flask up to the light scanning for deposits called urates. Urates are increased in gout and other rheumatic conditions, then commoner than heart attacks or cancers. A uric acid theory suggested those predisposed to produce more uric acid suffered from gout and rheumatism. The theory was correct for gout.

Urate chemistry lay on the cutting edge of science. A new compound, lithium, discovered in 1817, dissolved urates. Alkaline substances were thought to help gout or rheumatism, and this underpinned the popularity of spa waters. Berzelius suggested that spa waters might contain lithium. The great European spas quickly discovered their waters either did contain lithium or else they added it. In 1929, 7 UP started life as a lithium-containing drink.

Justus von Liebig, a young academic, returned from Paris, the epicenter of scientific excellence, to the University of Giessen in Darmstadt. He opened a chemistry laboratory. At the time, there was a chasm between inorganic and organic chemistry. Organic life differed from the inorganic universe. In 1830, Frederick Wöhler synthesized urea, an organic molecule in Liebig's laboratory. Urea's synthesis was portrayed as a death knell for vitalism, the idea there is something unique about human life that will never yield to the probing of materialist science.

Liebig became a superstar. In debates about cholera and contagion, his putrefaction theory was widely cited. Because organic molecules are more complex than inorganic molecules, he argued, they are unstable and more likely to decay. The decay of one molecule destabilizes the next producing putrefaction or fermentation. This was a poisoning process, something more understandable than the vitalism of germs. St Anthony's Fire is a recurrent epidemic that involves chemical poisonings from ergot on rye. In *Organic Chemistry* (1840) and *Animal Chemistry* (1842), Liebig outlined how everything from digestion to excretion and decomposition involved chemical reactions. Just as in the laboratory these were facilitated by catalysts, none of which needed energy or supervision.

Liebig's triumph led to a development of university posts in medicine and its related sciences across the German states. As the techniques linked to industry became more important, having a university that catered to subjects other than theology and law became a means of fostering regional development, just as later happened in America.

German sanitarians embraced Liebig's findings, setting up a clash with clinical medicine. In 1847 Ignaz Semmelweis, recently appointed to the obstetrical hospital in Vienna, having controlled for possible confounders, recorded a threefold higher rate of puerperal fever on hospital wards with doctors in attendance compared with wards where midwives attended the births. The data spoke loudly. Semmelweis, drawing from Liebig, thought that putrefying material under the fingernails of the attending doctors caused the contagion. Handwashing with chlorine bleach helped by removing the putrefying material. Leading doctors across Europe lined up to reject his ideas, explaining that puerperal fever was an epidemic not an endemic disorder. But German medicine was about to change.

The German Spring

Rudolf Virchow is often portrayed as the fount and origin of public health, or social medicine. He was born in Prussia in 1821. Supported by a military scholarship, he trained in medicine in Berlin, qualifying in 1847. At this point, the medical model remained more promise than reality and there were difficulties from America to Russia in working out how to distinguish between real doctors and quacks or charlatans.

In February 1848, Virchow was sent by the Prussian Government to Silesia to investigate a typhus epidemic. Untouched by reforms in Prussia, Silesia's population were mostly Poles. They were still serfs, or robots as they were known locally.

Virchow was shocked by Silesia's poverty and squalor, the vermin on the people, their poor diet, intemperance and licentiousness, insanitary towns and dwellings, and lack of morale. He noted a disease recently described in Italy, pellagra (rough skin disorder). The Catholic Church, it seemed to him, was keeping the people bigoted, stupid, and dependent. For Protestants, Catholicism induced submissiveness, fatalism, obscurantism, and mental bondage. The remedy was a dose of Liberalism. Get rid of serfdom. Make every man a property owner. Give him an incentive to produce goods that could be sold in exchange for other goods, and there would be a greater variety of food and a greater pride in work.

Along with many Prussians, Virchow regarded Slavs as inferior. He also distrusted the poebel, which "all too often lacks judgment and education and whose existence precludes peace and order." For liberal democracy to work, he suggested, the rabble had to be taken into society and be given civil, and legal rights. They also needed guidance. An activist medical elite would have to carry the burden of leadership and reform. Doctors should be the natural attorneys of the poor.

Virchow returned to Berlin in March 1848, convinced that the cause of the typhus epidemic was social:

> *Epidemics are simple: large warning signs from which the statesman can clearly read that a disturbance has occurred in the course of his people's development.*
>
> *Every widespread disease in the nation, be it mental or physical, therefore, shows us the life of the population under abnormal*

conditions and all we need to do is to recognize this abnormality and signal it to the statesman so he can dispose of it.

Medicine is a Social Science and politics is nothing but medicine on a larger scale.[11]

His return coincided with uprisings across Europe triggered by poor harvests from Ireland to Russia. Discontent was aggravated in Prussia by a censorship aimed at damping talk of unification and democracy, and a tax to fund railroad development. In France, artisans drove the revolution. In Prussia, an emerging middle class (bourgeois) wanted a seat at the table. When the military fired on a protesting Berlin crowd, Virchow took to the barricades.

Constitutional government seemed in the offing. Thirteen doctors were elected to the Berlin Municipal Parliament, including Virchow. All over Germany medical societies formed. An Assembly of Berlin Doctors formed with a mission to improve the conditions of the people and their doctors. Public health doctors at the time were paid a pittance by the local councils, who thought they had a right to offer medical views and even decide who their doctor might marry. Doctors pushed for liberal reforms to remove the bureaucratic restrictions on them and their ability to help the people.

Virchow believed in free trade to the extent of campaigning against laws abolishing quackery. If scientific medicine could deliver, he argued, there was no need for doctors to protect themselves with a guild or by licensing. The public would gravitate toward what worked and shun what didn't. Under his promptings distinctions between doctors and charlatans were abolished—temporarily.

When the 1848 Revolutions broke out, Karl Marx and Friedrich Engels rushed out a pamphlet, *The Communist Manifesto*. Population health was at the heart of this. In the 1840s, following in the footsteps of Villermé, investigative journalists in England like Charles Dickens, administrators

---

11 McNeely IF, *Medicine on a Grand Scale. Rudolf Virchow, Liberalism and the Public Health*, (The Wellcome Trust Centre for the History of Medicine, London) p 1.

like Edwin Chadwick, and doctors like William Duncan produced reports close to identical to Engels' *Conditions of the Working Class in England.* These overlapped with Virchow's "politics is medicine on a social scale," which did not mean that heart attacks have a political dimension or the personal is political. This was public health medicine.

Rather than workshops and artisans, as in France, influenced by Engels, Marx saw factories and their workers, a proletariat, as the emerging class and likely drivers of change. Unlike artisans (including doctors), who exercised discretion in applying their skills to produce goods, all the proletariat had was their labor. The proletariat were part of a productive apparatus. Once they became politically aware, they would become a revolutionary class.

Marx favored reversing the enclosure of the Common Lands that began in England over 200 years before. This was close to the core belief of Cabet's communists with their call for a return to primitive Christianity. Virchow, in contrast, favored extending private property. But both saw the state (the stranglehold of landowners) withering away, an interdependence of communities and individuals, the importance of education, a need to foster social harmony, the desirability of the unification of Germany, along with a removal of censorship, and universal suffrage.

A key dilemma of liberalism from Locke to Virchow was whether to let people decide for themselves to follow what the latest science showed about health and disease. To Virchow, it seemed inevitable that for a period the people would need to be guided by doctors using science to set them on an upward course. Virchow from the start, in line with Liberals from Locke to Obama, saw education and consensus as key. Marx, in contrast, like feminists later, saw people being excluded from a share in power even if they were educated.

Marx saw something else. The word capitalism had just been coined and pointed to something different to the Free Trade Petty and Smith had argued was a source of wealth. New machines and techniques were something people could make money from. To adapt Defoe: *estate's a pond, trade's a spring and technique's a river.*

After the 1848 Springtime of the Nations turned to Winter, disenchanted French communists emigrated to Nauvoo Illinois and set up an Icarian community there. In Prussia, rather than set up representative assemblies, reformers turned to rules and procedures to improve the functioning of the bureaucracy. Many Germans followed the Irish to America. Marx moved to London, where sustained by Engels, and by journalism, he wrote columns for the *New York Tribune*, and worked on the vista glimpsed in the 1848 Manifesto.

Virchow remained a member of parliament but turned to the laboratory and microscope. Xavier Bichat had helped create the medical model in 1800, when he located tissues as the seat of disease. In 1860 Virchow proposed the cell as the fundamental unit of the body and that all pathology would ultimately be cellular. This move laid the basis for bacteriology.

He described atherosclerosis. Today, a cholesterol paradigm claims lipids thicken arteries, causing heart attacks and strokes. Virchow thought the difficulty was not with cholesterol but arterial inflammation. This view dominated until 1960 and is influential again today. New evidence suggests statins help not by lowering cholesterol but by being anti-inflammatory. Smoking may be hazardous because of the inflammation it causes.

His reputation at this time was so great that his opposition to Semmelweis' theories about puerperal fever killed these views and Semmelweis. Virchow linked puerperal fever to atmospheric conditions, the mental state of women, and disturbances in milk secretion. He dismissed the idea that pathology examinations, of which he did a lot, might be a cause.

Virchow was given a chance in 1870 to practice medicine on a political scale. Berlin was then the foulest smelling capital in Europe. Its population was approaching a million. Sewage ran in the streets, carried away in carts by ladies of the night to fertilize nearby farms. Successive cholera epidemics put a premium on cleaning up the filth and smell.

Virchow was made overseer of the creation of a new sanitary system. Landowners who used Berlin night soil to fertilize their farms opposed the scheme. The landowners recruited Liebig to argue that the nitrogen from fecal material had a value beyond all description and that the canalization of Berlin would be a calamity for Prussian agriculture.

Sanitation demanded taxes. Would homeowners pay when they got nothing tangible for the money? Raising funds for Virchow's expensive project introduced the notion of taxation for public investment. The work took 10 years but made Berlin fit to be a capital city.

The sanitation scheme was an example of technocratic development that did not involve a redistribution of wealth. It made public health a business. Doctors, bureaucrats and industrialists began to consort at exhibitions laying out the latest in safe school desks, tools for meat inspection, or checks for food adulteration. It was accepted there should be a public health input to food and drugs quality, vaccination schedules, the collection of medical statistics, factory inspections, and a bureaucracy to implement the latest healthcare orders.

As this was happening other developments were afoot that were about to marry medicine and politics in ways that affect each of us to this day.

SOCIAL HEALTH

There were 39 German states in 1860, bound by a common legal and linguistic heritage, and growing trade links. Some were Protestant and some Catholic. The united nations of Britain and France appeared to stand in contrast to Germany, Italy, and America but all countries were unifying, putting in place national systems of government not possible previously.

In 1862 Otto von Bismarck became Prussian Chancellor. He engineered a war against Austria in 1866 and against France in 1870. Industrialization and improved road and rail networks enabled Prussia to mobilize more rapidly than France and win. Victory triggered the unification of Germany in 1871 under the Prussian Kaiser with Bismarck as Chancellor.

When a truce was declared with Prussia, a collection of socialists and republicans remained in control of Paris. They resisted efforts of the new French Republic to regain control. Marx celebrated the Paris Commune as a harbinger of a revolution that would bring the proletariat to power.

Bismarck took note because of a growing socialism in Germany and its links to medicine.

The medical complaints of mercury workers in Furth bring home the politics. Furth-Nuremberg was a center of the European mirror industry. The first Guild for Mirror Makers opened there in 1373. Their technique involved silvering the backs of mirrors with a mercury tin amalgam to improve the reflection. But the workers suffered. Few complained. The effects of their exposure were only detected if they visited a doctor with other issues or if a worker figured a new treatment, such as electrotherapy, might be worth trying. They could see in the mirror and in each other the flush, tremors, irritability, and madness mercury caused. The only remedy, however, was to stop working, which brought the certainty of pauperism and maybe death. The workers lied to officials out of fear of losing their jobs.

A link between mercury and ill-health had long been known at one level. At the same time it was widely used by physicians to treat syphilis and other conditions. It may have contributed to the death of Schubert and other composers and caused more of the clinical picture of tertiary syphilis than syphilis did. When the Furth Provincial Medical Association reported on mercury poisoning among mirror workers in 1861, Adolf Kussmaul, one of a new breed of university physicians, agreed with them. This was a game changer, perhaps in part because Liebig and others came up with alternate ways to silver mirrors. The use of mercury for silvering was banned.

In 1863 triggered by concerns over industrial health, a German Workers Association formed, which quickly went on to oppose the Franco-Prussian war.

Marx published *Das Kapital* in 1867. This moved decisively beyond the challenges facing artisans, like the mirror-workers, to the alienation of a new class condemned to factory work. He pointed to a new dynamic introduced by technology, a new source of capital. As he was writing, a German chemical industry was taking shape out of which spewed goods that no artisan could ever have made, novel goods not readily categorized under the heading of needs or wants. An industry with a research footing.

While he grappled with the issue of value, and the economic crises capitalism was prone to, Marx was more an anthropologist encountering a new tribe than an economist. What he saw was no longer just a matter of exploitation by capitalists but a transformation of humanity by technique. The mass-production of goods by machines made it seem like machines were inherently productive, just as it seems guns kill people, or drugs rather than doctors cure people. In the process our experience changes. Plunging a knife into someone is very different to pressing enter on a computer controlling a killer drone a thousand miles away. He could see no limit to our new fetish with technique.

A German Socialist party appeared in 1869. The socialists accepted the need to work with the state and its institutions to bring about change. They saw a proposed Factory Act as a test of whether the state would respond to the health and safety needs of workers. Industry argued its techniques were so diverse and growing so rapidly, it was not possible to legislate in a way that would protect their interests. Bismarck accepted the argument that money put into health and safety would be a tax on jobs, which given growing international competition was not in the national interest. The 1869 Factory Act designated factories as private property and so not subject to inspections. In 1875 the Worker's Association and Socialist Party became the Socialist Workers Party, later the Social Democrats, the main opposition party in the Reichstag.

Marx predicted Bismarck would try to provoke a revolution. Bismarck did enact a set of punitive Anti-Socialist laws in 1878 but Marx didn't predict the next step. Recognizing that insurance had stabilized risky trade routes and ventures, Bismarck put State-sponsored insurance schemes forward as a means to stabilize the state:

> *A policy aimed at strengthening the state should cultivate the concep-*
> *tion among the non-propertied classes, which form at once the most*

*numerous and the least instructed part of the population, that the
State is not merely a necessary but a beneficent institution.*[12]

He began with a Health Insurance Bill in 1883, the first steps toward universal health coverage anywhere. The insurance was compulsory. Virchow argued for voluntary coverage. Bismarck responded:

*Politics is not an exact science... I fully recognize the prominence
of the speaker[Virchow] in his field of expertise [but] since [he] has
amateurishly stepped out of his field into mine, I must say that his
politics strike me as lightweight.*[13]

This was followed by Accident Insurance (Workman's Compensation) and later disability bills in 1884. As Bismarck put it:

*the complaint of the worker is the insecurity of his existence; he is
unsure if he will always have work, he is unsure if he will always be
healthy and he can predict that he will reach old age and be unable
to work. If he falls into poverty, and be that only through prolonged
illness, he will find himself totally helpless being on his own, and
society currently does not accept any responsibility towards him
beyond the usual provisions for the poor, even if he has been working
all the time ever so diligently and faithfully.*[14]

The original proposal had the Federal Government contributing to the insurance pool. It also established workers' commissions to provide input on factory health and safety issues. The Social Democrats sniffed a political threat and opposed Federal funding. The Liberals opposed a program even Bismarck called State Socialism. A Centre Party opposed the expansion

---

12 Bismarck, O von, *Gesammelte Werke.* (Berlin, ,1929) p XII.

13 McNeely, I.F. *Medicine on a Grand Scale: Rudolf Virchow, Liberalism and the Public
Health* (The Wellcome Trust Centre for the History of Medicine at UCL, 2002.)

14 Reichstagsprotokolle, Bd. 082, 05.*Legislaturperiode 04.Session 1884, 9. Sitzung am
Donnerstag, 20.03.*1884 (Sitzungsbeginn: page 133), speech of Otto von Bismarck:
page 161 ff., page 165, Bavarian State Library, Münchener Digitalisierungszentrum
(MDZ).

of Federal power at the expense of States' rights. The Bill was passed but federal funding was scrapped and the input from workers to health and safety, which employers argued might heighten worker awareness of colliding interests, was eliminated.

Marx didn't live to see these changes. He died in March 1883. Virchow had campaigned for just such changes, but he voted against a welfare capitalism he viewed as fooling people into supporting the state.

Bismarck and Virchow did agree on the idea of *Kulturkampf* (Culture Wars). Virchow coined the term to characterize efforts to stamp out the influence of Catholicism and its 'cells' in every parish. While Bismarck was against Liberalism and Modernism, as the Vatican was, he had a Lutheran distrust of Rome and its new corporate risk management strategy, papal infallibility. Much of what the Vatican complained about, as Petty recognized in 1660, were features of modern life that flew in the face of traditional religious beliefs and sensitivities. The challenge for faith communities then and now is how to address modern realities. How to steer a course between Providence and Progress.

Bismarck's course brought medical revolutionary zeal to an end. Virchow had wanted to restrict the use of the word doctors but no other medical regulation. Health insurance needed medical certification and designated board-certified doctors to decide who should receive treatment. The scheme would control costs by controlling the doctors who decided who was sick and what treatment was needed.

American finance houses, meanwhile, impressed with Marx's analysis of the inevitable march of technique, with capital in its train, invested in technique. Marx's insights on the fetish nature of technique and alienation sparkle to this day. After his death, some on the left turned to a discourse analysis. This sociobabble mapped onto the later psychobabble of psychoanalysis and did no more to change society than psychoanalysis did to change patients.

VORSPRUNG DURCH TECHNIK

Later Marxist analyses of health link disease to inequality and call for a change in the social environment. British opposition to vaccination took the same approach; give us living conditions equivalent to those you enjoy, not vaccinations. The march of technique, however, was about to impact on health without creating the opposition vaccines did. And Marxism didn't adapt.

In 1875, as the new sanitary system was being built in Berlin, Robert Koch isolated a bacillus responsible for anthrax. With state sponsorship of his research, Koch moved from Frankfurt to Berlin and bacteriology was born.

Key to the new science was William Perkins 1856 distillation of mauveine from coal tar, so called because it could dye clothes mauve. The ability to extract dyes from coal tars and manipulate their chemical structure opened the prospect that everyone could now wear the colors of royalty or a multi-colored garment like Joseph once had. A new chemical industry began to reshape the industrial landscape of Europe with Germany at its helm.

Some of these dyes had additional properties. Some were analgesic (pain relieving), others were antipyretic (fever reducing). Did the fever reducing properties of willow bark lie in a chemical that could be isolated? Sure enough, salicylic acid was discovered. Instead of physicians giving quantities of bark or ground up foxglove where no-one could be sure what the dose was, with the patient as likely to be poisoned as benefited, it was now possible not only to produce new medicines but to standardize the dose.

Above all, in Koch's laboratory, Paul Ehrlich found these dyes stained human and bacterial cells. The action of specific dyes on specific cells fit precisely with Virchow's idea that the cell was the basic functional structure in the body. We could literally see whether a medicine was hitting its target. This allied to a new ability to manipulate molecular structures, made it possible to work out which bit of the structure was critical for which action. Structures could now be optimized for specific effects. Modern pharmacology was born.

Staining distinguished also between bacteria. Specific bacteria could be demonstrated in the phlegm of this patient with TB, the pus from that patient with anthrax or the feces from a cholera patient. This made it important for hospitals to have a medical laboratory to detect which germs a patient might have, to distinguish among blood cells on a blood film and to search for cancer cells in tissues surgically removed.

Ehrlich moved beyond Virchow's idea of a cell to the receptor, the lock for which a drug would be a key. One of his stains was methylene blue. A series of laboratory 'accidents' in which sputum from a TB patient was left on a heated surface and methylene blue was contaminated with ammonia led Koch in 1882 to the discovery of a tubercle bacillus.

Facing opposition to his claimed link between bacillus and disease, Koch elaborated principles that might underpin such a claim. First the illness should not be present in the absence of the bacterium. Second the illness should come after the bacterium is present. Third increasing the dose of the bacterium should be more likely to lead to the illness. Fourth removing the bacterium should lead to the resolution of the illness. The rules hold if the words drug and drug effect are substituted for bacterium and illness.

These principles involve challenge, dechallenge and ideally rechallenge (CDR). They apply to cause and effect generally. When Christmas lights had diodes, the set often failed after a year in storage. The trick was to unscrew each bulb in turn, until unscrewing one turned the lights on. If screwing that bulb back in turned them off again, it was certain that bulb was defective and could be discarded.

Cholera broke out in Hamburg in 1892. Koch recommended boiling water before use. Max Von Pettenkoffer, Koch's principal opponent, was a sanitarian. He opposed a quarantine. Banning trade to prevent cholera would be a bigger disaster than cholera itself. Von Pettenkoffer also thought boiling water would be useless. But it worked.

A few months later in the annual Public Health Meeting, the lessons from Hamburg were discussed. Von Pettenkoffer was viewed as losing the debate. He responded by drinking a broth of cholera bacilli from Hamburg water in front of a class in Munich. He survived. There was more to cholera than just the bacillus, he claimed. The constitution of the person, their overall health, nutritional status, and exposure to other contaminants could not be neglected. True though that may be, Von Pettenkoffer was swept aside by the force of history. There is nothing mystical about the force of history. It typically means more people stand to make a living out of the new way of viewing things than from the old way.

Among the people who came to work with Koch was Emil Behring, who helped isolate diphtheria and came up with an antitoxin. Behring and Ehrlich worked to enrich the antitoxin to make it clinically effective. Diphtheria was one of the greatest killers of children. It caused membranes to form in the throat that led to gruesome deaths by strangulation. One of Goya's most striking pictures, *El Garrotillo* from 1819, shows a father desperately trying to avoid his child being garroted by diphtheria.

The impact of diphtheria antitoxin was extraordinary. James Herrick reported in 1890:[15]

> *In the case of an attractive 7-year-old in whom the disease had invaded the larynx, I inserted a tube which gave relief for several hours; then it was evident that the tube was becoming clogged. The parents begged me not to let the child strangle. I explained the desperate nature of the trouble… they understood. The mother left the room, the father took the child in his arms, and with little difficulty the tube was removed. As the father uttered "Thank God" the child gave a feeble gasp and was gone. In memory I can still see the room, the exact location of the bed, the chair, the limpid child in the father's lap, the adjustment of the light.*

And Thomas Shastid in 1894:

---

15 All quotes cited in Healy D, *Pharmageddon*, (California University Press, Berkeley 2012).

Night after night, sometimes for a week in succession, I would be called to get up and go to some residence, there to cut up some child's windpipe therein to introduce a tube through which it might be able to breathe until it should be able possibly to throw off the terrible infection. Even then, not infrequently, the child died, because the false membranes continued to form—lower and lower, deeper and deeper, into the airways, until at length it had reached beyond the lowest extremity of our air passing tube.

Now compare these with Alfred Schofield in 1896:

I found the boy very ill, the whole back of his throat being like white velvet. I had never used the new remedy before but determined to try it to save the boy's life. I injected a small quantity under the skin of the stomach and watched the throat. I can only compare the marvelous result to the disappearance of snow beneath a hot sun. After the second dose, every trace of the membrane disappeared, and the boy soon recovered.

This was the first treatment for a scourge that took thousands of children annually. It made specificity compelling. It put a premium on getting the clinical diagnosis right because the antitoxin could be harmful. In the debate between biomedicine and social medicine, the sanitarians could not win this argument. As Behring put it:

While these views had their merits, now, following the procedures of Robert Koch the study of infectious disease could be pursued unswervingly without being sidetracked by social considerations and reflections on social policy. [16]

The new German research based pharmaceutical industry began looking to international markets. In the US and Britain, the medicines landscape was populated by proprietary brands, a set of elixirs and cocktails with secret ingredients that claimed to cure everything but were often toxic

---

16 Bloom SW, "The Word as Scalpel", *A History of Medical Sociology*, 20.

or ineffective. The new analgesics and antipyretics increased the pressure to standardize preparations. This fed into a development of pharmacopoeias of approved products. Pharmacists became the guardians of these drug classifications.

All modern medicines have a brand, generic and chemical name. Efforts to classify medicines are often frustrated by this. There still wasn't an agreed list of drugs for European markets in 2010. Around 1900 distinctions between chemical, generic and brand names preoccupied American pharmacists, who linked brands to quackery. Into this mix stepped a German pharmaceutical company, Kalle. They, and thirteen other companies, had produced a new antipyretic with 13 different chemical names. The generic name was acetanilide. Kalle distinguished their version by trademarking its brand name, Antefebrin. Sales boomed. Bayer followed by registering Aspirin and Heroin in 1898, names with greater resonance to this day than acetylsalicylic acid or diacetylmorphine.

The keepers of the flame had a dilemma. So much that was trademarked was worthless, but these compounds could not be ignored. For those who wanted medicine to be rational, branding seemed a violation. Antefebrin and other German drugs, however, were not medicines a pharmacist could compound in his pharmacy. Pre-made by a drug company, they threatened the livelihoods of pharmacists.

With the creation of a diphtheria antitoxin, Behring took a further step into the darkness of commerce. Almost immediately after the discovery was announced, public health services in New York and Chicago made it available for free. Behring, however, linked to the Merck Company in Darmstadt, took out a patent on the antitoxin. There was uproar. States like New York and Illinois has been getting antitoxin from companies like Mulford in Pennsylvania. Mulford now came up against the Merck patent. Mulford went to Court arguing that patents could not apply to a generally accepted scientific process. The legal case took a decade and resolved in favor of patenting.

Patenting had begun in Venice in 1494. In 1791 the new French parliament permitted drugs to be patented. Chemists and trade associations argued the rights of inventors should be recognized. Physicians and pharmacists argued their vocation was to treat the sick, not to make a profit. Patents, they predicted, would increase the price of medicines, which would be detrimental to public health. It would also confer state approval on certain drugs, offering their manufacturers a commercial advantage that could lead to injuries if the true hazards of the new drugs had not been fully recognized. In 1844 France reversed the 1791 law and removed medicines from the domain of patentable products.

In America, Behring was seen as an Antichrist. Matters were made worse in 1901 when he was awarded the first Nobel Prize in medicine. It was close to impossible for a sanitarian to be awarded a Nobel Prize, as the award hinged on making a discovery an individual could claim credit for. The rewards of science are skewed towards mechanism-based medicine and mechanisms lay a basis for patenting and inputs as likely to lead to wealth as health.

Magic Bullets

Methylene blue was the progenitor of antipsychotics and antidepressants. Ehrlich showed it stained both malarial cells and nerve cells, leading him to try it as a treatment for malaria and others to try it for mental illness. It clears malaria parasites from the blood but doesn't cure. It unquestionably tranquilized mental disorders but this was ignored.

The malaria results led Ehrlich to chase other drugs. A series based on arsenic had effects in the test tube on the syphilis treponema. This led to Salvarsan in 1910. Despite unease about a drug for an immoral disorder, discovered by a Jew, and a weak action, Salvarsan became the biggest selling drug in the world. When World War I broke out threatening supplies, the US government, over-riding German patents, instructed US companies to make it.

En route to Salvarsan, Ehrlich created the concept of a Magic Bullet. The specificity of these interventions appeared to promise a new efficacy with a minimum of collateral damage. In practice, Magic Bullets created 'adverse events', the unintended collateral effects of a drug.

The mystique of specificity can be dangerous. Specific interventions—to lower cholesterol or clear blockages from arteries—can do more harm than good. We can live with most germs and elevations of blood pressure and may even need them. Clinical efficacy needs wisdom. Surgery is a mutilation. The intentions that lead to this mutilation and the relationship within which it happens are key to what the action means and its outcomes. Similarly, giving a medicine is an act of poisoning. The intentions of the poisoner and our awareness that we are being poisoned and to what end are key to the outcome.

Specificity however sells drugs. Its rhetoric can penetrate our views of ourselves to a greater extent than specific treatments cure ailments. In mental health, for instance, aside from the specific effects of a drugs such as penicillin for tertiary syphilis, the antipsychotic and antidepressant derivatives of methylene blue are non-specific tranquilizers. Their designation as antipsychotics and antidepressants however is all about specificity, as is the idea they correct imbalances of serotonin in depression or dopamine in psychosis. This is marketing not science or medicine. A marketing that has transformed how we view ourselves.

ACCIDENTS AND SYSTEMS

When God was in Heaven and monarchs on their thrones, inexplicable events like plagues were seen as stemming from our sins or as governed by Providence. There were also rare or random events that were difficult to fit into any narrative, referred to then and now, as Acts of God. These were accidents. In the case of accidents, such as my horse bolting and your child being run over and killed, I would be held responsible. I would have to forfeit goods or money to the equivalent value of what had been lost. An eye for an eye and a tooth for a tooth.

The first hint that some occupational accidents might happen regularly came in 1662 from John Graunt's figures, which threw up a constant string of deaths linked to building work in London. As the politics of industrial health played out, Compensation Acts were passed in Germany and then

Britain, America and France to support workers injured in workplace accidents, unless the owner could show the worker was drunk or otherwise brought the event on themselves. These put a premium on ensuring workplaces free of hazards.

These acts brought two scenarios into view. Banana skins affect individual workers but if a mine collapsed, or a chemical factory exploded, hundreds might be killed. The worst ever mining disaster happened in 1906 in the North of France, when over 1000 miners lost their lives. Mining disasters were a regular feature of our new industrial societies. While the system rolls over the deaths and injuries of individual employees, when hundreds die, questions get asked about the meaning of the events. The mine owners talk about accidents. Workers and their families are more likely to talk about murder.

Another set of occupational events cannot be labelled accidents. Industrial work exposes employees to lead and mercury, respiratory disorders linked to the mining of coal, slate or asbestos dust, and heavy labor leads to arthritic disorders.

The burden in these instances remained on the worker to demonstrate a causal link. A psychosis or tremor can be tied to mercury in workers making mirrors or hats because it clears when the person leaves work. What about exposure to lead, which:

> *could not be attributed to the gradual onset of the effects of a particular occurrence, but was an intoxication which had developed over a number of years as a result of constantly handling white lead, it was a chronic disease caused by continual exposure. This… must be regarded as an occupational disease, the nature of which is unalterable even if… the Defendant failed to meet the regulations and make the necessary provisions to avert danger. Diseases arising gradually out of the effects of industrial production are however not accidents but the common and foreseeable drawbacks of an inherently unhealthy industry which must be taken into account by everyone participating*

in that industry. The Accident Insurance Act does not provide for insurance against such diseases or invalidity resulting from them.[17]

Lead poisoning in children knocks points off their IQ and makes them hyperactive and antisocial. There is a link to poverty in many instances. Children had higher body lead if they lived in slum dwellings with lead in the paintwork. Those who grew up in these settings were more likely to fail in life. But not everyone who grows up in poverty fails. Is the role of medicine to campaign to alleviate poverty or to pinpoint issues about poverty, such as the presence of lead in paint, that can compromise performance and can be remedied?

Or tuberculosis? Around 1900, North Wales had the biggest slate quarries in the world. When the death rate from tuberculosis was falling in Britain, it was increasing in these quarries. Repeated enquiries heard that quarrying gave the workers silicosis, a lung disorder caused by inhaling silica. Did silicosis make TB more likely? Local doctors said the condition was down to poor diet: the modern housewife spent too much time at school and her only domestic skill was the ability to use a tin opener.

Silicosis does predispose to TB. But, just as the mirror workers in Furth fifty years earlier took their chances with mercury, so Welsh quarrymen kept quiet about their chest condition. There was no other employment in the area.

You don't have to silver a mirror or go down a mine to appreciate the psychology and politics here. When medical treatment goes wrong, short of being invalided, many of us opt to cope. Speaking up, if there is no remedy, marks us as losers, and the herd leaves losers behind. The injured worker or patient is like a dog barking at a passing caravan.

With a drug and an injury there is an extra twist. Unless a doctor assigns causality, we will be unable to get anywhere. And, if he didn't intend to hurt us, a doctor is unlikely to concede that he did in fact injure us. Bystanders will side with the likely winner rather than loser, and we are always more likely to lose.

---

17 Cooter R, Luchin B, *Accidents in History* (Clio Medica Amsterdam), 184-5.

By 1900 it seemed that for modern industrial states to work there had to be a degree of shared responsibility, but in practice everybody takes steps to avoid responsibility. There are a few systems where we put our lives in the hands of someone else, like a pilot, with a relative confidence borne from the fact that if we go down, she does too. Most systems are more like medicine, where the prescribing doctor has little to lose if we go down, and little incentive to make things as safe as possible.

For the loser in industrial or medical events, beyond the injury an identity is destroyed just as if acid had been thrown in a face. Once marked in this way, the only people who understand are those similarly marked but not even losers like the company of losers.

Histories

An accident also means something incidental in the sense that having arms, or a scarred face, is incidental to rather than part of the essence of being human. But while who we marry is incidental to life, it may be central to the meaning of our life. There are happy and unhappy accidents. Our history, the story of who we are, hinges on accidents in this sense. The Liberal narrative of progress assumed most accidents are happy. Marx saw non-accidental forces driving things forward. Max Weber was conflicted.

Born in 1864, Weber celebrated the role of Liberalism in the creation of modernity in *The Protestant Ethic and the Spirit of Capitalism* (1904). This tackled a quandary William Petty grappled with; how can a Christian justify making money? Weber put the evident progress Protestant states made compared to Catholic ones down to entrepreneurs seeing their success as a sign of God's favor. Education, contracts, and the rule of law freed individuals to drive progress. He also, however, recognized that by 1900 liberalism had transmuted into a progressivism that had moved closer to socialism.

Although plagued with ill-health like Marx, Weber viewed science and health as domains free from the corruption of politics. But strikingly in 1919 he noted that politicians, like doctors, must stoop to a certain amount of evil in order to bring about good. Like doctors on a grand scale, they may have to persuade us to take our medicine.

We were all becoming ever more entwined in a bureaucracy. While bureaucracy ideally created a level playing field which should contain power and make life fair, the good bureaucrat efficiently carried out orders whether they agreed with them or not. Just as Marx saw factory techniques universalizing, for Weber the rationality of bureaucratic technique meant it too would universalize. Where Marx was optimistic about the potential of new physical techniques, Weber feared that, even if run by angels, the impersonal rationality of administrative procedures would conflict with the needs of the individual.

He tried to pull liberalism and socialism together hoping socialism might protect liberalism from exploitation by the rent-seeking of those who held capital, while liberalism might save socialism from a bureaucratic overgrowth that risked imprisoning us in an Iron Cage.

Keeping our balance on the tightrope between the alienation that stems from new physical techniques on one side and behavioral techniques on the other requires a solid sense of identity. The sense that people might be perfectible was fractured in the 1870s with Cesare Lombroso's *L'Uomo Deliquente* which described psychopaths—individuals whom neither religion nor education could save. In the 1890s, the return of hypnosis, a recognition of multiple personality disorder, and the madness of crowds, further clouded the liberal horizon.

Added to this, the new nation states underpinned by industrial and bureaucratic techniques that would always seek to globalize, indeed become totalitarian, seemed to be on an inevitable collision course.

On June 28, 1914, Gavrilo Princip assassinated Franz Ferdinand of Austria in Sarajevo. There was nothing accidental about this, but just as dislodging a single stone can trigger an unintended avalanche that sweeps away everything in its path, Princip's actions triggered a maelstrom of events that may as well have been random.

The War confused the German Left. The proletariat were not supposed to support a spat between capitalists. Feminists were confused by the failure of women to oppose the nightmare. In October 1918, a communist uprising in Germany helped bring the War to an end. But both liberals and socialists combined to put communism down and execute its leaders. Like doctors, socialists had opted to work with the system. Weber died from influenza in 1920. The alliance he sought between liberals and socialists never materialized.

While Russia's 1917 communist revolution succeeded, it was not because the proletariat rose up. History, which Marx viewed as predictable, had begun to look like a bad dream. An Institute for Social Research opened in Frankfurt in 1924. Its leading figures, Theodore Adorno, Erich Fromm, Max Horkheimer and Herbert Marcuse, looked to marry Marx with Freud who, like Marx, saw the unfolding of history in term of a dialectic driving from within, and who claimed to be able to interpret fetishes and dreams.

In 1925 in *The Trial*, and a year later in *The Castle*, Franz Kafka introduced us to the nightmare of a perverse bureaucracy capable of combining the impersonality of rational procedure with the vindictiveness and narrow-mindedness of village life.

Denn heute gehört uns Deutschland und morgen die ganze Welt.

4: THE BUSINESS OF AMERICA

Whatever hardships settlers had taming the wilderness, in America food was untainted, air fresh and water pristine. The frontier gave people a place to live free of the constraints of others. It was a land of individuals—once the tribes were wiped out. And, in New York, small though it was, America had a cautionary Old World tale.

The Europeans, who brought smallpox, tuberculosis, and dysentery with them, had to cope with Yellow Fever when it hit New Orleans, Philadelphia, and New York from 1793 to 1806 killing thousands. It caused jaundice, compromised coagulation, bleeding into the gut and black vomiting. Endemic in the Caribbean, it wiped out a French army in Santo Domingo leading Napoleon to sell Louisiana to the United States in 1803.

When cholera struck Europe in 1831, Americans hoped it would not cross the Atlantic. On its arrival in New York in 1832, efforts to activate a Board of Health failed for the reasons that led to Charles I downfall. Doctors raising alarms and reporting cases were branded as unpatriotic. Quarantines might save lives but certainly interrupted business. Cholera was also capricious. It did not travel up or down the Mississippi as Yellow Fever had. In later outbreaks, it appeared in parts of the country thousands of miles apart with no one able to explain why. A plague had never travelled by rail before.

In an 1845 tract *Sanitary Condition of the Laboring Population of New York*, John Griscom described squalid and overcrowded tenements in which prostitution and venereal disease thrived. He coined the phrase "cleanliness is next to godliness," adding that "ventilation is not just a moral but a religious duty". Providence created what would be Eden, were it not for our sins. The need was to ensure that man's natural capacity for virtue and health was not corrupted by the inequities of social organization.

New York set up a Metropolitan Board of Health in 1866 that finally got to grips with cholera. The driving force behind this was Elizha Harris, a medical doctor. He framed sanitary science as a wealth creating segment of the political economy. But standard medical practice had failed in the face of cholera. As a consequence, where doctors had been licensed as medical practitioners in all States by the 1830s, by the 1840s medical licensure had bitten the dust everywhere except New Jersey.

Healthcare populism rushed in. A vogue for self-help made growth industries of herbalism and botanicals. Americans outdid Europeans in seeking the benefits of hydropathy, mineral waters, spas, and fitness centers. The Reverend Sylvester Graham became famous for advocating vegetarianism, the use of bran, exercise, and bathing. Industrial empires were made from new healthy foodstuffs such as cereals. There was a focus on mastication, dieting, and vitamins when they were discovered. An interest in organic foods stirred. Homeopathic practitioners, Christian Scientists, Seventh Day Adventists, osteopaths, chiropractors, and electrotherapists made greater inroads into the American health market than anywhere else.

The way the story is usually told American physicians, faced with challenges to their role, turned to Paris to learn more about the new medical model. With the emergence of Koch's laboratory in the 1880s, Berlin became the place to visit. Hewing to this path, in 1910 American medicine arrived back on the mountain-top from which it had been displaced. A cadre of elite East Coast physicians did visit Europe. From the 1860s, however, America had a greater influence on Europe than the other way around. It had also worked out how to distinguish between doctors and others in the healthcare space.

MILITARY MEDICINE

The first American contribution came in 1846, when William Morton used ether to anesthetize a Boston patient undergoing surgery. Anesthesia spread triggering debate. Some argued a depressing agent would depress other functions militating against recovery, others that dulling the pain of surgery could not be morally right.

The critical issue was a novel ethical one. Anesthetics kill. If with anesthesia less people die because the surgeon can do a better job, still some people die from the anesthetic itself. Could a doctor, whose duty it is to save life, intentionally jeopardize that life by administering anesthesia? Can evil be done even though good might result? Is the apparently morally better path, or the path that produces the better outcomes, the more ethical? For many, the 'natural' course of action must be better. Compared to bleeding or purging, which mimicked nature's ways of healing, anesthesia was a triumph of technique.

American innovations in another theater of operations built on this. For a decade before the Civil War, the input of physicians to the US Army had been reduced to save money. When war began, physicians split between North and South leaving a meagre medical input to each side. The military recruited young men with little training and fewer preconceptions.

Initially on the back-foot, the North eventually not only mobilized troops, factory production, and transport, but also a health system. Jonathan Letterman, a doctor, was appointed to manage the medical lines of supply. He organized ambulances equipped with dressings and medicines to remove troops from the battlefield, and treat them quickly. He set up stations for triage, which gave rise to the concept of First Aid. Both sides agreed to use a Red Flag for medical cover and to regard medical personnel as non-combatants. This laid the basis for the later Red Cross and Geneva Convention.

After initial stabilization, troops were removed to Field Hospitals for surgery and then by rail or other transport to General Hospitals in the area. By the end of the War the North had over 130,000 beds in more than two hundred hospitals, including floating hospitals on the Mississippi and off the Carolina coast. Professional nurses were recruited. The needs for ventilation, isolation, and specialization led to single story pavilions spread across a campus. These offered cleaner conditions than were found in the hospitals America had in Philadelphia, New York, and Boston. Disinfection was the order of the day before it had been accepted in Europe.

The first ever use of mass firepower with efficient rifles led to limb fractures, traumatic amputations, and chest wounds. Fractures were treated with immobilization and a new method, plaster of Paris. An emphasis was put on amputation, which anesthesia made possible. Naval blockades left the Confederates short of drugs including chloroform, but Julian Chisholm invented an inhaler that reduced the amount of chloroform needed by 90%. Morphine was used liberally for pain relief. Toward the end of the war, it was administered by the just invented hypodermic syringe, which helped spread morphinism after the war.

Benjamin Howard invented a technique to close penetrating chest wounds that quartered death rates. Gordon Buck reconstructed a face, the first step in the creation of plastic surgery. By the end of the War America had the best surgeons in the world.

Despite these efforts there were 600,000 cases of dysentery and gut problems led to 37,000 deaths in the first year. Typhoid claimed a further 27,000 lives. More soldiers died from disease than from combat in a war that took close to 2% of the population.

American innovations were adopted by Prussia in the Franco-Prussian War in 1871. When Japan opened to the West in 1871, it sent physicians to Germany who brought back American medicine. When Japan declared war on Russia in 1904, the difference showed. The Japanese boiled and sterilized water for drinking and treatment. They banned alcohol and prostitution. They had First Aid stations and evacuation lines to hospitals. They deployed typhus vaccine along with diphtheria and tetanus antitoxins. They were the first to lose more men to combat than to disease in a modern war, and they beat the Russians.

The network of military facilities vanished quickly after the Civil War, but American cities began to build hospitals to cater for a growing group of urban casualties. In 1873 there were 178 hospitals. By 1923 there were almost 5,000 focused primarily on surgery, making hospitals the domain of allopathic rather than homeopathic or complementary medicine.

The War laid a template for urban healthcare. After infections, muggings or being hit by carriages were the commonest cause of death and injury in cities, escalating further with the first automobiles. These casualties led citizen associations to lobby for street lighting, a police presence, urban ambulances, and casualty departments, later called accident and then emergency departments. The idea of training civilians to administer First Aid emerged.

For urban ambulance cover to be effective, hospitals needed to be coordinated in a system as they were in the Civil War. American and British hospitals in the 1860s were voluntary hospitals, set up by philanthropists or religious groups. When hospital building began after the war, a tension emerged between voluntary and state systems. Urban casualties lie on a fault-line between state and non-state medicine. Voluntary hospitals were not located according to an urban or national response system. Private medicine, like private enterprise, is supposedly more efficient than public medicine. In peacetime the Army is a metaphor for waste and inefficiency. In War it's just the opposite.

At this point, European hospitals offered expert generalism rather than specialization. The message Americans took from the Civil War was that treatment and innovation benefit from specialization.

Since 1800, techniques have been a greater driver of history than supposed great men. But technique comes with risks. In the case of a technique like anesthesia, there are the inherent risks. The technique can also shape enterprises in a way that can expose us to hazards—seducing us into anesthesia for cosmetic surgery for instance. The benefits of technique can also make its hazards disappear.

War and its Discontents

George Stephenson launched the first steam powered rail engine in England in 1825. 'The Locomotion' triggered a burst of rail laying and train building everywhere. Railroads rapidly became the biggest industry in America, helping knit the country together, playing a major role in the Civil War and shaping occupational medicine and law.

In 1841, Nicholas Farwell lost an arm when a locomotive derailed. Farwell sued the Boston and Worcester Railroad. Chief Justice Shaw's verdict argued Farwell had assumed the risk of injury when taking on a job at an agreed wage. Other legal cases ruled out compensation if there was any contribution from the employee to the injury. An employer had to be responsible for the entire damage before an employee could be compensated.

The Civil War changed how these issues were viewed. New military techniques led to new injuries. While these injuries might have a contribution from the prior health of the soldier or the mistake of a colleague, injuries are intrinsic to the job of soldier. Recognizing this, the US government created aftercare for veterans. The railway, mining and lumber industries followed suit, employing company doctors to screen workers before employment, assess and treat injuries when they happened, and after a Great Railroad Strike in 1877, to certify workers for pensions.

Even before the War, train crashes left victims, some of whom were paralyzed, blind, or deaf, but without visible injuries. What to make of these 'traumatic neuroses'? Neurosis at this point did not mean a psychological problem. It meant there was something wrong with the nerves of those affected, even if just as with whiplash injuries there was no clear damage. Many physicians believed the potential for compensation from injuries like these would lead some to "set out on a broad road of imposture and dissimulation". Others blamed the shock of the event; "the vastness of the destructive forces, the magnitude of the results, the imminent danger to the lives of a number of human beings and the hopelessness of escape." But without evident harm, it was not possible to be compensated.

The Civil War shaped these issues also. 'Nostalgia' had first been noted by French physicians during Napoleon's campaigns. There were thousands of cases in the Civil War. The debate about nostalgia took a distinct turn in 1871 in the American Journal of the Military Sciences, when Jacob

Mendes da Costa reported on a case of 'irritable heart'. William Henry H had enlisted in 1862, apparently in good health. He admitted to being anxious before the Battle of Fredericksburg. Afterwards he had pains in his chest and palpitations and was unable to move. The symptoms recurred during military duties, especially while on the march. After being wounded at Gettysburg, he was incapacitated and confined to bed.

Da Costa could find no evidence of a structural change in WH's heart, no murmurs, nor irregularities of his pulse. Might the disorder be 'functional', arising from an irritability conveyed to the heart by the recently discovered sympathetic nerves? Da Costa's syndrome came to mean chest pains without a cause. It remained a neurosis until in 1991 Japanese physicians described *tatso tsubo* syndrome, also called broken-hearted syndrome. Shocks, mediated through the sympathetic system, are now known to cause this, with a physical change visible on scans.

As Da Costa's syndrome took shape, the Connecticut physician George Miller Beard coined the term neurasthenia to cover similar states involving fatigue and malaise. Neurasthenia was a nervous weakness revealed by our increasingly frenetic way of life. Beard used electricity to treat it as Mesmer had used magnetism. He blamed the poor results some reported on their failure to choose the right patients, to follow his guidelines, and to understand the nature of electricity.

In the Russo-Japanese War, the Russians offered proximity treatment for a new condition they termed shell shock. They believed this was a physical disorder. Proximity treatment is now the standard approach to battlefield stress. The Russians also recognized evacuation syndromes, and the possibility that disability might be feigned.

The traumatic neuroses raised medical and political considerations. These complex clinical pictures can make it difficult to tell how much a prior constitution or pre-existing disease has contributed to a disorder. Just exactly which consequences of an injurious event is an employer, or the military, responsible for? Is there a difference between a conscript and a professional soldier? The military have a longer history of grappling with these issues than health insurance or workers compensation schemes.

THE EMBRACE OF TECHNIQUE

The conventional story is that the flimsy base of American medicine, exposed by cholera in the 1830s, led to its disestablishment. After decades in the wilderness, American doctors discovered biomedicine thanks to the Carnegie Foundation who supported Abraham Flexner's 1910 review of American medical education. Discussion of the Report almost immediately referred to its classic status but its detailing of a lack of laboratory inputs to American hospitals and medical education is tedious. The sections on the medical education of women and African Americans are more interesting.

The report is billed as triggering the release of $300 million from the Rockefeller Foundation (over 20 years) to turn the laboratory deficits around. This money is pitched as capitalizing American medicine. Flexner feeds into a narrative that the heroes of biomedicine have been lionized, despite doing little to advance our health. Contributions from the social sciences, in contrast, have been minimized when in fact infections like tuberculosis were vanishing long before drug treatments emerged.

American medicine certainly changed around 1900 but it had little to do with Flexner. The Civil War brought a new America into view, a country of growing cities and railroads, huge factories and industrialization, and a growing navy and military. A country whose rhetoric spoke to the management of its people in a value-neutral scientific way.

In 1865 the American Social Science Association (ASSA) was founded:

> *To guide the public mind to the best practical means of promoting the Amendment of Laws, the advancement of Education, the Prevention of Crime, the Reformation of Criminals, the Progress of Public Morality, the adoption of sanitary regulations... it will aim to obtain by discussion of the real elements of Truth, by which doubts are removed, conflicting opinions harmonized, and a common ground afforded for treating wisely the great social problems of the day.*[18]

---

18 Bloom S.W., *The Word as Scalpel*, 25.

The ASSA was followed by the American Associations for Anthropology (AAA), Economics (AEA) and Political Science (APSA). One input to these developments was a push across the Western world toward applied knowledge rather than philosophy. This was activist and advocacy oriented. Another input came from the growth of social statistics in the 1860s on wages, housing conditions, and the structure of families. The data suggested areas for reform and became a template for social science input to policy.

After the War there was a growth in universities, rivaled only by Germany. The new State universities were less hidebound than English and French Colleges, which still majored on the classics. An abundance of academic posts meant that those with dissenting views had other institutions to go to, from which they could return if they turned out to be right.

These were the settings needed for the creation of a new science, sociology. The first sociology lecture was given by William Sumner in 1876. Before medicine was funded by the Carnegie or Rockefeller Foundations, the social sciences began to receive funding from the Russell Sage Foundation and the Millbank Memorial Fund.

While the new sciences traced a lineage to Europe, mentioned Auguste Comte in France who created the term social science, as well as Karl Marx, Herbert Spencer, Emil Durkheim, and Georg Simmel, Americans embraced the idea of bringing data to bear on society, an approach that later led to opinion polling and cultural events like the Kinsey Report.

One of the key sources of data stemmed from school inspections which began in the 1880s, in the wake of Education Acts mandating school attendance. These inspections revealed a picture of concern not just about individual children but about the national condition. Many children had visual, dental, orthopedic, and other defects. Many were engaged in child labor. Just as the Kinsey Report did for sex, these inspections created an image of what childhood should be. They also set a precedent for the idea of annual medical check-ups, which became grist to the health insurance mill. Along with inspections of Army recruits, they made the condition of the nation a political concern.

Meanwhile in 1911, Frederick Winslow Taylor's *Scientific Management* proposed analyzing work into its components. Standardizing the methods, tools, work settings and time workers took would both increase competitiveness and solve labor relations. Taylor's workers were required to work to Guidelines. And a new function became explicit, that of a supervisor or manager to ensure Guideline compliance. *Scientific Management,* pilloried in Charlie Chaplin's movie *Modern Times,* functioned more as a symbol of where we were headed than as a manual on how to run a factory.

John Watson's first article on behaviorism in 1913, with its call to ignore the inner life of subjects and focus on manipulations that affected behavior, however, did hold open the prospect of a future scientific management. There were approximately 300 psychologists in America in 1913. By 1930 there were 3000—more than the rest of the world combined. America also produced more academic psychology literature than the rest of the world. This focus on the science of behavior suggests a need to find common ground in the most pluralistic society on earth.

In 1910 stimulated by French school inspections, Alfred Binet developed the first intelligence tests. IQ tests were included among the tests Robert Yerkes and Louis Terman used in screening American troops enlisting for the Great War. Some psychologists dismissed testing as applied rather than real psychology. The test results, however, mapped onto Bell Shaped Curves. This seemed to point to a distribution of intelligence in the population. Large numbers of people suddenly seemed below average, with apparent differences between races. The results fed into debates about race, immigration, and eugenics.

The advocates of scientific management, industrial psychology and a new breed of physiologists were offering to manage the problem of worker fatigue. Fatigue was code for slackers. Psychologists were also offering to make education and family life more 'scientific,' offering their input to school inspections, child guidance clinics, and aptitude testing to match pupils to later education and careers. These developments had as great an impact on American and global healthcare as any change in the biomedical sciences.

Changing Cultures

The culture of health can change because a treatment makes a difference as anesthesia did in 1860, diphtheria antitoxin in 1895, or antibiotics in 1940. If treatments work, people vote with their feet and healthcare facilities open or shut without any engineering of cultural change. Cultures also change when a new view offers more livelihoods than an old one. In the case of the germ theories that emerged in the 1880s, the new pathways of contagion created opportunities on main street. Tradesmen and retailers marketing their wares spread ideas about germs and made Koch and Pasteur household names.

There were, for instance, new markets for water filters, for bathroom suites with white china fixtures, along with tiles or linoleum on walls and floors to replace carpets, drapes, and privies. These needed plumbers to install them. Dust emerged as a vector of infections putting a premium on cleaning tools and reagents and adding to the argument for replacing curtains by blinds and wallpaper by paint. Flies came into focus, spurring an interest in gadgets to shield food, followed by food wraps. Meat and milk needed inspection. Hygiene contributed to the later growth of the plastics industry, and gadgets from vacuum cleaners to fridges.

There was a boom in the market for disinfectants. The American Public Health Association in 1885 ran a survey of disinfectants, finding that *Pasteur's Marvelous Disinfectant* didn't cut the mustard. If APHA didn't point to flaws in their products, manufacturers put out adverts claiming their disinfectant was APHA endorsed.

Newspapers thrived on stories from the frontline in the war against germs. The bugs sold copy in a way filth never could, and disinfectants were good sources of advertising revenues. Municipal and state health programs, insurers, women's clubs, all began advertising, borrowing from the patent medicine advertisers. A market for Domestic Guides emerged. The *Ladies Home Journal* appeared in 1883, and *Good Housekeeping* in 1885.

Managing germs was one of those areas where everyone wins. To invert Upton Sinclair's famous dictum, it is easy to get a man to understand something, if his salary depends on it. Most of the ideas about germs were wrong. We all teem with germs. We would die without them. Efforts to make everything hygienic played a part in later polio epidemics that began in New York in 1916. The use of paint rather than wallpaper almost certainly contributed to the poisoning of children, as paint came laced with lead. And plastic now fills our oceans.

The language of germs was a babble as far removed from real germs as the babble about serotonin was from real serotonin a century later. Everyone, even complementary therapists could write books and preach about natural ways to manage germs, as they do for serotonin now. It's not always the usual suspects who are making money out of new arrangements. A culture is captured when the words fly up, but the meaning remains below.

Germs became women's business. Up to 1848, the home had been a place where men and women worked together. But while many women were still sent down mines after that, worked in poorly paid factory jobs, or as domestic servants, as men began to work in factories their wives remained at home. The home became a woman's domain. She was the Health and Safety Executive, the sanitary officer, and the person responsible for ensuring 'accidents' didn't happen. Gendered ideas of pink and blue began to take hold.

Germs inserted themselves between Providence and Determinism. When epidemics were sent by God, there was a concern that having a technical answer might encourage moral decline. If venereal disorders for instance were caused by microbes, having a treatment might encourage wantonness. But while the spread of germs by toilet seats did become a way to explain away liaisons, far from leading to moral randomness, the germ concept slotted easily into a model that made the universe appear lawful. It mapped onto evolutionary theories and the struggles the fittest needed to win to survive. Getting infected was not an accident. It was lawful not exceptional. It was also no surprise that the poor and immigrants would be seen as the repositories of germs.

Tuberculosis

In this groundswell of changes, what is now thought of as biomedicine played little part other than to provide iconic images of aseptic surgical theatres and surgeons wearing face masks, and scrubs. But, everything was changing.

Up to 1850, deaths from tuberculosis (TB), the White Plague, ran at over 400 per 100,000 people. This was 20 times the death rate from AIDS in the United States in the 1980s or from opioids now, and 10 times the Covid death rate as of July 2020. After 1850, the death rate began to decline except in urban tenements. By 1880 New York was the second largest city in the world; its TB death rate stood at 800 per 100,000. TB was thought to be hereditary, becoming manifest in conditions of defective ventilation, poor light, stress, and overwork. A first sanatorium opened in New York State in 1880, designed to reverse these stressors.

This wisdom was upended in 1882, when Koch isolated a tubercle bacillus. Hermann Biggs, newly qualified from Cornell and Bellevue, headed to Berlin to learn more. Biggs came back to a post as a pathologist for New York City endorsing the idea that TB was communicable but not highly contagious. This made it preventable. The bacillus mandated a municipal diagnostic laboratory. Biggs set one up in 1892, the first in the world. He also campaigned to have New York hospitals confine TB patients to a special ward rather than have them mix with other patients. He offered the free diagnostic testing of sputum.

He pushed to make TB notifiable. This ideas was as shocking as the ideas of blood tests for and notification of AIDS in the 1980s. Aside from Scandinavian notifications for syphilis, no other disease was notified anywhere. Biggs proposed compulsory notification of all cases in public institutions. When he tried to extend the scheme in 1897 to private patients, New York physicians argued he would cause panic, nervous breakdowns among those notified, and ruin to the boarding house business. Besides, was this test anything more than a laboratory artifact?

Biggs did an end run around his colleagues. He tied free sputum testing to notification. His lure worked. He was helped by the fact that diphtheria antitoxin appeared in 1895 and he also provided tests for diphtheria and the antitoxin for free. He was aware that when "the public demands, it usually gets what it wants; the problem then is to get the public to desire this additional health conservation machinery." He proved adept at managing the media, encouraging colleagues to write pieces for newspapers, making sure they stuck to human interest and avoided statistics. Some wrote letters creating artificial disputes, keeping the argument going by writing under two different names. He ran free public lectures and events handing out illustrations of tubercular lungs and other 'literature'.

His biggest asset was Lillian Wald, a nurse, who in 1893 took over a house on Henry Street on Manhattan's lower East Side. With colleagues, and supported by philanthropy and later insurance companies, Wald set about offering a public health nursing service. Domestic visiting had begun in Britain in the 1860s, offering sanitary advice. It had some support from medicine as long as it was a part-time activity supervised by middle class women. It was resisted once there was a hint of professionalization.

Wald and her colleagues bought into Bigg's new vision that "the greatest enemy of mankind is man himself." What he and they were offering was not traditional sanitarianism. The focus was not on the environment but on people and what they did. In creating the role, Wald and her colleagues found they had more autonomy than hospital nurses and could do many things doctors otherwise did. They held clinics and focused on ways in which people transmit germs. They also wrote many of the newspaper stories.

By this time, Biggs had identified the phenomenon of carriers, people with an illness but not suffering obviously. In 1903 he pushed for and got compulsory detention powers to help the management of TB. Billed as a sanatorium, Riverside hospital opened on North Brother Island for among other things the detention of willfully careless consumptives and its most famous case, Typhoid Mary. This legislation means that, to this day, TB patients can be detained, the only condition besides mental illness for which this can happen.

TB is as hereditary as schizophrenia. What is inherited is a predisposition to the infection. It was common for family members to sleep with an affected relative believing body heat would be helpful. The new understanding prompted a turn to isolation, a ban on spitting, and a mobilization of the community. A Pennsylvania TB Association formed in 1894, becoming a National Tuberculosis Association in 1904. It supported testing and notification. Frustrated at a lack of comparable progress in Germany, in 1891 Koch wrote to Biggs "I wish to cite the example of the free American people who of their own free will accepted the limitation of their own liberties in the interest of the public health."

Within a few years 90% of New York cases were being notified. The annual US mortality rate from TB, 212 per 100,000 in 1905, had dropped to 75 in 1925. In 1950 just as streptomycin was entering clinical care, it had dropped to 29. The changes came neither from traditional sanitarianism nor biomedicine but mostly from a managed, almost military, medicine

THE PROGRESSIVE ERA

When William McKinley was shot in 1901, Theodore Roosevelt became President. He had played a part in the Spanish American War as the commander of the Rough Riders, a unit that deployed Gatling Guns as an offensive weapon used from horseback. In line with the image of someone who solves a problem with a novel technical approach, Roosevelt's Presidency was viewed as progressive as was the era from 1900 to 1920. This was Turgot's Idea of Progress writ large, a belief in the merits of intervention and of science, and a willingness to trust experts.

With the growth of industries linked to physics and chemistry, new electrical goods, plastics, explosives, dyes, rubber products, artificial fibers, and automobiles came on the market. In an open market, competition should drive prices down. Faced with falling profits, the new manufacturing companies banded together in cartels. A cartel presents the world with apparent competition when companies in fact coordinate prices and marketing, creating de facto monopolies.

In America both Republicans and Democrats were committed to competition, which implied trust-busting. This led to a Sherman Anti-Trust Act in 1890, a Clayton Anti-Trust Act in 1914 and the creation of a Federal Trade Commission (FTC) to take action against the unlawful suppression of competition. In practice every move the FTC took was gutted by the US Supreme Court. Anti-trust acts were used to break up unions rather than companies.

Anti-trust rhetoric, however, made American consumerism a political force that eliminated socialism. The first department stores began to appear in American cities after the Civil War. Jane Addams, Josephine Lowell and Florence Kelley set up a National Consumers League in 1899 to promote safety and reliability through thoughtful purchasing. Louis Brandeis, an activist lawyer and later Supreme Court judge, crystallized the issues when he referred to the plain people of America. America has the man on the street, the consumer, rather than a working or middle class. The practical way for citizens to shape industries was through concern about prices, the artificial forces that might keep these high, and the conditions in which goods were made. Every purchase in the market was a vote.

These votes however can be captured as the Chicago meat-packing industry demonstrated. Around 1900, using the new rail network and abilities to refrigerate food, and setting up assembly-lines before Henry Ford did, Big Meat companies created factory farming. This option was inconceivable up till then. It eliminated a swathe of artisans like butchers and laid the basis for what twenty years later became the fast-food industry. The silk-workers in Lyons would have recognized what was happening, although this was on a scale not even Marx could have imagined. With a comparable warehouse and internet exercise that targets convenience, Amazon today has eliminated many of our town centers. Our sympathies may lie with booksellers and being able to trace our food, but as with the gladiators our 'votes' decide who dies.

Companies also turned to marketing around 1900. Marx had seen that growing capacities to produce would in time supply all our needs and companies would then have to tap into our wants. The experts on understanding what people might be persuaded to want were the nineteenth century manufacturers of proprietary remedies. As Claude Hopkins, the author of *Scientific Advertising* in 1923, put it "the greatest advertising men of my day were schooled in the medicine field." Their skill lay in persuading the public that Carter's Little Liver Pills, Lydia Pinkham's Vegetable Compound, Clark Stanley's Snake Oil Liniment, or Coca Cola would restore health or beauty, resolve halitosis, conquer fatigue, and ward off calamity.

The proprietary medicines' market both exemplified and defied conventional views of the Free Market. In the 1830s an advertising war broke out between two Samuel Lees, both from Connecticut, who produced Bilious Pills. Far from leading to market collapse, this dispute spurred demand for Bilious Pills. Other proprietors joined in with their own brands. Managed the right way, competition could increase sales without prices falling. Advertising was key to this. In 1800 there were 200 newspapers; by 1860 there were 4000. In 1800 there were roughly 100 over-the-counter proprietary medicines listed in New York; by 1860 there were over 1500 countrywide. By 1900 thousands of compounds were being advertised in a trade worth hundreds of millions of dollars.

The advertisements marketed lifestyles. The key ingredient was the branding on the bottle rather than anything in it. The money came from huge mark-ups. The selling price might be a hundred times the cost of production. Marketing does the same today when it gets us to believe that the latest App or designer label in addition to doing what it says on the tin will soothe the vague discontent at the heart of our lives. As the sales of bottled water show, differentiating between products hinges on encapsulating our wishes in a brand, and saturating us with this message, rather than with details of what we are buying.

Linked to the development of marketing, and to counteract a new investigative journalism that was hell-bent on scrutinizing corporations, a new public relations industry was also born. This honed new skills from getting a story in first, to generating doubt and playing on the psychology and politics of identity. Before 1940 the new science of psychodynamics had more effect on American business than on American medicine, perhaps because Edward Bernays, one of the creators of this industry, had great brand value as Freud's nephew.

Anti-trust actions aimed at encouraging entrepreneurs and nimble companies. In the case of medicine and pharmaceuticals, along with regulatory actions, they paradoxically incentivized corporate development. Only a bigger company can support marketing and regulatory departments. And if bigger companies are going to compete, they need to eliminate waste and promote efficiency. Rather than enter a market, they aim to control it.

Intervening

The era was a golden one for the press. Growing advertising revenues for everything from bathroom fittings to patent medicines, the emergence of magazines like *Good Housekeeping* or periodicals like *McClure's*, and transport networks that crossed the continent, led to a boom in sales. The press fostered a national consciousness, an extraordinary achievement given the difficulties Europe now has in repeating the trick.

Sandwiched between the advertisements in newspapers and periodicals were articles by a new breed of investigative reporters exploring the difficulties farmers, workers, women, and immigrants were having in an increasingly national economy. Plus, there were new characters and situations to describe. In a tradition that took inspiration from Mark Twain and Jack London, these reporters went down the mean streets. They sketched in a cast of hustlers from party bosses, to racketeers, reformers, and captains of industry doing deals in red light districts, oil refineries, slums and smoke-filled hotel rooms. The spirit of the era was caught by Louis Brandeis, a defender of the right to privacy but also an advocate for transparency, with the phrase "sunlight is the best disinfectant".

Ida Tarbell's exposé of Standard Oil was an early investigative classic. Charles Beard began a tradition of deconstructing the American constitution the way scholars had deconstructed the Bible, claiming it was anti-democratic in its failure to contain the powerful. These 'muckrakers' raised the specter that in this New World of corporations bigger than

States, backroom deals among CEOs could gain control over government. Promoting competition and free enterprise was about political freedom as much as economics

For a decade, a newly formed Chemical Bureau within the Department of Agriculture had pushed for action on food adulteration. Concerns had developed, just as they had in Britain and France, that a disaster from a growing list of adulterants could cause the market to collapse. An anti-adulteration act could help markets grow.

The first move was triggered by vaccine contaminants. The success of diphtheria antitoxin in 1895 created a new biologics industry. In 1901 samples of antitoxin contaminated with tetanus led to the death of 13 children in St Louis, while 9 children in New Jersey died from contaminated smallpox vaccines. This led to passage of a Biologics Control Act in 1902.

In early 1905 Samuel Adams, an investigative journalist, ran a series of articles in *Colliers Weekly* about the claims made for and the actual contents of the most popular patent medicines. His alarming articles provoked no immediate action.

A few months later, *The Jungle*, an Upton Sinclair novel about Chicago meatpacking plants changed everything. Sinclair aimed at alerting the public to an industrial transformation taking place. Instead, like Marx writing *Das Kapital* in 1867, he pointed to the profitability of the new way of doing things, helping consolidate them. But an incidental message in the book, that dead bodies were ending up in the food chain, caused uproar. As Sinclair put it "I aimed for the public's heart… but by accident hit it the stomach."

Bodies in the meat, the Chemical Bureau predicted would cause the food industry to collapse if something was not done to maintain consumer confidence. Roosevelt intervened to ensure the passage in 1906 of a Food and Drugs Act, designed to prevent the manufacture, sale, or transportation of adulterated, misbranded, poisonous, or deleterious foods, drugs, medicines, or liquors. In the case of medicines, prevention meant listing the ingredients on the label.

There were efforts to ban misleading therapeutic claims for medicines. The Supreme Court however held that, whereas the ingredients of a medicine were a matter of fact, claims as to the benefits of drugs were a matter of opinion. The public was entitled to the facts. The new Food and Drugs Agency was not entitled to interfere with the right of members of the public or their doctors to form their own opinions.

The Act was designed to support trade rather than to suppress it. Its thrust was that science could support progress. Those wedded to the wisdom of markets expected that putting as many facts as possible in the hands of consumers would be a win-win proposition. The consumer would only buy quality foods and drugs, leading to better companies, greater employment, and more trade. Before the Act, for instance, Heinz had one tomato ketchup among many. Most ketchups used several chemicals to stabilize the mix. After the Act, Heinz sales outstripped others on the back of its promise that, using ripe tomatoes in clean factories, it avoided adding benzoate of soda as other manufacturers did. Just as in Britain in 1875, businesses found ways to use the new Act to their advantage.

The Act went into effect just as new dyes displaced mercury and lead as food colorants and stabilizers. The notion these dyes might give rise to chemical sensitivities or hyperactivity in children are modern but, seeing images of nerve cells picked out by methylene blue, it was difficult to think we could get away with using these 'drugs' in our food without other effects. Along with regulating food, drugs and cosmetics, the Chemical Bureau set up a laboratory in which Dr. Bernard Hesse examined the 80 dyes then in use in foods and came to the view that sixteen were possibly safe but only seven should be permitted.

There is unquestionably a story of progress from 1871 when the first British Food and Drugs Bill was enacted through to 1962 when the capstone of all Food and Drugs Acts was put in place. An increasing focus on specificity led to steady increases in therapeutic capability. This is not the same thing as better care, and it would also be wrong to assume we knew more about therapy in 2006 than we had done in 1906.

If an agitated patient went into an asylum anywhere in the Western world in 1870, the staff knew to avoid meat and to feed him milky broths. As he settled, meat might be re-introduced keeping an eye on whether it activated him. Meat-eating wasn't the cause of the condition but 150 years ago, doctors, nurses, and families knew more about the effects of food on us than we know now. In addition to the pharmacopoeias, a slew of books like Dr Hume Simons' *The Planters' Guide & Family Book of Medicine* (1848), outlined the astringent, anodyne, aperient, cathartic, diaphoretic, diuretic, emetic, emulcent, expectorant, narcotic, refrigerant, sialogogic, and stimulant effects of a range of foods and herbs. These foods do what people in 1848 said they did, but today most of us have lost a feel for the effects our foods have on us—in part because they are so processed.

We have gained and lost knowledge. A Slow Food movement has rolled back some of what was done to us. But there is no sign of a Slow Medicine.

BIG MEDICINE

Before 1900 health was not a Federal issue. A National Board of Health formed in 1879 was disbanded with its functions taken over by the Marine Hospital Service, underpinned by the only Federal Health Act, a National Quarantine Act. This was passed to block entry to the country of persons suffering from loathsome or contagious diseases, idiots, and insane persons.

The Spanish American War in 1898 raised the Federal profile in health. Defeating Yellow Fever was critical to US military success. No one knew how Yellow Fever was transmitted. Hoping to show it was not contagious, Stubbins Ffirth in the early 1800s slept in the sheets of people who had died from it, and swallowed their black vomit, but didn't catch the disease.

Mosquitoes had been under suspicion since Ffirth noted that unlike smallpox or measles, chilly weather put an end to an epidemic. By the 1890s, mosquitoes were back on the radar as the British conceding bacteriology to the Germans staked out parasitology, winning the second Nobel

Prize in medicine in 1902. But controlled exposure to mosquitoes turned up nothing, and nothing like a bacterium could be found in blood.

In August 1900, hemmed in by an order not to use troops who had not given consent, a US Army medical team decided to let themselves be bitten by mosquitoes. One died and another nearly did. Their efforts nailed down the mosquito as a vector despite the continuing mystery of the missing bacterium, later shown to be a virus. These efforts have gone down in history as an example of heroic self-sacrifice in the cause of science. The success transformed the Marine Hospital Service in 1912 into the US Public Health Service.

The first mission of the new service was to nail down the cause of pellagra, a disease Virchow noted in Silesia 60 years earlier. Pellagra began with dermatitis but ended in madness or dementia. It appeared in the American South around 1900 and spread rapidly among the poor, women, and African Americans. Medical opinion fingered a germ as the cause, but nothing showed in blood, stools, or other bodily fluids.

Using epidemiological methods, a PHS team under Joseph Goldberger in 1916 pinpointed diet as the cause. Pellagra occurred where poverty dictated diet. But even though the data was compelling, this claim made little inroad against the germ theories. It was too vague. Was the dietary component a deficiency or a toxin? It took the isolation of the B vitamins a decade later, and a demonstration that B1 could prevent pellagra, to settle the issue.

While these breakthroughs were happening, and men were celebrated because of them, preventive medicine was created. The women behind it have been written out of history. Josephine Baker was one of the second generation of women doctors. She used Lillian Wald's public health nurse network in the summer of 1908 to see if she could reduce New York's high infant mortality. Between them they reduced deaths per week on the lower East Side from 1500 to 300. Baker pushed for the creation of a Bureau of Child Hygiene within New York's Department of Public Health. This was set up in 1908 and she ran it for the next 15 years, by which time every state had its own bureau.

In these 15 years, Baker mapped out the elements of infant and maternal health, key to a twentieth century increase in population. She flew beneath the public health radar. The prevalent idea was: "if it's not something we quarantine then it's not public health." Baker focused on well-babies and keeping them well. The greatest mortality was in the first four weeks of life. The brief therefore was to track down all pregnant women and give them the input women now get from antenatal care, along with home visits after a birth to ensure the new mother knew what was needed in terms of hygiene and breast feeding.

Later work ranged from eliminating diarrheal disorders, head lice, and trachoma to reducing the 90% death rates in foundling hospitals. Where diarrheal and other disorders needed either breastfeeding or pure milk in the first year of life, Baker showed that foundlings could get perfect milk but still die for lack of the milk of human kindness. Fostering halved the death rates. Sensible hygiene and human contact gave children in lower East Side tenements better survival rates than the children of the wealthy on the upper East Side. This confounds any simple linkage of inequality to ill-health.

Aiming at replicating nationally what Baker was doing in New York, Senator Morris Shephard began Congressional Hearings that led to the Sheppard Towner Act. He was faced with doctors saying that Baker's program was immoral. It was clearly God's will these children died. Others complained that keeping children well would be bad for medical business. Infant and maternal health was so off the medical radar at the time that the administrative support for the hearings came from the House Committee on *Labor*. The hearings came to life when Baker pointed out: "It's six times safer to be a soldier in the trenches in France than to be born a baby in the United States."

Biggs, her boss, had used the term preventive medicine before her, but in a semi-quarantine sense. Baker created the idea of a medicine that prevents people from becoming ill. The War raised the specter of cannon fodder replacement and she was wily enough to sell saving babies to ensure future troops. Within a few years official documents promoted infant health in both Protestant and Catholic States with even Russia becoming as pronatalist as the Catholic Church. Once the idea caught hold, no country could afford to be left behind. Historians conjure up a pronatalist zeitgeist to account for the single biggest advance in health ever. They don't explain how it happened.

Women won the vote successively in American States starting with Colorado and Federally in 1920. Their new power translated in 1921 into the Sheppard Towner Act, a first-ever Federal social security bill. In response to evidence that 80% of women received no antenatal care and higher than necessary infant mortality rates, the Act put in place prenatal and child health centers. These were staffed by women doctors. Public health nurses visited women for hygiene and childcare issues. There were provisions to combat infectious disease, improve occupational safety, and inspect schools to make them more hygienic.

When the Sheppard Towner Act was drawn up, the American Medical Association (AMA) supported National Health Insurance. By 1921 when it passed, AMA was against insurance. When Sheppard Towner came up for renewal in 1926, AMA termed it unsound in policy, wasteful, unproductive, and tending to promote communism. It was not renewed. It re-emerged in Roosevelt's Social Security Act in 1936. In 1921 45 of the 48 State Directors of Child Welfare were women. In 1936 only 12 were women.

Meanwhile, as Baker noted, the focus moved from having children to having well-behaved children. There had always been difficult children who mostly grew out of their problems but "nowadays if a child is anything but a little robot he is taken to a child psychologist to have the cause discovered… We are in danger of making the bearing and bringing up of children such a complicated process that many women are afraid to undertake it."[19]

---

19 Quote from SJ Baker (1939), *Fighting for Life* (New York Review of Books).

Clinical Medicine

Medicine was changing. It was throwing up complex cases that were a job for more than one person. This led Richard Cabot, a Boston physician, in 1905 to set up a first Department of Social Work in Massachusetts General Hospital (MGH). Previously, doctors visited people in their homes and treatment took place there, including in some cases operations. By 1900 office practice was becoming the norm with patients visiting consulting rooms. The expectation of a good clinician was that, while bringing the latest science to bear on a case, they would also have a grasp of the individual and their situation. Now there was a growing likelihood a doctor would have no feel for the patient's social situation. Many thought this was hazardous for both patients and medicine's soul.

Cabot organized for social workers to ensure dietary and other hygienic aspects of a patient's life were as systematically assessed as their blood films. While there was a growing amount of multidisciplinary work within medicine with physicians and surgeons consulting each other about cases, and generalists consulting specialists, bringing social workers to the table changed the meaning of multidisciplinary.

In 1909 Cabot established weekly Clinico-Pathological Conferences in MGH. These became a central part of hospital life. The Boston Medical and Surgical Journal (later the New England Journal of Medicine) featured these conferences from 1924. The focus was on diagnostic puzzles. Based on a clinical presentation, with the possible extras of laboratory results and X-rays, the audience was asked to engage in a process of differential diagnosis. In some cases a postmortem or surgical result might reveal the correct verdict. This was the natural extension of the medical model that had begun in Paris a century previously. It has a drama celebrated in television series like *House*.

The conferences led to an awareness that just as postmortems often spoke to what patients could live with rather than what they had died from, X-ray and laboratory abnormalities might be incidental rather than diagnostic. Diagnosis could not be reduced to reading an X-ray. Tests helped clinicians know if a symptom of sore throat might stem from diphtheria, a streptococcal infection, or neither, but the tests could be wrong. Given that diphtheria antitoxin can pose its own risks, a child with ambiguous clinical features but a negative laboratory test for diphtheria posed a clinical challenge. Treat and perhaps kill the patient with something that could never have done them any good, or stick with the test result and take a gamble on the patient dying? These are not easy issues as Cabot found to his cost. Diagnostic acumen took its place alongside traditional wisdom as key clinical skills.

Medicine was moving into new domains. The exploration of the living machine threw up more questions than answers. In a patient with leg pain on walking, X-rays may show almost normal blood flow to their legs, while other patients with blocked arteries might have little difficulty in walking. Many patients with blocked arteries can be helped by graded walking, but their X-rays almost demand operations. These operations can make things worse. What might be biologically plausible and what is right for a patient are different things.

When all tests are negative, is the problem in the patient's mind? In office practice, a doctor may diagnose a patient as the diagnosis provides a means of negotiation between doctor and patient, considering a step into the business of therapeutic poisoning. The stakes get higher in hospital medicine where the interventions are more drastic, and specialists rarely see the outcome of their interventions.

Cabot's records from 1895 to 1915 show that many of those who came to him had learnt to speak a clinical language and to engage with the diagnostic process. While diagnosis involved a detachment from the patients' experience, this was not viewed as alienating. Even when the verdict was grim, knowing what was wrong could offer benefits. His patients talked about locating problems in their trachea or bronchioles or alveoli, just as American patients today talk about their dopamine and serotonin levels. They think this language is one of progress but it is often a language of rhetorical gestures rather than meaning.

Finally, when a patient saw Cabot in his office, they would hand over money. Up till 1900, there had been little point having health insurance because medicine could do little to save anyone. As surgery extended its reach and people survived, this was changing. It was common practice not to bill in cases where the person might be unable to pay, especially if they could not be helped. Wealthy patients were charged a premium to cover those who couldn't or didn't pay. Cabot was one of many doctors around 1910 who thought health insurance might be a better method of handling payment issues.

Historians viewing these exchanges talk of a carriage trade. They see elite physicians ensuring their consultation business continued rather than engaging with wider social issues that might lead business to dry up. There is no celebration of clinical medicine. It is viewed as an imperial power, contributing less than hygienic measures. Cabot confounds all this. He was seen by older doctors as drifting away from clinical medicine, and by others as dangerous because he created medical social work and favored health insurance.

Health Insurance

The American Medical Association (AMA) formed in 1847, following in the footsteps of the British Medical Association (BMA). AMA was a small operation up to 1900 but between 1900 and 1910, before the Flexner report came out, it grew from 8,000 to 70,000 doctors. Doctors in private or group practice are businesses. A body representing them is a Trade Association rather than a Trade Union. Trade Associations tend to be conservative.

When it came to health insurance, the main need before 1900 was for casualty insurance. The first insurance plans began in the early 1850s. After the Civil War over 60 organizations offered coverage for injuries linked to rail or steamboat travel, mining, and other industries. As in the case of nervous travelers, insurance generally aids the growth of a new sector perceived to be risky. In the 1890s the issue of sickness and disability coverage arose, with several plans on offer. In 1911 the Western Clinic in Tacoma offered the first prepaid plan for lumber mill employees at 50 cents per person per month.

Economists at the University of Wisconsin set up the American Association for Labor Legislation (AALL) to lobby for workers compensation. In 1915 AALL, with the support of AMA, produced a draft Health Insurance Act, offering a sickness benefit. They claimed it would reduce poverty by reducing disability and encourage accident and sickness prevention in workplaces. But employers, who had accepted the idea of workman's compensation to manage legal liabilities, didn't see the benefit of sick pay for employees. The unions were also ambivalent, preferring the idea of mutual fund support rather than a federal scheme. And while both Germany and Britain had introduced health insurance to blunt the appeal of socialism, there was little socialist presence in the United States. There was even less after 1914, when Henry Ford surprised everyone by doubling the minimum wage in his factories to $5 a day. Other companies followed suit.

The AALL scheme also ran into problems with the major life insurance companies, Prudential and Metropolitan. While collaborating with Josephine Baker, Lillian Wald persuaded Metropolitan that her visiting nurses could save lives. This would save Metropolitan money on death benefits. By 1912 Metropolitan was paying for 1 million visits per year and claiming the scheme had reduced death rates of policyholders by 12% per year, saving the company up to $2 million per year.

The new health insurance bill offered a death benefit to cover terminal illness and funeral costs. This compromised life insurance business models. The companies lobbied against the bill. Their lobbying brought a new entity into view, dubbed The Money Trust by Louis Brandeis. Members of the Boards of Prudential and Metropolitan, sat on the Boards of other major financial institutions, and helped to turn large sections of the business community against health insurance, Brandeis argued. While groups like the Freemasons and Illuminati, operating under conditions of secrecy because of state censorship, had existed before, these visible connections among financial institutions provided evidence that a group, not restricted to national boundaries, might shape events around the world.

In 1910 AMA thought insurance could bring more people into the medical tent. But America was at the height of a hospital building boom. There seemed no end to the number of hospitals being built. America had more general hospitals than the rest of the world combined, equipped with X-ray facilities and equipment for interventions that could not be delivered at home. Hospitals had become a must have for urban centers to attract business and development money. All had a notional commitment to the charitable care of (white) people who could not pay. Against this backdrop, AMA became wary that, rather than letting the market grow, insurance would lead to 'capitation'. Physicians would have to compete for contracts to offer a service to a specified number of people for a fixed price. Opinion swung toward decapitating health insurance; against what AMA now called socialized medicine.

For Richard Cabot, social medicine meant the necessary adjustments we need to live in urban (social) situations, such as engaging in vaccination programs and employing social workers. For Herman Biggs, social meant a medicine that required an administrative (management) input. For AMA social suggested something hostile to the spirit of free enterprise and voluntary effort, where doctors would have to act as medical police.

But the world was changing. In 1914 America declared war on drugs, with the passage of the Harrison Narcotics Tax Act. This introduced prescription-only status for opiates and cocaine to control the supply of these drugs. Their use had been increasing since the Civil War. Prescription-only status meant the drugs could only be legally obtained from a doctor. This was the clearest instance of 'medical policing' anywhere in the world.

The medical certification that went with workers' compensation schemes also involved policing, as did public health nursing, more developed in America than anywhere else. And in American healthcare, communities were more active in the policing of infection, aided by advertising and a new public relations industry, than could be found anywhere else.

Medicine had become the Business of America.

THE INTERVENING YEARS

We might have foreseen it
The triumph of calculation
The atom calculated
By its chances.
What can I know? What must I do?
What may I hope?
And what are my chances?

We ought to be able to survive it.
Out of the unknown activities
of unknown agents
Mathematical numbers emerge. The last
Invisible world
of the buyers, the sellers, the planners —
We ought to be able to survive it.

George Oppen
Wheelers & Dealers: The Theory of Games

5: THE BUYERS, THE SELLERS, THE PLANNERS

A century of medical advances was put to the test in August 1914. Disease had led to the greatest loss of life in war previously. A combination of better understanding and vaccines meant that typhoid, typhus, tetanus, diphtheria and dysentery killed comparatively few in the Great War.

Nearly 20 million troops were wounded, making wound control critical. Gangrene, common initially, became rare. Over half a million amputations stimulated the development of orthopedics, prostheses, and rehabilitation medicine. Surgical tools from theatre lighting to retractors and mobile X-ray units came into use. Intravenous saline infusions helped manage shock and the just developed blood typing made mid-surgery blood transfusions possible.

Face masks became an enduring image of the War as Nitrogen Mustard gas was used in the first chemical warfare. Death could come from anywhere, even from the skies.

Psychiatric casualties numbered in the millions. Early on, the sheer difficulty in executing so many men prevented armies from following standard procedure and executing soldiers who for no obvious reason would not fight. Initial opinions divided between seeing these behaviors as malingering or neurological damage caused by explosions. The officer class was affected, challenging ideas that only those of poorer stock or women got nervous disorders. By the end of the War, concepts of traumatic neuroses and nostalgia crystallized into shellshock. As Charcot had said thirty years earlier, men could become hysterical.

Using combinations of persuasion and electrotherapy (faradism), leading British hospitals produced rates of recovery from shellshock that have probably never been bettered. This electrical input was, like Mesmer's magnetic force, something that had an ambiguous relationship to recovery.

Psychoanalysis played no part in these recoveries. The War though made Freud, perhaps because his nephew Edward Bernays was central to the development of a public relations industry in America after the War. Americans were quick to realize the value of embodying messages in the new cinematic medium emerging in Hollywood, laying the basis for a propaganda industry closely linked to military needs ever since.

The cause of these neuroses was one thing, the payment of a pension another. A favorable pension ruling was more likely if, for instance, fits were diagnosed as 'true' rather than 'functional' epilepsy. Where the focus was on function or trauma, a soldier's history of delinquent behavior or his family's history of nervous conditions could lead to an emphasis on a vulnerable pre-existing constitution. This might leave him without a pension.

All sides provided hospital beds on an extraordinary scale. Britain put in place more beds than its National Health Service has now for a population double the size. Prussia alone had as many beds as Britain. These hospitals were run by women physicians and surgeons, while men were becoming hysterical at the front.

Preventive Medicine

The Great War reinforced the lesson of the Civil War that systems count. As George Newman, Britain's first Chief Medical Officer writing to Britain's first Minister of Health in 1919 put it:

> *Whatever the case before 1914, the experience of war had demonstrated beyond all question that industrial hygiene forms an integral part of the practice of Preventative Medicine.* [20]

---

20 All quotes from Newman G, *An Outline of the Practice of Preventive Medicine*. (His Majesty's Stationery Office, London, 1919). See text: samizdathealth.org/shipwreck/

Newman was a Quaker, as Josephine Baker was. He too had worked on infant mortality before the War. When he visited New York to meet Herman Biggs, he offered her a job. But in line with the seamless writing of women out of the script that began once the War ended, he doesn't credit her. She stuck with New York's Irish (Tammany) way of doing things.

Biggs and Newman wrote reports after the War. Neither mention each other or compare their countries, even though America and Britain had similar healthcare systems, with both endorsing a Liberal combination of free market and progressive policies distinct from the more centralizing tendencies of Germany and France. While America contemplated health insurance, in 1910 Britain put a National Insurance Act in place, part of a push to establish a national Health Department. Three decades later, America and Britain had very different systems with Germany and France somewhere in between.

Britain's population had grown from 3.5 million in 1600 to 33.5 million in 1910. Only 10% lived in cities in 1800, but over 80% did in 1910. America's population had grown from 3.5 million in 1800 to 80 million, of which 60% was still rural. In both countries, birth rates and infant mortality were falling. Measles, tuberculosis, rheumatism, and venereal disease were becoming a greater threat than epidemics.

After the War, the focus switched from sanitation to encouraging individuals to develop their physiques and increase their powers of resistance to disease. Public Health became something sanitary engineers did; it removed nuisances. Preventive Medicine was what doctors did, aimed at making individuals fitter. It brought heredity, nurture, nutritional status, habits, and occupation into the frame. Alarming data on the condition of the national stock had begun to flow in from school inspections, inspections of army recruits, and in Britain from Health Insurance claims. Many were physically impaired, suffering from preventable disease and unfit.

The people needed to become health conscious. As Newman put it:

The practice of preventive medicine involves... far-reaching personal and social considerations, which affect not only the habits, occupation,

*and susceptibility of the individual but the capacity, security and
even the existence of the nation.*

He didn't quite say in order to get the nation's fighting stock in good
shape but:

*Workers in preventive medicine must not find themselves unprepared
with their plan of campaign or an adequate survey of the terrain
until the enemy has published his ultimatum and it is too late.*

Biggs and Newman covered identical ground but Newman's brief to
talk about the nation make his wording more politically revealing. This
lack of fitness, he argued, undermined the stability of the State. The task of
growing a sound and healthy race must begin with mothers and children.
If we permit ourselves to provide for the unguided propagation of a population of poor physique marked from birth with the stigmata of alcohol,
venereal disease, or mental deficiency, we shall discover we are building on
false foundations.

The industrial revolution, he said, had been a tragedy for children.
Hardship, cruelty, disease, and early death had placed an indelible mark
on them. While inspections had shown 80% of schoolchildren were free of
obvious disease, the rest were in poorer shape than anyone thought.

We needed new school services to produce:

*A citizen educated in hygiene, possessing a health conscience, and
trained in personal and social habits to avoid infection, to remove
or ameliorate the conditions predisposing to disease…, and to understand that the individual body in health is the first line in the defense
against disease.*

Insurance claims showed people missing work because of bronchitis,
indigestion, dyspepsia, and above all fatigue, which had clear economic
implications. Newman linked fatigue to heart failure, alcohol abuse and
anything that made workers less fit, including physical defects like flat
feet, club feet, poor teeth, poor sight, and indigestion. Indigestion was

manageable by avoiding too much tea, bolting food, irregular meals, incomplete mastication, constipation, and swallowing air.

References to dental health and poor teeth recur throughout Newman's and Biggs' reports in ways that seem as quaint as a focus on swallowing air. But this was a time when Henry Cotton, the superintendent of the Trenton Asylum in New Jersey, had begun removing teeth and other organs to cure madness, claiming hidden infections were the source of all medical disorders. Along with preventing alcoholism, good teeth were seen as a gateway to health and fitness at work.

Mothers were central to health. "To use up or damage women by setting them to hard wage labor in mill and workshop is probably the greatest human waste a nation can practice," Newman said. Letting women drink while pregnant was misguided as was failing to screen for congenital syphilis. Other conditions leading to feeble mindedness in the infant such as insanity or epilepsy in the parent, the effects of consanguinity, or physical injury to the fetus needed to be managed. Asserting that feeble-minded women were more fertile and the transmission of their conditions "a racial malady," he argued, the state needed to encourage worthy and discourage unworthy parenthood.

We also permit conditions of life and labor which either create lunacy, he said, or exacerbate traits of feeble-mindedness, low intelligence, psycho-neurosis, and neurasthenia to produce lunatics whom we incarcerate at a huge cost. Except for changes of life in women, these contributory factors could be managed through eugenics, stress management, control of alcohol intake, and increased fitness.

This was a different medicine to anything that had gone before. For the first time, a few people were in a position to review the state of the national garden and envisage removing the weeds and selecting the right plants to build on. A vision of transforming the ugliness of an unkempt nature into the beauty of a well-kept garden took shape, just as sensibilities about the physical world were moving in the opposite direction.

The management of the national garden involved, in Newman's view, eliminating the wastefulness and confusion in well-meant but arbitrary medical care. "Hospitals are dotted around with little regard for the needs of the population… with absence here, redundance there… representative government here, capricious control there." A coordinated network was needed, while avoiding the evils of bureaucracy.

With doctors, "There has been an immense growth of knowledge and a revolution in the public duties of medical men," Newman noted, "and it was now the purpose of a scientific scheme of national health to reduce caprice, chance and surprise to a minimum." In the sphere of national health, physicians couldn't just do what they wanted.

Anyone managing the health of the nation today would have a plan for cancers, and heart attacks. Biggs makes no mention of these. For Newman, cancers and heart attacks were rare. Heart conditions he was confident began with infections early in life, with some linked to alcohol or occupational stressors. In a footnote he notes a reported link to tobacco.

The Americans meanwhile were about to take the radical step of prohibiting alcohol. For Biggs, an epidemic of polio in New York in 1916 featured prominently. Epidemics were supposed to be a thing of the past. For Newman polio didn't register. The influenza pandemic of 1918 affected America more than Britain, perhaps linked to greater aspirin use. Newman regarded influenza as something that could be managed with a good nasal drill.

Other non–infectious disorders like rickets came on Newman's radar. He was skeptical of reports that Vitamin D might be a cure. Getting children to exercise in the open air would do as much for rickets as giving Vitamin D.

Finally, unlike Biggs, Newman had the colonies to consider. While Ireland was slipping out of the Empire's grasp, there was still a need to manage India:

> *The effects of [managing malaria and yellow fever] will be as far reaching as those of any discoveries ever made in medicine… I believe we are on the eve of the occupation of the Tropics by the white man. If this be so, then great civilizations, in the course of time, will develop in tropical regions.*

Preventive medicine put eugenics on the map. The Scandinavian countries were the first to adopt eugenics. In 1927 in Buck v Bell, the US Supreme Court endorsed laws supporting the sterilization of women likely to pass on feeble-mindedness. This position was supported by progressives including Theodore Roosevelt, Louis Brandeis and Oliver Wendell Holmes who in the Buck case stated, "Three generations of imbeciles are enough." This judgement underpinned the sterilization of 50,000 women.

Germany had a consensus in favor of preventive medicine and eugenics before the Nazis campaigned to restrict tobacco use, alongside traditional campaigns to eliminate alcohol and prostitution. From the mid-1930s onwards, Germany implemented a Copernican Revolution in health policy. Instead of the State revolving around the individual, the individual would revolve around the State. This vision embraced the elimination of those who could not contribute to the efficiency of the Volk, whose genes might pollute the national stock, or whose lives were not worth living. Thousands of the mentally ill and mentally handicapped were eliminated with medical assistance and later in gas chambers before others were eliminated. Health policy gave us the Holocaust.

THE COSTS OF MEDICAL CARE

After 1920 the trajectories of American and British health services diverged. The British loss of nearly a million young men produced the first hints of the aging population profile that concerns health planners today. The need was to warehouse the medically indigent, the war wounded and the elderly infirm. Workhouses were rebadged as State Hospitals.

America had more acute care hospitals than the rest of the world combined. Their focus was on workplace and automobile casualties, and obstetric services. A steady rate of tonsil, adenoid and appendix removals, hysterectomies, varicose vein stripping and growing rates of breast cancer surgery kept the operation afloat. These hospitals had few medical beds. Cardiology and coronary care units only appeared in the 1960s.

By 1930 70% of American hospitals were private where only 12% of European ones were. While these hospitals claimed they would treat medical conditions regardless of ability to pay, they offered treatment of acute illnesses, not accommodation for the medically indigent. By 1950 most American doctors were specialists, whereas only 10% of Europeans were

Facing rising costs of care, in 1927 AMA and Metropolitan Life established a Committee on the Costs of Medical Care (CCMC). Echoing Newman, CCMC thought medicine should be preventive and American medicine lacked a system. CCMC embraced group practice, begun by the Mayo Clinic. This built on the idea that medical developments meant that optimal treatment might require the collaboration of several specialists. A group had three or more doctors working together to provide a comprehensive service. Mayo began seeding group practices across the mid-West.

The final CCMC report endorsed hospital care, which its public health members labelled a recipe for runaway costs. It endorsed group practice, which AMA, the home of individual practitioners, labelled medical soviets. AMA branded CCMC a tool of the great Foundations, public health officialdom, social theory, even of socialism and communism.

Everyone agreed, though, there was unmet medical need: "The ordinary layman lacks the knowledge to define his own medical needs and can rely only on the expert opinion of medical practitioners and public health authorities." Not even the wealthiest were getting enough medical input. "The amount of care which people need is far greater than that which they are aware of needing, and greater than that for which they are able to pay under present conditions."[21]

A parallel Ogburn report concluded that:

> *A considerable proportion of the people in this country are still suffering from a multitude of preventable defects, disabling diseases and minor ailments. An unnecessary toll of millions of dollars is imposed on the nation annually, thousands of human beings are*

---

21 Starr R, *The Social Transformation of American Medicine* (Basic Books) 263.

needlessly destroyed and there is widespread suffering, inefficiency and disability. Knowledge is at hand to prevent this… it is not being utilized. Human life in this country is wasted as surely in times of peace as in war.[22]

Choice of Care?

In 1920 American railroad, mining and lumbering companies had a million employees in employer medical programs. These offered early treatment of industrial injuries, assessment of workers prior to hire, and some disability compensation. Employees were not always happy at payroll deductions for the services of company doctors but faced with rising medical costs it was something.

Across the board, American physicians were hostile to corporate hierarchies and efforts to commercialize practice beyond simple fee for service. Any system that made a profit offering medical services as commodities, they claimed, was likely to injure the public. Medicine was starting to offer real benefits, but many still argued the core of the medical act lay in a relationship rather than in techniques. What happened to patients should not be determined in a laboratory.

The economic crash in 1929 left impoverished Americans facing soup kitchens. US hospitals however worked out a way to survive. Justin Kimball, vice-president of Baylor University, came up with a scheme for prepaid hospital insurance. For $6 a year, the plan offered 21 hospital days. This created a Blue Cross network. While anyone who could pay the premiums could join Blue Cross, the new network sold the scheme to employers as a group plan. Make it a perk of the job and it would ensure the fitness of their workforce. Without obviously discriminating against anyone, this immediately ruled out the elderly, the infirm, the unemployed and the chronically ill.

Blue Cross was marketed as the American Way. Just as Equitable Life in Britain had done in 1762, the scheme played on the responsibility of a

---

22 Bloom SW, *The Word as Scalpel*, 59.

provider to look after himself and his family and offered itself as a discrete way for the middle class to get the comforts of privilege. Private healthcare was the Way of Democracy, and a test of America's desire for continued self-government. Metropolitan Life followed suit. Doctors saw Blue Cross and Metropolitan keeping medicine under physician rather than government control.

Noting that a government insurance system would spread risks more efficiently, CCMC still favored private insurance on the basis that America was more affluent than Europe. Blue Cross more forcefully argued "that the provision of health care under the government would be the most extravagant experiment the taxpayer has yet been forced to support. He would pay not alone in money, but in his own health, and in the health of those dependent on him."

In America, Metropolitan offered grants to support special fracture units. In Britain, in contrast, appeals to health insurers to support fracture facilities got nowhere. Orthopedic surgeons found that saving money did not seem to motivate insurers:

> *They [insurers] simply say that so far as they are concerned, it is a question of finance, and the premiums are so regulated that they cover even the most expensive case. Any attempt... to reduce the period of incapacity would merely mean that employers would press for a lower premium and the Insurance Company would be no better off than before. We cannot hope, therefore, for help in the way of securing improved treatment from Insurance Companies.*

Here is a central issue of medical economics: How to ensure what works gets funded, while other novelties don't. America's insurance industry produced the fracture clinics Britain's orthopedists wanted. America, however, also spent more on Iron Lungs for polio victims and later brain scans with no benefit to patients from the investment, than Britain where the scanners had been invented. These difficulties led Britain's wealthy orthopedic surgeons to ally with the Labour party in the 1940s to push for a National Health Service, thinking a state aided rather than state-controlled service would give doctors what they wanted.

While the relationship between doctor and patient was lauded in America as being at the heart of medicine, by 1920 family doctors were vanishing. The closest most people could get to a generalist was a hospital internist. Britain, meanwhile, was on its way to creating a family medicine system run as businesses even after incorporation in a National Health Service. This system was prized by British doctors and patients for 50 years as giving something like a marital relationship.

Big Medicine

When elected President in 1932, Roosevelt moved to create a Social Security Act "to provide sound and adequate protection against the vicissitudes of life." He told his cabinet to explore maternity benefits, accident, unemployment, old-age, crop, and health insurance.

This aroused Republican opposition. George Chandler from Ohio said: "With unemployment insurance no-one would work; with old-age and survivors' insurance no one would save; the result would be moral decay, financial bankruptcy and the collapse of the republic." John Taber claimed: "Never in the history of the world has any measure been brought in here so insidiously designed as to prevent business recovery, to enslave workers, and to prevent any possibility of the employers providing work for the people."[23]

AMA opposition forced Roosevelt to drop universal health coverage. The final Act supported maternal, child and public health through the Public Health Service. When Roosevelt and Congress created the National Institute for Health, as part of the later War effort, AMA had no objection to State chemistry and State biology.

---

23 Cited by Truman in 1952, see: trumanlibrary.org/publicpapers/index.php?pid=2255. Both cites in Arthur Schlesinger, *The Coming of the New Deal,* (Houghton, Mifflin, Harcourt, New York)311.

At the end of the War, Roosevelt, who had been crippled with polio from 1921, was diagnosed with coronary artery disease, and malignant hypertension. His death from a stroke put these new disorders on the map.

Harry Truman, a believer in Big Medicine, succeeded him. Truman supported a Burton-Hill Act which led to a wave of State hospital building. He supported public health, maternal and child health programs, and funded a National Institute of Mental Health (NIMH). He proposed a universal health coverage in which citizens were free to choose their doctors, and "doctors had the right to expect higher average earnings than they had received before."

AMA campaigned against Truman's Bill, spending $5 million ($50 million in 2020 terms), then the most expensive-ever lobbying campaign. Their messages were "keep politics out of medicine" and maintain the public's right to choose their own doctor. AMA pointed to the Soviet Union's introduction of free healthcare for all. Against a developing Cold War, they spun socialized medicine as an Un-American perversity.

The failure of Truman's Bill and the success of Blue Cross tempted private for-profit insurers into the market. To compete with the non-profit Blue Cross, these schemes introduced deductibles in packages billed as covering major medical expenses but discouraging frivolous use. The few prepaid group plans were not well placed in this market, but they survived to re-emerge in the 1980s.

Meanwhile in 1948, Britain's Labour Government started a single payer, universal coverage, National Health Service (NHS), paid for by taxation. The British Medical Association opposed this. Aneurin Bevan, the Health Secretary, said that to manage doctors' objections he had stuffed their mouths with gold. Once embedded in the new system, however, doctors became its biggest defenders.

NOT SO BIG PHARMA

In 1935 Gerald Domagk and colleagues in the German pharmaceutical company, Bayer, working with azo dyes, developed Prontosil, sulfonamide. This was the first sulfa antibiotic. It was lifesaving for streptococcal infections, producing miraculous recoveries in women with puerperal fevers, and children with septicemia. Over the next twenty years sulfa drugs gave birth to the sulfonylureas, which were the first non-insulin treatments for diabetes and from these came the thiazides, which became the leading diuretics and antihypertensives.

Bayer patented sulfonamide and all related molecules. It lost control of the new market, however, when Ernest Fourneau, France's leading pharmacologist, realized sulfanilamide, which Bayer had ignored because it was not a dye, was also an antibiotic.

The new antibiotics captured American attention with the hospitalization of Franklin D Roosevelt Jr. for a life-threatening infection in November 1936. His response to Prontosil led to newspaper accounts of the new miracle drug. Therapeutic nihilism went out of fashion overnight. While many doctors remained cautious, others tried the new drug for erysipelas, scarlet fever, meningitis, cellulitis, otitis media, pneumonia, gonorrhea, and tonsillitis. People going into hospital or undergoing operations were treated prophylactically. There was little sense anything could go wrong.

In response to a request for liquid sulfanilamide, in 1937 Harold Watkins, a chemist working for Massengill in Tennessee, dissolved the drug in diethylene glycol. He shipped Elixir of Sulfanilamide around the country. Weeks later in Tulsa, several dozen people presented to their doctors with severe abdominal cramps. Some stopped urinating, became comatose, and six died. One doctor, James Stephenson, made a link to sulfanilamide and alerted the AMA, which had greater standing on medicines then among doctors than did the FDA.

FDA heard about developments on the grapevine, sent an agent to Tulsa, and pressured Massengil to recall the drug on a technicality: the product was misbranded. An Elixir is alcohol based and diethylene glycol is not an alcohol. Without the misbranding, FDA could have done nothing. There were 107 deaths.

Sulfanilamide was a universe apart from the over-the-counter panaceas that concerned regulators, whose adverts combined scientific claims, testimonials from satisfied patients and celebrity endorsements. As the Twenties Roared, weight-loss drugs became big business. Alarmed by "anti-fat fraud… fabulous sums are spent on these fakes since the female skeleton became the fashion," the Federal Trade Commission (FTC) challenged Raladam Co., over its adverts for Marmola. This weight-loss compound was made from desiccated thyroid gland extracts and laxatives. The FTC wanted Marmola adverts to mention it should be taken under medical direction. Raladam appealed to the Supreme Court in 1931 and won, on the basis that anti-trust statutes only outlawed trading practices that were unfair to a competitor. Deceiving consumers was not illegal.

Roosevelt's government tabled a new Food and Drugs Act in 1932. This stalled in committee. In the wake of sulfanilamide, in March 1938, a Wheeler-Lea Act gave the FTC a brief to tackle injuries to or fraud on consumers rather than just acts that disadvantaged other companies. FTC took and won a new action against Raladam. In June 1938, Congress passed a Food, Drugs & Cosmetics Act.

Up till then, FDA handled drugs in the same way as food. It pushed for accurate labeling and checked for adulteration. The new Act required drugs be safe to use under the conditions prescribed or recommended in the labeling. But what did this mean?

For drugs like sulfanilamide or barbiturates, companies argued, consumers would need a correspondence course in medicine on the label to be able to use them. How do you tell a layman a barbiturate is contra-indicated in nephritis? How does a company explain that the medical decision might be to use it despite a contra-indication? And a change to the label every time a new side effect was detected would cost, industry claimed, millions of dollars.

It was not clear how to produce the right label for drugs like sulfanilamide. FDA had been blocked from regulating company claims for the benefits of a drug in 1907. In medical practice, the onus was on doctors to decide when to use a medicine and when not. Of the 107 sulfanilamide fatalities, 105 had been on prescription, many of them questionable. FDA therefore didn't have any great faith in medical discretion. Making a drug 'prescription-only', however, solved the claims-of-benefits difficulty, and allowed companies to skip putting medical details on the label

Companies argued for the right to say which drugs would be prescription only. This would contain costs and avoid socializing medicine, they said, and avoided bureaucrats saying what treatments people could have? Aiming to increase sales and reduce liabilities, Merck switched everything to prescription-only except "about a dozen commonly used household drugs". Many commonly used medicines became prescription-only with less information on their labels than before.

FDA tried to restrict prescription-only status to drugs recognized as needing medical supervision. Pharmacists also pushed for clarity. Senator Hubert Humphrey, a former pharmacist, and Congressman Carl Durham introduced the Humphrey-Durham amendments in 1951, restricting prescription-only status to drugs needing medical supervision.

Ethical Pharma

Before 1940 America had a roaring trade in proprietary medicines but not a pharmaceutical industry. Hundreds of low-profit, small-firms, or branches of chemical companies, produced analgesics, herbals, mercurials and arsenicals some of which had been treatment staples for centuries. A few companies like Sharp and Dohme, and Mulford and Sons had moved into the production of vaccines and sera. The discovery of insulin in 1922 led to a move into hormone preparations, such as desiccated thyroid glands, and sex steroids extracted from animal urine. A market in vitamins was growing.

After the 1938 Act, some companies switched to a self-proclaimed 'ethical' manufacturing of drugs for medical use. E. R. Squibb was the biggest of these, Pfizer one of the smallest. These companies imported sulfonamides under license from Europe. In the early 1950s, when some

US companies discovered tetracycline antibiotics, they initially licensed them to other companies for marketing. When companies realized that with other companies holding a license on the same drug, they were marketing against each other, this changed.

All was changing. As part of the war effort, Roosevelt capitalized the research on which industry would draw when he endowed the National Institutes of Health (NIH). The Nazi threat led to an influx of scientists from Europe funded by government money poured into research. In June 1941, an Office of Scientific Research and Development (OSRD) was established to co-ordinate projects from the building of a nuclear bomb to the production of penicillin. OSRD channeled more than $500 million into over 2000 projects. A Public Health Services Act in 1944 established a budget to continue these research programs in the NIH or universities around the country after the War.

The War put a premium on antibiotics. A compelling candidate drug, penicillin, had been isolated from the pencillium mold and demonstrated to be safe by Howard Florey and Ernst Chain in Oxford. The issue was one of scaling up production. OSRD picked Merck and Pfizer, because they had deep-vat fermentation facilities, used by Pfizer to produce citric acid for food and soft drinks. In late 1943 large quantities of penicillin came on-stream, and it was released into general use at the end of the War.

Meanwhile, Japanese success in the Pacific cut off supplies of quinine for malaria. The alternative, Atabrine, caused severe side effects. Supported by OSRD, James Shannon in New York's Goldwater Memorial Hospital persuaded colleagues to send him researchers keen to avoid the front-lines. One of these, Steve Brodie, transformed research on drug effects by measuring drug and metabolite levels in blood, and showed that soldiers were being given doses of Atabrine that were too high.

At the end of the War, Julius Axelrod, a technician from a non-profit laboratory asked Brodie if phenacetin, an analgesic, could cause methemo-globinemia. Aniline, a breakdown product of phenacetin, could do so. Did phenacetin lead to aniline in the blood? Brodie's way to answer questions like this was with new techniques in this case spectrophotometers and spectrophotofluorimeters. Phenacetin did produce aniline. Another of its metabolites was acetaminophen (paracetamol). Brodie and Axelrod had discovered a new drug.

Shannon was made Chief of the NIH after the War. He took Brodie with him, who took Axelrod. Making use of new techniques like radio-labeled drugs, Brodie, Axelrod, and a slew of visiting scientists, such as Arvid Carlsson, created modern neuroscience, the basis for a later generation of drug development. Many were awarded Nobel Prizes.

Patents were another factor that laid a basis for the growth of pharma. While penicillin helped manage gram positive infections like pneumonia, there was still a premium on developing new antibiotics especially for gram negative infections caused by e coli, the cholera bacillus, and above all for tuberculosis.

In 1943 Albert Schatz and Selman Waksman at Rutgers University discovered that a group of actinomycete soil organisms produced streptomycin. In collaboration with Merck, this was tested in mice and then in the Mayo Clinic where its credentials as the first drug to benefit TB were confirmed. In September 1948, the patent office granted Patent No 2,499,866 for streptomycin.

This patent was remarkable in three respects. First it violated an understanding that products of nature could not be patented. Waksman argued that microbes don't produce antibiotics naturally; they only do so when cultured in an artificial medium. This claim was wrong, but the patent office didn't check it out.

Second, patent law required an element of genius. Patents were granted to inventors rather than skilled mechanics. Chasing streptomycin was an obvious thing to do in the wake of penicillin. In the wake of streptomycin, companies geared up to mass screen potential drugs by technicians (and later by robots). A new US Patent Act in 1952 lowered the bar, requiring only that the *average* doctor or microbiologist looking at an experiment claimed to support a new drug's benefit should not be able to predict the result.

Third, the patent on streptomycin was a patent for streptomycin. It was a *product* patent rather than a *process* patent. Up till then, industry had operated with patents on processes; if another company found a different way to make a drug, they too could take out a patent.

Several drugs related to streptomycin, aureomycin produced by Lederle, and terramycin produced by Pfizer were patented soon after. Pfizer found that aureomycin was chlortetracycline and terramycin was oxytetracycline, and the core tetracycline compound was also an antibiotic. Five different companies claimed priority on tetracycline, which was on its way to being a $100 million-a-year cash cow. When the companies stopped barking, the deals done behind the scenes became grist to the mill of Congressional hearings.

The realization that companies could exploit the monopoly possibilities of the patents by marketing their own drugs, so that every advertising dollar would produce a return to them, led to a dramatic vertical integration of the industry. In 1940 there had been several hundred largely local companies, none accounting for more than 3% of the market. A decade later 15 companies controlled 80% of a rapidly growing US market. By 1960 pharmaceuticals offered the greatest return on investment of any industry in America.

THE LONG DECADE

Between 1946 and 1960 America was focused on the Cold War and investigating communist and homosexual infiltration of the government and the media.

Medicine in contrast was a focus for optimism and openness. Cortisone and the steroid hormones came on stream in 1947, leading to oral contraceptives in 1957. Nitrogen Mustard drugs appeared for cancer (1947), antipsychotics (1952), tranquilizers (1955), anticonvulsants (1955), diuretics (1955), antihypertensives (1957), antidepressants (1957) oral hypoglycemics (1957), and lipid lowering drugs (1960) followed. Death from infection became rare. Mental hospitals began to empty. Unwanted pregnancies were about to plummet even as love became free. The stigma of disease began to lift.

Spearheaded by Roosevelt in 1938, the March of Dimes mobilized private philanthropy to conquer polio with a vaccine in 1954. This kick-started a vaccine business.

Even the thorny question of drug brands was put to rest. For both doctors and patients, a brand name drug from Merck, such as the antihypertensive Diuril, or the antidepressant Tryptizol, counted for as much as having a Hoover or Mercedes in other walks of life. Ethical brands seemed to have a basis in reality, rather than marketing.

In 1947 the infectious disease part of the Public Health Service (PHS) was reborn as the Centers for Disease Control (CDC). Roosevelt's stroke, and Eisenhower's later heart attacks, put the male heart in the frame and the PHS turned to the epidemiology of heart disease. Preventive Medicine saw beriberi, pellagra, syphilis, rheumatic fever, endocarditis, rubella, and congenital problems as the causes of cardiac conditions, but something else seemed to be going on. Overall mortality rates had dropped from 1900, but while the rate of decline among women continued, male life expectancy stalled. Lung cancer, coronary heart disease and duodenal ulcers came into the frame as new causes of death.

No one had studied heart disease before. The PHS opted to take a town of around 50,000 people, recruit a sample of 6000, select those with no obvious cardiovascular disease between the ages of 30 and 59 and follow them for 5, 10 and 20 years. Vlado Getting, the State Commissioner of Health for Massachusetts, offered Framingham. The study began recruiting in 1952 and reported in 1957.

America was then the leading producer of tobacco in the world and Britain the leading consumer. James I of England opposed tobacco when imports from America began, writing a pamphlet about it in 1604, and taxing imports. Charles I increased the taxes. German research in the 1930s flagged tobacco's risks and the Nazi government restricted its use. American insurance companies also linked smoking and mortality. Consumption, though, continued to escalate.

Two British studies in 1947 pointed to a six-fold rise in lung cancer rates from 1930 to 1944. Deaths from lung cancer in Britain overtook deaths from tuberculosis in 1950 and were the highest in the world. Was lung cancer caused by influenza, tar on roads, fumes from car exhausts, or smoking? In 1950 studies by Ernst Wynder and Evarts Graham in America, and Richard Doll and Tony Hill in Britain suggested smokers were sixteen times more likely to get lung cancer than non-smokers. These articles had no impact other than to trigger a $5 million research grant to AMA and a $500,000 grant to Britain's Medical Research Council from the tobacco industry to research the true causes of lung cancer.

Doll and Hill began tracking a cohort of 40,000 doctors. In 1954 they showed elevated cancer rates among smokers compared with non-smokers, a fall in risk in those who quit smoking, and a link to heart attacks. Cuyler Hammond and Daniel Horn in America confirmed the link to cancer.

In America, jobs and profits were at stake. In Britain, the NHS depended on tobacco taxes. While many British and American doctors gave up smoking, AMA remained agnostic. The British Minister for Health acknowledged a link while chain-smoking through a press conference. By 1964 there had been 7000 articles on the links between smoking and lung disease. A US Surgeon General's Report embraced the findings, put a health warning on cigarette packages, and banned cigarette advertising on television.

While epidemiology had picked out cigarettes as the cause, the tobacco octopus squirted epidemiological ink into the water to cloud the picture. Could tobacco really cause cancer when life expectancy had been rising progressively with increases in the sales of cigarettes? Maybe the cancer prone were more likely to smoke. Why could no-one show smoke causing cancer in the laboratory? Epidemiology offered correlations not causes, they said.

These maneuvers laid a template for the way the lead, nickel, asbestos, coal gas and other industries handled later epidemiological challenges. It is too simple to blame a private manufacturer's conflict of interest, in that Britain's nationalized coal gas industry responded the same way. This was corporate risk management, not unlike the response of the Vatican Corporation to later claims of child abuse.

CDC now bill the turnaround in attitudes to smoking as one of the greatest public health achievements ever, but this turnaround didn't come from government. While lawsuits and research helped, it was Californian consumers in San Luis Obispo and Beverly Hills who turned things round by banning smoking in public places like restaurants. It took 50 years from the first articles to a significant drop in smoking rates.

Cancer and dementia feature today the way tuberculosis did in the nineteenth century. One in two of us is liable to be diagnosed with cancer or dementia. One reason for this is we live longer. Increased screening for cancers and cognitive impairment also raises awareness of these disorders without establishing if they are more frequent. The message that cancer and dementia are degenerative disorders implies that the removal of death by infection has revealed underlying cancer and dementia rates that have been invariant since the Greeks. It's the luck of our genes if we get cancer. Finding a cause is not the issue. Finding a cure, which can only come from the pharmaceutical industry, is.

The link between lung cancer and smoking, however, put environmental triggers in the frame as causes for cancer. Richard Peto and Richard Doll in 1981 estimated that 75-90% of cancers are preventable. Song Wu and colleagues modeling environmental and genetic inputs also concluded in 2015 that 70-90% of our cancer risk lies in environmental factors.[24] In addition to the 30% of cancers smoking caused, Doll estimated that diet might cause up to 35%. But diet is more difficult to investigate. We can't stop eating.

The first Framingham results in 1957 implicated cigarette smoking, raised blood pressure and obesity as causes of heart attacks. Saturated fats showed up as a minor risk. This coincided with Merck's development of chlorothiazide, which, just as it was about to be marketed under the trade name of Diuril as a diuretic for heart failure, was found to be

---

24 Wu S, Powers S, Zhu W, Hannum Y, *Substantial contribution of extrinsic risk factors to cancer development*. (Nature, 2015), doi:10.1038/nature16166

antihypertensive. The Framingham findings, and the launch of Diuril, came together with an increasing turn to medical check-ups for health and life insurance, and actuarial evidence that raised blood pressure was a risk for premature death.

Fresh from success on the infectious disease front, and with new weapons emerging, victory in the war against heart disease and cancer was confidently expected. The new challenge seemed more exciting that eliminating deaths from Road Traffic Accidents that were as numerous as those from cancer or heart attacks. Besides which, seat belts faced push-back from automobile makers and the experience of Prohibition stymied alcohol restrictions.

Not So Silent

Medicine has always had textbooks, but the 1950s saw something new. Leo Meyler's *Side Effects of Drugs* in 1952 became the first book to deal with the hazards of drug treatment. Donald Hunter's *The Diseases of Occupations* was published in 1955.

James Wilson published *The Principles of Teratology* in 1959. Congenital conditions had referred to difficulties arising in labor. Hints of something different came from children born in Hiroshima and Nagasaki, from the effects of rubella infections, and from vitamin A deficiencies. Wilson, working at the University of Rochester in New York, and others grasped the moment to establish a Teratology Society in 1960.

The PHS' turn to epidemiology led to liaisons with the new National Cancer Institute and other arms of the NIH that put air and water pollution on the map as contributors to disease. Chemical, steel, electrical, and other industries relied on industrial hygiene studies that began in the 1920s, largely funded by industry. Laboratory animals were dosed with suspected pollutants to establish if there was a threshold dose below which injury was unlikely. Studies typically issued recommendations centered on ventilation, washing after shifts, and other ways to keep exposures below threshold levels. The threshold was a rough measure that paid as much heed to industry costs as it did to biology and medicine.

Industrial hygiene studies looked for evident poisoning from acute exposure. The new epidemiology linked chronic low-level exposure to lead or sulfates in air or polychlorinated biphenyls (PCB), vinyl chloride and above all DDT in food and water to cancer, bronchitis, emphysema, and reproductive abnormalities as well as the disappearance of bird populations. The concept of a threshold value below which toxic substances were safe came under attack. Crops dusted with DDT fed to hens or cows, for example, led to increased concentrations in milk and eggs and ultimately breast milk, and the consequences of exposure were often delayed. While dusting troops in war with DDT was safe, DDT wasn't harmless.

As Rachel Carson put it in 1962:

> *All these facts—storage at even low levels, subsequent accumulation and occurrence of liver damage at levels that may easily occur in normal diets—caused FDA scientists to declare as early as 1950 that it is "extremely likely the potential hazard of DDT has been under-estimated". There has been no such parallel situation in human history. No one yet knows what the ultimate consequences may be.* [25]

Many were concerned about the environment before Carson, but *Silent Spring* was a tipping point. Up to 1800, we had cut down forests, wiped out animals for the sake of it, and seen nature as something to be mastered. After 1800 a new sensibility emerged. By 1962 a limitless wilderness appeared increasingly fragile. Reports from Japan of methyl mercury poisoning from fish at Minimata intertwined our health with the health of the planet.

An Unintended Revolution

Henry Beecher was a medical officer with US troops landing on Anzio Beach in Italy in World War II. Used to civilians routinely asking for more pain relief than was advisable, Beecher faced wounded soldiers who asked for less and got by on saline when the morphine ran out. Context seemed key. In civilian life, a wound is a disaster. In War, it's a ticket to safety.

---

25 Carson R, *Silent Spring* (Penguin Books, 1962) 38.

Beecher returned to a Chair in Anesthesiology in Harvard. From this base, against the current of the times which favored specific treatments, he persuaded the military, NIH, and others that placebos needed exploration. He set about recruiting a team.

Louis Lasagna was the only child of Carmen Boccignone and Joseph Lasagna who met in New York although both came from Viarigi, near Milan. She became a seamstress. He went into the restaurant business. Louis was born in 1923. The family moved to New Jersey and Louis went to college in Rutgers and medical school in Columbia. After qualification, he moved to Johns Hopkins in 1950 as an instructor in pharmacology.

When Lasagna heard of Beecher's work, he visited Boston in 1952. Beecher took to him, and secured army funding claiming Lasagna was uniquely qualified to advance this new field. The lab worked on psychedelics because the US military were convinced the Soviets had built factories beyond the Urals to make the just-discovered LSD, which they would drop into the drinks of diplomats or generals to get military secrets from them. LSD may in fact have been used by either the US or French military in the town of Pont-Saint-Esprit in 1951 to see if an entire town could be disabled. These were heady times.

Beecher's team had to be vetted. Their psychologist, John von Felsinger, refused, claiming this was McCarthyism, as did Beecher's secretary, giving the team a mixed security profile. Their reports were sent to the Pentagon by armed courier, briefcase manacled to his wrist. At least once, the Pentagon called to ask for a second copy. Beecher responded: you told us to destroy everything after we sent it, what happened to the first one? "It's lost in the Pentagon somewhere."

Lasagna's work involved assessing the analgesic effects of morphine and nalorphine and the effects of hypnotics. In blinded studies patients had pain relief or fell asleep—on placebos. These studies led to a 1954 Lasagna article *A Study of the Placebo Response*, which has ever since been among the top 30 cited articles in medicine. Up till then, some people were thought to be placebo reactors while more mature people weren't. Lasagna showed that clinical staff who thought they could pick out placebo reactors—younger, women, less educated, troublesome—were invariably wrong.

The impact of this article was huge. The *Lancet* offered an adulatory editorial entitled *The Humble Humbug*, a phrase that gained wide circulation as a title of a *Readers Digest* article. The *Journal of the American Medical Association* (JAMA) carried a Beecher summary "The Powerful Placebo".

Some could see nothing novel. Doctors had always given placebos. Some, like Richard Cabot, argued that deception was unethical. Others figured it necessary. Some argued that for two millennia doctors had obviously been giving nothing but placebos. No-one expected a placebo that 'worked'. One that had pain-relieving or hypnotic effects. Deciding if a drug worked had become more complicated. Rational treatment was going to involve more than just giving a specific drug for a specific indication.

In 1954 Lasagna moved back to Hopkins to the first ever post in Clinical Pharmacology hoping to put the new discipline on the map. Beecher wrote "I [will] watch your future career, for if it is anything like your performance here, it is bound to be spectacular." Lasagna continued to work on hypnotics, analgesics, placebos and on clinical trials.

It was the best of moves and the worst of moves. For a century, German pharmacologists had tweaked the structures of molecules to make different compounds. To study the idiosyncrasies and interactions of new drugs in clinical settings, clinical pharmacology (therapeutics) seemed needed. Lasagna was one of its fathers, but the baby never thrived. There are still some clinical pharmacologists and journals of clinical pharmacology, but most doctors figure they understand therapeutics.

Lasagna had a winning personality and his work on placebos and reactions to psychedelic drugs made him a natural person for the media to turn to explain a phenomenon thrown up by the Korean War. When captured US troops appeared on television denouncing the United States; brainwashing came into view. Unaware the West was doing more brainwashing research than anyone, the public were alarmed. *The Manchurian Candidate*, later a movie starring Frank Sinatra, crystallized the new threat. Lasagna was well placed to explain it.

In the 1950s television was entering homes across the continent and with topics like these to talk about, Lasagna became the first media doctor and for a period likely the most famous doctor in the US. *The New York Times* and *New Yorker* turned to him to write articles on issues from brainwashing to fears about the Atomic Bomb.

When Arthur Kallet and Harold Aaron of Consumer's Union started *The Medical Letter on Drugs and Therapeutics*, they approached Lasagna for medical input. This was aimed at physicians, a complement to *Consumer Reports*, offering a first assessment of Good Drugs and Bad Drugs. Within a year there were 12,000 subscribers. Along with the continued success of *Consumer Reports,* a consumer movement was beginning to be heard.

Lasagna had an ability to cut to the heart of things. Facing tobacco claims that the link to lung cancer was dubious, most people who smoked didn't get lung cancer, he responded that this was like automobile makers claiming car crashes never killed anyone because most people driving cars didn't die. When industry dismissed reports of strokes and clots among some women using the first oral contraceptives, he was clear he had seen a flood of young women dying from strokes and this just didn't happen normally. In television debates about contraception, he insisted women would and should use them but that there were risks. On one side, industry spokesmen denied any hazards. On the other, physicians claimed not enough was known to use them. As he was to find, the middle-ground is a difficult piece of medical ground to occupy.

The Framingham Study by this time had produced a tenuous link between cholesterol and heart attacks. Cholesterol was well known to be present in atherosclerotic plaques lining the arteries of people dying of heart attacks. Virchow described these plaques in the 1860s. His hunch was that inflammation caused plaques. In contrast, Ancel Keys, a physiologist, became an international figure in 1955 on the back of claims a diet rich in lipids caused atherosclerosis. This was picked up and promoted by businesses who saw a chance to substitute margarine for butter, corn oils for other oils, skimmed milk for real milk, and other dietary changes without any solid evidence this would make a difference.

Lasagna billed the cholesterol story a fad. The contrast between the immediate changes in diet based on no evidence and the resistance to change in the face of the evidence linking smoking to heart attacks was striking. As with the germ theories, lowering cholesterol created jobs. Stopping smoking didn't. Now it seems that just as zealous adherence to germ theories led to increased rates of mental handicap because of lead in paint, and to polio epidemics, so the cholesterol mania may have given rise to our obesity and diabetes epidemics through increased consumption of trans fats and refined sugars.

Framingham put a premium on lipid-lowering drugs. Richardson-Merrell submitted Triparanol to FDA in 1959 as the first cholesterol lowering drug. People who liked high cholesterol foods could eat them without worry provided they took Vitamin Triparanol. Ancel Keys featured in 1961 on the front cover of Time Magazine at the height of Triparanol's marketing campaign.

In August 1961 reports linked Triparanol to cataracts. Earlier observations linked it cataracts in animals, and stillbirths. Even though company reporting to FDA turned out to be felonious, an FDA reviewer E. I. Goldenthal could still see: "This compound is causing toxic effects including eye damage, liver changes, loss of sexual function and suspected deaths at low doses." He was overruled by his boss, Frank Talbot, who said: "My thinking was that here was a drug purporting to lower cholesterol. We were dealing with a highly lethal disease state… this drug might be helpful in dealing with a number one killer of men." Merrell withdrew Triparanol but Ancel Keys and the cholesterol bandwagon rolled on.

Meanwhile in 1958, Evan Thomas from Harper Brothers, who was resisting company pressure to bring out a book on the new medicine, met Lasagna and wrote "I really like this guy Lasagna. Why not get him to write a book. He's good."

Lasagna had a ringside seat at the 1959 Congressional Hearings on the pharmaceutical industry. This produced material for *The Doctors' Dilemmas* covering the new medicine. Published in March 1962, it was reviewed by Beecher in breathless terms:

> The Doctors' Dilemmas *has my awed admiration. I cannot think of anybody in this country or Europe who could have written this book other than Dr Lasagna. I'm sure it will lead to a great deal of discussion in the areas that he has dealt with so beautifully.*

Mike Gorman, a leading health lobbyist, sent it to President Kennedy, billing it as "the best book about medicine I have ever read,… erudite, wise, witty, and exceedingly balanced." He told Lasagna "Kennedy read [it] with great relish… and used the chapter on the AMA in some of our task force discussions on medical care for the aged and on mental health."

In England, the book's front cover stated "in one of the frankest books ever written by a physician Dr Lasagna examines his profession from Hippocrates to Salk, describing its follies, fads, frauds—and achievements." Writing a book about the follies of your profession is tricky. A *Lancet* review said: "The book has quite a good index though for no obvious reason."

The Doctors' Dilemmas captures pharmaceutical marketing, shady practices, and overblown claims in a chapter on "The Drug Industry and Medicine Avenue". But Lasagna did not see industry as an evil empire. He was more scathing about AMA and doctors. Graduates from his medical class were asked in 1962 to list the most important medical issues. They mentioned the population explosion, public health in underdeveloped countries, cancer, but most answered socialized medicine, the need to prevent a welfare state and getting the government out of medicine. Two years later a poll of US doctors showed them more likely to vote for Goldwater than Johnson.

On March 7, Lasagna spoke in Britain about Medicine and Pharma. Among changes required of industry he listed a proliferation of identical drugs from different companies whose marketing concealed this, along with company failures to test for toxicity and to reveal the results of their tests. Doctors meanwhile needed to change their incomprehension of industry. Most of them also were *prima donnas* who were not keeping up with the science behind clinical practice—clinical pharmacology.

It was important that medical and industry minds met, or Government would legislate. More involvement from an incompetent FDA would not help. Medicine could up its game. Industry should employ more academics. It should eliminate the excesses of competitive marketing and advertising should embrace reality: "Drug A is just about as good as Drug B, but there is no evidence that it is better. It may suit some patients."

On March 15, President Kennedy addressed Congress on the importance of protecting consumer interests. He outlined rights to safety, to be informed, to choose, and to be heard in the areas of drug safety and effectiveness, transportation, financial protection and regulation, housing costs, quality, and information. Drug safety and effectiveness received the greatest emphasis. America didn't do socialism, but it had consumers whose every purchase was a vote and votes should not be wasted:

> *As all of us are consumers, these actions and proposals in the interest of consumers are in the interest of us all. The budgetary investment required by these programs is very modest—but they can yield rich dividends in strengthening our free competitive economy, our standard of living and health and our traditionally high ethical patterns of business conduct. Fair competition aids both business and consumer.*
>
> *It is my hope that this message… can help alert every branch of government to the needs of our consumers. Their voice is not always as loudly heard in Washington as the voices of smaller and better-organized groups—nor is their point of view always defined and presented. But under our economic as well as our political form of democracy, we share an obligation to protect the common interest in every decision we make.*[26]

In 1962 America had the best life expectancy in the world. It slipped below the average for the developed world in the 1970s and has since dropped further despite spending more on health than any other country. Americans were told life expectancy was still rising but just not as fast as elsewhere. Since 2015, it has been falling.

Kennedy echoed Louis XVI in 1789 in talking about spreading the benefits of new opportunities and empowering more people. Like Lasagna,

---

26 *Public Papers of the Presidents of the United States,* John F Kennedy, (1962) 242-243.

he was more concerned with AMA than with the new industry which seemed Silicon-Valley-like to be changing the world for the better. A draft drug safety act sat in his office. Events were about to transform this draft into an Act that changed healthcare globally.

6: ACCIDENTS OF BIRTH

Medical books are monuments to the frailty of the human body and the wonders of medicine. They terrify us when discussing even the most trivial of disorders, which they portray as likely to lead to imminent death. But when they discuss the merits of remedies, they soothe us as though we are destined for immortality.
Montesquieu, cited in Pinel 1800

When Louis XVI addressed the French Parliament in June 1789, he was a similar distance in time from the discovery of machines that radically changed industry as John Kennedy in March 1962 was from the discovery of new 'machines' impacting on health.

A medicine is a chemical and information. The chemicals cost little to make. They are unavoidably hazardous. Information about when and how to use them and what can go wrong can transform a chemical into a medicine. Before 1962 doctors treating us generated this information. Since then, randomized controlled trials (RCTs) have standardized medical products. We are the material on which RCTs work. Without our involvement trials cannot generate anything. Our involvement in trials which helped us greatly in the 1960s, however, is now deployed against us, especially those whose responses to treatment don't suit the needs of the system.

Any encounter between two people is multifaceted. In addition, the information that arises in settings where one is distressed and seeking answers, and another wants to help, can be biased in many ways. It makes sense to think that drawing conclusions from many patients and doctors rather than just an individual case might even out biases. It makes even more sense to think that taking 200 patients and randomly assigning 100 to treatment X and 100 to treatment Y, designed so neither doctor nor patient can tell the difference, with observers recording responses on a pre-agreed schedule without getting emotionally involved with the subjects, would give even more objective information.

This is what RCTs are billed as offering. They give rise to supposedly pure data, which can be interrogated statistically, equivalent to handling knowledge in isolation chambers. Pitting data against bias, RCTs appear to offer a path to objectivity.

RCTs also had, for many doctors, a supreme virtue, which is that it would be easier for a camel to get through the eye of a needle than a homeopathic remedy to get through an RCT. But this position contains a weakness. If medicine has lost the authority to say we don't need RCTs to say that claims of cures based on nothing are bunkum, something has gone wrong. Similarly, while science is about data, hewing to process is also what bureaucrats do or anyone who lacks the authority to make a judgment call.

The Sorcerer's Apprentice

In 1906 the American Medical Association (AMA) created a Council on Pharmacy to undertake controlled trials of new drug treatments. The carrot for companies was AMA would only advertise treatments that carried its seal of approval. These trials matched cohorts of patients, with one getting the index treatment and the other not. AMA were offering control by authoritative input rather than just the views of a jobbing clinician.

By 1935 it was clear that even distinguished clinicians needed controlling. Harry Gold, a physician in Columbia University, studying the effects of drugs in angina, found patients gave him different histories to the one they gave the researcher, giving him an insight on the delicate dance between mesmerizers and mesmerized. As patients we are highly sensitive to cues from our doctor and offer answers we think she wants. To manage this, Gold introduced placebos, keeping both researcher and patient blind to their treatment. He called his new design 'double-blind'. Gold's placebos were inert substances, a far cry from the placebos Beecher was soon to see on Anzio beach.

The road to randomization started with Ronald Fisher, an English mathematician working at an agricultural laboratory in the 1920s. The judgment of horticultural professionals was the gold standard as to whether a new grain or fertilizer was superior to previous ones. Far from doubting these judgments, Fisher depended on them to frame judgments mathematically.

Many factors could bias the assessment. The new fertilizer might get a light, drainage, or soil benefit the comparator didn't. Standard agricultural trials controlled for known confounders much as drug trials did, by matching patches of ground in which the treated and comparison grains were put. But what if there were confounders no-one knew about?

Fisher realized that randomly assigning fertilizer to patches of ground could control for both known and unknown confounders. Light, drainage and soil factors would be the same in each group just as age, sex and ethnicity ordinarily are in a medical trial now. This had to be true for unknown confounders also.

The only thing that could then get in the way of a true result was chance, and chance could be assigned a value. If we clip a coin, we can make it come up heads 19 times out of 20. If a tail turns up once in twenty, we don't doubt that the coin has been clipped. If we know what we are doing, we can expect the true result 19 times out of 20. Statistical significance for Fisher meant we knew what we are doing. "A phenomenon is experimentally demonstrable when we know how to conduct an experiment, which will rarely fail to give us a statistically significant result." No clinical trials in medicine meet this criterion.

Jerzy Neyman and Egon Pearson at University College London took a different approach to experiments. They turned to the work of Carl Friedrich Gauss who in 1809 tackled a difficulty astronomers had when measuring stars. They rarely got the same result twice. Did the different readings come from different stars, or from errors (poor telescopes) built into the act of measuring? Measuring errors, Gauss argued, would distribute randomly around a mean in a Normal Distribution curve or confidence interval. If a measurement fell outside this interval it likely came from a second star. Every measurement has a confidence interval around it. The more precise our measuring abilities, the tighter the interval.

Gauss' insight was developed by Pierre Simon Laplace and their combined inputs to central limit theorem, least-squares optimization, and linear algebra have underpinned progress in the physical sciences. Combined with randomization, later advocates of RCTs in medicine argued confidence intervals offered state of the art rigor.

Confidence intervals work for measuring stars. Diabetes, breast cancer, asthma and most diseases, however, comprise up to 50 different superficially similar conditions. Even if the illness is identical, one person's heart rate may increase on a treatment that causes another's to decrease. One may become drowsy where another is sleepless. Taking the mid-point of a confidence interval as a best guess as to where a star is makes sense. The midpoint on a sedation scale or pulse rate in response to treatment doesn't make the same sense. Confidence intervals are now used to describe clinical trial results rather than statistical significance, but their use does not mean they have a basis in medical reality.

When discovered in 1944, streptomycin was put into standard trials to assess its effects on TB. These trials balanced known confounders and established that it could help but the investigators also saw patients that quickly became tolerant and some had hearing loss.

Short of money to supply the drug, Britain's Medical Research Council (MRC) made streptomycin available through a trial. Tony Hill was the MRC's statistical adviser. Invalided out of medical school by tuberculosis, he studied statistics instead. The 1930s medical statistics world was tiny. Hill was well connected and appears to have been a popular and plain-speaking lecturer.

Hill loosely credited Fisher with the idea of randomization and used it to control for the subtle ways clinical researchers steer likely responders into favored treatment groups. The patients were randomly allocated to streptomycin or no treatment. The trial confirmed streptomycin and randomization had benefits but missed the problems of both. There was no obvious need to turn to RCTs after this and most trials remained standard trials.

This trial made Hill the key figure on the MRC clinical trials committee. Michael Shepherd from London's Institute of Psychiatry became the secretary and undertook the first RCT of the kind that happens today. Shepherd compared the effects of reserpine to placebo in patients with anxious depressions. This trial found reserpine beneficial for anxiety and depression. Today reserpine is universally viewed instead as causing depression, on the basis that it can also cause agitation and suicide.

If the clinical world operated like Fisher's notional fields, so that the fertilizer that works in this field will work in the next one, or like Gauss' stars so that we can be sure how many stars we are seeing, medical RCTs would tell doctors how to treat the patient in front of them. Trials don't. It's often down to chance whether a drug that has been shown to work in an RCT will be of any use for the person in front of a doctor. Doctors likely know less about how to treat us and how to respond if things go wrong than they did 50 years ago.

Despite this, the RCT had taken its first steps toward becoming medicine's hadron particle collider. It would reveal what therapeutic agents were really made of.

A Simple Twist of Fate

Shepherd took a sabbatical at Johns Hopkins University in 1956. There he met Lasagna. Both men were born in 1923. They got on despite contrasting styles. Shepherd was aloof and drew lines in the sand. Lasagna was sociable and worked to find areas of agreement. Shepherd's insistence that RCTs trumped clinical knowledge embroiled him in disputes that derailed his career. Lasagna was a pragmatist.

Both attended a Conference on the Evaluation of Pharmacotherapy in Mental Illness in Washington DC in September 1956. This 1000-delegate meeting running from early morning to midnight across 4 days was convened in response to the discovery of chlorpromazine, the first antipsychotic, in 1952. Chlorpromazine flooded into America in 1955. Its tranquilizing effect on psychosis was so remarkable no marketing was needed to encourage psychiatrists to prescribe it. A year later with asylums emptying, and a new psychiatry emerging, the task was to build on this foundation.

Chlorpromazine's benefits were clear. No trial was needed to persuade anyone. Still, there had been so many failed treatments across medicine that controlled trials were a topic at the meeting. Lasagna had emerged as the leading figure in America on trials, because of his work on placebos. By virtue of his contacts with Shepherd he was one of the few who knew anything about randomized trials. In a meeting with all the grandees of psychiatry present, he was one of the top three contributors to the proceedings. Senior figures from NIMH and elsewhere tried to recruit him from Hopkins.

For Shepherd, who disliked medical enthusiasms, RCTs delivered better evidence of what drugs did than individual clinicians could. Lasagna took a softer view: clinical trials were important but clinical observation was too. Even though chlorpromazine had undeniable effects on patients, clinicians running trials were astonished to find that patients on placebo might have identical motor side effects and that putting televisions on back-wards made a difference to chronic patients. As Lasagna remarked, they were in a "Mush Zone" and "brother, you need some controls."

Few at this meeting doubted that intensive psychotherapy was the next best thing to meeting God. But the new placebo discoveries seemed to offer a bridge between the world of pharmacology and psychotherapy, as did lysergic acid diethylamide (LSD), discovered in 1948. LSD appeared to aid psychotherapy rather than act in Magic Bullet fashion like chlorpromazine. Besides when a placebo was powerful enough to replace physical treatments, psychotherapy didn't seem to lose out by being equated with placebos.

The papers given at the 4-day meeting covered 662 closely printed large pages. For drug trials to be useful, most thought criteria for illnesses would be needed. One person's schizophrenia might not be someone else's. Rating scales would be needed to quantify and objectify drug responses. All agreed these were a dumbed down clinical interview, but if expert wine tasters can map the features of a wine on key dimensions, could not clinicians do the same? Lasagna's use of rating scales to test hypnotics and analgesics persuaded many it was possible to objectively study internal mental states.

The meeting was in part about containing the larger-than-life Nathan Kline. Based in New York, Kline had discovered the psychotropic effects of reserpine and was later to discover one of the first antidepressants. In the wake of chlorpromazine, huge amounts of money were allocated to NIMH on the back of his advocacy. As Shepherd put it:

> *I went to hear him talk to a congressional committee in Washington in 1955… He was full of what the Americans call pizazz. He made these congressional characters feel that if they didn't take this on board they were doing the gravest disservice to the American nation since King George III with the British Army.*
>
> *It was a wonderful performance. He undoubtedly played this enormous role. There were his counterparts in this country [UK], people like [William] Sargant but Sargant was restrained by the system. I remember thinking at the time that if you had behaved in that flamboyant manner with television appearances, the girlie magazines, the whole business… you'd have been drummed out of the profession.*
>
> *His private practice was like something out of a Hollywood movie. It was hardly describable but this is what you paid for… He became famous and a rich man in a way that is inconceivable here… I went with him to a television studio to listen to him give a*

> *talk and it was like listening to an advertising agent… Others have*
> *clambered on the bandwagon since but Kline made the bandwagon.*[27]

Kline's verdict on the new fetish with trials was that the field risked engaging in a rabbit-out-of-the-hat trick. To pull a rabbit out, you have to slip it in, in the first place. This is what criteria and rating scales would do—with a twist: not only would the public be fooled but the magician would fool himself as well.

Ed Evarts of the NIH noted that but for an accident of history, rating scales, diagnostic criteria and controlled trials could have shown chlorpromazine was beneficial for dementia paralytica (tertiary syphilis), a disease that looks identical to dementia praecox (schizophrenia). The field would have set off down a route of producing more tranquilizers when antibiotics were the cure. An academic apparatus risked getting in the way of finding the real answer. Seventy years later, the treatment of schizophrenia has made no advances on chlorpromazine.

Fritz Freyhan criticized a naïve faith in technical objectivism:

> *the time, we hope, has not come when the clinician abdicates, and*
> *the rating-scale takes over as a judge… While one can easily spot*
> *the… shortcomings of non-experimental studies, it appears to be*
> *tremendously difficult for multidisciplinary groups to acknowledge*
> *limitations and sterility in rigid experimental design.*

Meanwhile, frustrated with drugs of dubious benefit, in a 1956 paper on hypnotics, Lasagna crystallized an issue that was to marginalize clinical observation in ways that would later horrify even Shepherd:

> *It is unfortunate that the Food and Drug Administration cannot*
> *take regulatory action against a drug whose efficacy for the condition*
> *for which it is offered has not been demonstrated. Adequate toxicity*
> *data are required from manufacturers before introducing new drugs;*
> *similar requirements as to effectiveness should be included in our*
> *federal statue. It appears to be an accepted fact that toxicity and efficacy*

---

27 *Shepherd Interview* on samizdathealth.org/shipwreck/

cannot each be considered separately in vacuo as it were. Is it such a horrendous leap, therefore, from the present position to one where respectable, reliable evidence that a drug's therapeutic potency must be provided by the manufacturer before the compound is released?[28]

Hill's new RCTs seemed to him like just the hurdle to keep drugs of dubious benefit off the market. No-one could have anticipated the consequences of putting this hurdle in place.

PRESENT AT THE BIRTH

Four weeks before the 1956 Washington Conference, Senator Estes Kefauver was in Chicago bidding to be the Democratic Vice-Presidential candidate. As a sponsor of the 1950 Celler-Kefauver Act that beefed up Clayton Anti-Trust Act scrutiny of mergers and monopolies, Kefauver was the keeper of the Anti-Trust flame in American politics.

Growing corporate power was a hot card fueled by a post-War increase in mergers and industry consolidation. Where 50 years before, some railroad companies were bigger than State governments, by 1950 General Motors was fully a fifth the size of the entire US government. Its CEO could claim that what's good for General Motors was good for America. Or as Kefauver saw it: "Every day in our lives monopoly takes its toll. Stealthily it reaches down into our pockets and takes part of our earnings."

Kefauver was up against a new charismatic candidate, John F Kennedy, whom some viewed as too Tammany, too close to organized crime, too far to the right, and Catholic. Kennedy had momentum and it required old style political arm-twisting to derail him. Kefauver's campaign was coordinated by Bill Haddad.

William F Haddad was born in Charlotte, North Carolina in 1928, the eldest of five children, to a father from Cairo and a mother from Kiev.

---

28 Lasagna L, "A study of hypnotic drugs in patients with chronic diseases." *Chronic Diseases 3* (1956), 122-33

He joined the merchant navy at the age of 15 and became the youngest American GI in World War II. After the War he became a journalist before joining Kefauver's team in 1954. When the Democrats lost in 1956, he helped run Kennedy's 1960 Presidential campaign, despite misgivings, and the choice of Lyndon Johnson as a running mate. When Kennedy won, Haddad was drawn into the Camelot apparatus and in this role was a founder of the Peace Corps. He later ran for Congress, before assisting Robert Kennedy in 1968.

He also ran a 400-person consultancy firm. He became a Vice-Chairman in the DeLorean automobile company in 1979. John DeLorean wanted to be the first businessman to become President of the United States. After that, Haddad became CEO of a pharmaceutical company.

Asked what he did, he usually said investigative journalism. He worked at the *New York Herald Tribune* before moving to the *New York Post*. His talent for breaking stories led in the 1960s to the then biggest ever fine against the pharmaceutical industry. Some years later, based on leads, he warned the Democratic Party six weeks before the Watergate break in.

After losing to Eisenhower and Nixon in 1956, Kefauver returned to his anti-trust roots. As a champion of the consumer, and believer in entrepreneurs rather than corporations, he spotted an opening when his staff showed that versions of the same antibiotic, marketed by different companies, had identical prices, sometimes up to 1000% of the manufacturing cost. Administered (rigged) prices were a tell-tale sign of corporate collusion. There was also evidence of company backhanders to doctors to prescribe more expensive on-patent drugs. As Chair of the Senate Anti-Trust and Monopoly Subcommittee, in December 1959 Kefauver began Congressional Hearings on pharmaceutical price fixing that have been celebrated, in part because of the media reporting, which Haddad coordinated.

Branding seemed key to rising drug costs. Pharmacists once tailored pharmaceuticals based on a doctor's prescription. This bespoke tailoring had some chance of taking individuality into account. But by 1950 most prescription medicines came as brands in ready packaged doses, like off the peg garments. Many popular brands involved drug combinations, especially combination antibiotics. These came in a fixed ratio, the dose of neither of which might be quite right for a patient. It was a profitable business but not rational medicine.

Distinctions between branded and generic drugs came into view. Some companies like McKesson's made compounds at a fraction of the market price but did no selling. Why not sell all drugs as generics? The new miracle drugs were patented, and companies claimed they needed to recoup their research costs. Still, it seemed, the money was going into research on doctors and what they could be enticed to prescribe rather than on producing novel drugs. Where was the research in sticking two antibiotics together to produce a new brand?

Frederick Meyers, a University of California professor of pharmacology, stated that "most of the program [in drug research] has come from European and British researchers." The work done by American firms aimed "to exploit and market" these foreign products but "mostly to modify the original drug just enough to get a patentable derivative." Kefauver's staff produced figures to show that out of 77 countries surveyed, 28 allowed product patents and in these countries the prices of drugs ranged from 18 to 255 times higher than in process patent countries. Both American-made and European-made drugs cost less in Europe than America.[29]

As with any industry, Pharma had its share of shady sales practices. It dumped defective drugs on foreign markets rather than destroy them. It gave kickbacks to doctors, bought medical opinions, hid safety data, lied openly in advertisements and took shocking risks. It sent detail-men (drug-reps) to doctors. Companies portrayed these as educators, supporting a busy clinician. Critics saw glad-handing and bribery by 'professional' friends.

Drug advertising was also booming. Walter Griffith of Parke Davis told Kefauver "the ethical pharmaceutical industry of this country" had turned out "3,790,908,000 pages of paid journal advertising" and "741,213,700 direct mail impressions". Some of these were clearly misleading. One

---

29 For all quotes see Harris R, *The Real Voice* (Macmillan, New York, 1964)

antibiotic advert, for example, featured two chest x-rays giving the impression of clinical improvement when the x-rays came from two different patients neither of whom had had the antibiotic.

Few people at this point could distinguish marketing from sales. Dale Console, the Medical Director at the Squibb Institute put it this way: "If an automobile does not have a motor, no amount of advertising can make it appear to have one. On the other hand, with a little luck, proper timing, and a good promotion program, a bag of asafetida with a unique chemical side chain can be made to look like a wonder drug."

Arthur Sackler embodied the new marketing. Sackler was born in Brooklyn in 1913. In the 1930s, when it was easier for a Jew to get into medical school in Germany than the United States, Sackler got in. Coming from a relatively poor background, he worked his way through College by getting commissions on selling adverts for business schools to student newspapers. After qualification, at the outbreak of War, he had an option to do his service in a hospital on the home front—either psychiatry or obstetrics. He picked psychiatry and was based at the Creedmore hospital in New York. He was joined there by his brothers Mortimer and Raymond who studied medicine in Britain.

Sackler set up a Medical and Pharmaceutical Information Bureau in 1948 to co-ordinate the placement of stories about drugs in newspapers and periodicals. Two years later, he became Chairman of the Board of William Douglas McAdams, which became the biggest agency advertising pharmaceuticals on the back of accounts for Librium launched in 1957 and Valium in 1960. McAdams helped make these the best-selling drugs in the world and Sackler very wealthy.

Sackler was already wealthy enough to help Raymond and Mortimer, when they ran into trouble with Senator Joseph McCarthy in 1952 for refusing to take a loyalty oath. When Creedmore requested their resignations, Arthur set his brothers up in the Glutavite Corporation, a company that sold l-glutavite, a combination of monosodium glutamate (MSG) and B vitamins, as a cerebral tonic. Without submitting them to FDA for approval, McAdams pitched these claims in adverts to doctors in the *Medical Tribune*.

He also bought Purdue, Frederick & Co., a drug company established in 1892. By 1952 it was only doing $22,000 worth of business a year. It had the rights to water-soluble chlorophyll, the mainstay of photosynthesis. This was then newly isolated and marketable as an elixir of life but didn't sell. Nor did Pre-Mens, a combination of ammonium chloride and caffeine for premenstrual tension. He struck gold, however, with a British laxative, Senokot, which became a million-dollar compound.

In 1959 Sackler set up the *Medical Tribune*, a free circulation newspaper supported by advertising which ran features on medical issues aimed at doctors. Written engagingly, it reflected mainstream medical views. In addition, Sackler's view was that patients were not getting the full benefits of the breakthroughs tumbling out of drug companies, because information about new drugs was not circulating. The brief of the *Medical Tribune* was to make the information more accessible than standard journal articles, often before approval.

The listed *Medical Tribune* address in Manhattan was an empty office. The *Tribune* operated in the same building as McAdams whose senior personnel wrote many of its editorials and features. The rules of the American Association of Advertising Agencies (AAAA) banned Agencies from controlling media outlets. McAdams resigned from AAAA.

Sackler came to Kefauver's attention because of Henry Welch, the head of FDA's Antibiotic Division. Welch edited two journals *Antibiotics* and *Chemotherapy and Antibiotic Medicine*, published by the Washington Institute of Medicine (WIM), which paid him a modest honorarium for his work. Five Nobel Prize winners were on his editorial board. WIM went bankrupt and MD Communications, a new Sackler company, took over in 1952. The journals began accepting articles on drugs before approval. In editorials, Welch promoted combination drugs as a next step forward in therapeutics. The journals also carried multi-page, multi-color glossy adverts, a Sackler invention. Among the advertisers were Pfizer, primarily a manufacturer of antibiotics, whom Sackler had persuaded into marketing.

Welch's honorarium was supplemented by a fee for every advert and all reprints sold. One industry insider joked they'd have to build a warehouse for the reprints Henry shipped them. Commenting that his FDA salary ($17,500) paid his income tax got Welch fired.

A Congressional Hearing in 1958 on the role of the FTC in the control of false and deceptive advertising of medical preparations had found that neither the FTC nor the FDA knew who regulated *prescription* drug advertisements. There were only two doctors in FTC, while FDA saw its brief as monitoring the labeling of drugs, not advertising. Sackler marched through this gap in oversight.

Another Sackler innovation was company-sponsored educational supplements for which companies paid more than they did for adverts. Spotting opportunities in this new market, Sackler set up journals in psychiatry, sexual medicine, and other areas.

While advertising and sales played a part in making a General Motors or a Mercedes brand, there was a basis for these brands in what marketers call the fundamentals. With Merck's Diuril and Tryptizol in 1959, doctors similarly thought you would get what you paid for. But from 1960 on, pharmaceutical brands increasingly reflected what marketers call sentiment.

For Sackler, it was raining money. He became a collector of art and a sponsor of medical schools and art galleries. He contributed to the Democratic Party and was invited to Lyndon Johnson's inaugural ball in 1964. Haddad's sources described him as someone even the drug companies found slippery. Lasagna, who was a member of Kefauver's backroom staff, knew Sackler. He suggested Kefauver meet Sackler privately. Sackler's later on-the-record testimony contrasts with Kefauver's grilling of pharmaceutical company executives.

Lasagna hadn't expected to testify. He did so after a joke backfired. Mark Nickerson, one of the most significant American pharmacologists, was supposed to testify. Kefauver's team asked Lasagna if Nickerson would be a good witness. Lasagna joked that he should be because he had had to appear before the House Un-American Activities Committee. Nickerson was nixed and "in a moment of madness I agreed to go on unprepared as a witness in his place."

He testified that drug manufacturers had created a "pharmaceutical numbers racket," bringing out new drugs to make existing ones seem obsolete even though the new ones might be inferior. The key was misleading advertising. But his central testimony was about efficacy. FDA had no procedures in place to ensure a drug worked as promised. If a drug didn't work for a condition for which it was marketed or worked less well than an available product, then it was inherently unsafe.

This idea caused confusion. In addition to antibiotics, the Hearings centered on analgesics, hypoglycemics, tranquilizers and steroids, each of which has an obvious effect. Upjohn's new oral hypoglycemic, tolbutamide, clearly lowered blood sugar. Chlorpromazine tranquilized. A short-term hypoglycemic or tranquilizing effect is a beneficial effect but in the early 1950s severely arthritic people who took cortisone got up from their beds and walked, but the effect was not sustained, and some were worse off having taken the drug. A beneficial effect and effectiveness are two different things.

The confusions became obvious.

> **Sen Kefauver:** *It is our understanding that FDA has had a very satisfactory experience in evaluating the efficacy and safety of antibiotics and diabetic drugs, is that so?*

> **Dr Lasagna:** *Yes sir.*

> **Sen Hruska:** *If that is true, why do we need another law?*

Hugh H Hussey, Chair of the AMA's Board of Trustees, made it clear that AMA's "Trustees objected strenuously to [an effectiveness] provision on the ground that only the practicing physician can judge the efficacy of a drug and he should not be deprived of the use of any drug by a government ruling or decision."

His testimony mirrored Lasagna's:

SEN KEFAUVER: *If you want a drug to be efficacious before it is marketed, why not make that a condition as to placing it on the market?*

DR HUSSEY (AMA): *It seems to me it is a condition under existing practice before it is brought to market.*

SEN KEFAUVER: *But if that is what the law means now, then why do you object?*

Safety was the legal requirement not effectiveness. If effectiveness is to be an aid to safety, consider this. Upjohn's tolbutamide was licensed by FDA because it clearly lowered blood sugar, but in a later RCT it led to more deaths than another hypoglycemic, metformin, or a stimulant to lose weight, or diet alone. Is tolbutamide effective? It takes time to run a trial that has a real-life outcome like death. The tolbutamide trial took 5 years. This is not practical for companies trying to get a drug on the market. Using RCTs to determine effectiveness is not the quick fix it seemed in 1962.

The Kefauver Hearings had run into sand when Lasagna went to London in March 1962. He believed doctors had avoided disastrous regulation. Both Lasagna and Kennedy saw AMA as a bigger stumbling block than Pharma, who had their sins but were the most profitable industry in the country, contributing to giving Americans the best life expectancy in the world. Kennedy was trying to get Medicare through Congress and did not want to antagonize Pharma.

Stories by then had begun to circulate in Germany about a scarcely credible hazard on a sleeping pill—birth defects. The defects were also beyond belief. Babies were born limbless or with useless flippers (phocomelia) where limbs should have been. Chemie-Grünenthal, the drug's makers, so successfully fought any linkage to their baby, thalidomide, that in March 1962 even Kefauver had heard nothing. Richardson Merrell applied to market it in the United States. As late as June 1962, they were still mailing samples of thalidomide to American doctors to run controlled trials.

On July 15, 1962, the thalidomide story hit the *Washington Post* in an article framed by Morton Mintz to make Frances Kelsey of FDA appear the heroine. "This is a story of how the skepticism and stubbornness of a government physician prevented what could have been an appalling American tragedy—the birth of hundreds or indeed thousands of armless and legless children." All Kelsey had done was to use the 1938 Drugs Act to refuse to be hurried into approving an application to market the new drug. She regarded the safety of Mer-33, as unproven, even though this drug came with a placebo-controlled trial demonstrating its effectiveness and safety, the first ever drug to do so.

On August 13, *Newsweek* ran "Tragedy from a Pill Bottle—some sad lessons learned", complete with photographs of Widekund Lenz, who had discovered the thalidomide link, pill bottles, armless babies, and FDA commissioner George Larrick, flanked by Frances Kelsey. The message was: "The shocking discovery that thalidomide has caused the birth of deformed babies has led to a hard look at the way new drugs are put on the market. How can we be sure disaster will not strike again?" There was a panic. Richardson-Merrell's cholesterol lowering Triparanol had just been pulled from the market and legal cases were piling up.

Kefauver's bill was recast. Even though the safety of thalidomide was the issue, not its effectiveness as a sleeping pill, the main feature of the 1962 Amendments was to switch the language of the 1938 Act from the Safety of drugs to the Effectiveness and Safety of drugs. Wherever the word Safety appeared in 1938, it was twinned with Effectiveness in 1962.

In evaluating effectiveness, Democrats wanted a preponderance of the evidence to point to effectiveness. Republicans wanted substantial evidence of effectiveness. Lasagna and Walter Modell offered adequate and well controlled studies carried out by experts to demonstrate effectiveness. The regulations later specified this meant RCTs. In practice this came down to two RCTs. There seemed every reason to think that if one RCT showed a drug worked, any other RCT would too. The experts believed that the knowledge RCTs generate was universal. There was no sense that, as later became clear, only 50% of trials might show a drug works or that 'works' has multiple meanings.

The Lasagna and Modell formula allowed the new Act to pass through both Houses of Congress and be signed into law on the same day, October 10, 1962. Photographs of the signing show Kennedy at his desk in the Oval Office with Kefauver standing behind him, handing him the pen he uses to sign the Act. Hubert Humphrey is on Kefauver's right, a beaming George Larrick on Humphrey's right, with Frances Kelsey beside him. With the Act signed Kennedy stood up, and reaching over, handed the pen to Kelsey.

In addition to an effectiveness criterion, the bill mandated animal testing of drugs for toxicity, gave FDA control over prescription drug advertising, and introduced informed consent provisions. At the last minute, it dropped a proposed tightening of patent provisions.

Lasagna had introduced consent forms in Hopkins to inform patients they were participating in a study of a new drug. Prior to 1962, a company could study a drug and, if it decided to proceed, could send the file to FDA expecting approval within a year. After 1962, because of informed consent FDA were involved before any patient was given a drug. Overnight the duration of FDA's notional involvement with a drug went from one to five or more years—a boon to company complaints about regulation.

As someone interested in monopolies, Kefauver was intrigued by prescription-only status where "He who orders does not buy; and he who buys does not order." We cannot protect themselves against the monopoly element inherent in trademarks or patents for prescription drugs. We are totally dependent on another consumer, the doctor, not to be influenced by marketing. Doctors can choose whether to give us the latest branded drug or an older, more effective, and less expensive one; we can only do as prescribed.

Thalidomide had been available over the counter in Germany. German doctors were not inhibited in recognizing its harms, as they might have been with a drug from which they made a living. But in the face of the thalidomide disaster, retaining prescription-only status seemed to make sense.

Prescriptions contributed to a sense that new drugs would be confined to disease states. But far from constraining the pharmaceutical industry within a medical framework, after 1962 approval to market a drug for lowering cholesterol, osteoporosis, or erectile dysfunction enabled companies to sell conditions. A point at which they geared up to re-engineer the medical marketplace to suit their product. By 1990 this re-engineering had become a fine art with Lilly able to recast anxiety as depression and Abbott to recast manic-depressive illness as bipolar disorder to make them Prozac and Depakote friendly disorders.

By constraining companies to market their drugs on prescription for diseases, and demonstrate efficacy through a new invention, the RCT, Kefauver put doctors firmly in company marketing sights. Companies now had to understand doctors better than they understood themselves. No-one in 1962 had any sense companies might be able to do this.

Had companies not been required to demonstrate effectiveness for disorders, we might have ended up with fewer diseases. The first antidepressants would have been marketed as tonics, or stimulants. St John's Wort, an herb with SSRI properties, is sold over the counter as a tonic for burn-out, but to get Prozac we must be diagnosed as depressed. The statins might have been marketed as making our arteries young again, rather than for a supposed cholesterol disorder. The bisphosphonates aimed at restoring youthful bones rather than treating osteoporosis. Doctors would have been duly skeptical about such claims.

The 1962 Amendments produced a shape-shifting effect on RCTs. Claims they offer gold standard medical evidence now abound. They are the standard through which companies make gold and this is down to an accident of history that took a poorly understood technique, made it mandatory, and created a mantra about gold standard medical evidence.

The effectiveness criterion underpins FDA's proud boast that since 1962 regulation has been based on science. The claim gave rise to a myth that 'scientists' from FDA keep the public safe. The myth is found everywhere.

But not since the Wizard fooled the citizens of Oz into thinking he was keeping them safe have we been so misled.

Under the 1938 Act, companies brought antibiotics, diuretics, antihistamines, hypoglycemics, anticonvulsants, steroids, antihypertensives, antipsychotics, minor tranquilizers, analgesics, antidepressants, stimulants, oral contraceptives, chemotherapies, and other effective treatments on the market without an RCT in sight. It is doubtful if we have had as many effective medicines licensed since 1962, and likely we have had more relatively ineffective drugs.

The effectiveness requirement is enshrined in regulation to contribute to safety. Under the 1938 Act it was impossible to discuss safety without efficacy. For example, sulfonamides were dangerous but in view of their effectiveness in saving lives, it was clear they should be allowed on the market. A hypnotic shouldn't cause peripheral neuropathy, and the 1938 Act kept thalidomide off the market for this reason. Since 1962, if some benefit is demonstrated, a drug like ropinirole can be brought on the market for restless legs syndrome, even though it causes gambling, sex addiction and personality change.

An effectiveness criterion that ensured we achieved effective treatments is one thing but if drug 'effects' are accepted as a stand in for effectiveness, and doctors fail to spot the difference, that is quite another thing.

On August 5, three weeks after the thalidomide story broke, as politicians and staffers were working on a new draft of Kefauver's Bill, the world woke up to the death of Marilyn Monroe from a barbiturate overdose.

Shortly after the 1962 Act was signed the *New York Times* got hold of the fact that Lasagna had lobbied for thalidomide's approval when it was being held up in FDA:

> *Dr Louis Lasagna, the former New Brunswicker who teaches at Johns Hopkins School of Medicine comes to the defense of the drug thalidomide in an editorial in the current issue of Medical Tribune, an independent medical newspaper. This was reported in the New York Times last week. He points out that if Marilyn Monroe's physician had been able to prescribe that drug instead of barbiturates, she*

might still be alive, that's because thalidomide is the safest sedative discovered to date. It won't kill animals or humans even in big overdoses. Lasagna who recently authored 'The Doctor's Dilemmas' used the movie queen's death from the overdose from sleeping medicine to make his point in the editorial that too severe laws against new drugs would seriously curb research. He feels that thalidomide is too valuable a drug to be lost despite the tragic apparent consequences of its use in early pregnancy.[30]

In a 1960 RCT, thalidomide worked as a sleeping pill and was safe. It sailed through the mechanism later put in place to ensure it didn't happen again. Lasagna had run the trial and had brought it to the attention of FDA as evidence thalidomide should be licensed.

George Larrick stepped down as commissioner of FDA in 1965. The pharmaceutical industry Blue Sheet reported that:

a sigh of relief was heard in industry quarters when Lasagna, whose name was rumored to have been seen at the head of a list of candidates, indicated he was not running. The lively Hopkins pharmacologist and author told 'The Blue Sheet' the job had not been offered to him and anyhow his special expertise was in a limited part of FDA's broad responsibilities. He was quoted in other quarters as feeling that a man would need to have his head examined to take the job.

THE PENDULUM SWINGS

With Richard Doll, Tony Hill had run the 1950 and 1954 epidemiological studies of smoking and lung cancer. He incurred the wrath of Fisher, a pipe smoker, who thought claims of a link to cancer were preposterous. It was more likely those predisposed to cancer took up smoking, he claimed. Tobacco-makers supported him. Hill's research had no impact.

---

30 See Lasagna L. "Letter to New York Times September 2nd in response to article on August 26 1962."

In contrast in 1965, when Hill delivered a lecture, "Reflections on the Controlled Trial," RCTs were everywhere. He noted they had invaded the:

> *the patter of the salesman: 'a double-blind trial on 22 patients has shown that XYZ is the wide-spectrum antibiotic of choice.' What would doctors have made of that 20 years ago? One may doubt whether it would have been a good selling point. Clearly it is thought [today] to be so.*
>
> *[F]requently with a new discovery, a new technique, or a new theory of disease, the pendulum at first swings too far… Given the right attitude of mind, there is more than one way in which we can study* **therapeutic efficacy**. *Any belief that the controlled trial is the only way would mean not that the pendulum had swung too far but that it had come off its hook.*[31]

He might have said, "Stop fetishing RCTs." By then Lasagna also thought relying solely on RCTs was wrong and began trying to put the RCT genie back in the bottle. His goal in adopting RCTs had been to cast doubt on claims that the latest panacea worked. Had RCTs been restricted to this, they might have contributed to safety.

But, by 1965 RCTs were transforming FDA from an agency with little option but to tolerate a certain amount of irrationality into one that saw itself as based on science, and able to promote rational therapeutics. The impression grew that RCTs demonstrated treatments worked, when RCTs aren't necessary if treatments really do work.

Twenty years later, FDA licensed Prozac on the back of two positive trials and at least three negative ones, as the regulatory criterion of two positive trials had been met. Regulation had reverted to the application of bureaucratic rules rather than engagement in science. The mantra of science-based regulation, Cheshire cat-like, remained.

There are now tens, perhaps hundreds, of thousands of trials in therapeutics, while there are likely still less than one thousand trials in surgery,

---

31 Hill AB "Reflections on the Controlled Trial." *Annals Rheum Disease* (1966), 25, 107-113.

even though RCTs are better suited to an evaluation of clean surgical strikes than they are to evaluating the effects of 'Magic Bullets' that impact on every system in the body. While the practice of surgery has made dramatic strides over the last 6 decades, the drug treatment of many conditions has gone backwards.

RCTs and Hypnosis[32]

Demonstrating a chemical can be a medicine is a different matter to demonstrating it can be a fertilizer. In either case, RCTs necessarily focus on a single primary endpoint. Paying heed to just one outcome is not an issue with a fertilizer, but it self-evidently is with a medicine where every one of a chemical's hundred effects needs attention. It is acceptable if a fertilizer kills a small proportion of ears of corn in an increased overall yield. This is not acceptable in medical practice.

Clinical practice once embraced heterogeneity and tailored treatment to differences. RCT based practice acts as though heterogeneity doesn't matter. Many drugs put some to sleep but cause others sleeplessness; some gain while others lose weight. It is psychotic to map these effects onto a confidence interval, and claim drugs have no more effects on weight or sleep than placebo. Telling patients any weight or sleep changes they think they have are all in their mind is gaslighting.

Paying heed to just one of a hundred things going on is the essence of hypnosis. Good care involves close attention to the individual. In trials, the patient might turn blue and grow feathers, but, because of the focus on a primary outcome, hypnotized investigators don't notice this. This is especially the case when, for the sake of objectivity, anecdotal accounts of what happened to individual patients are ignored.

The mantra that RCTs can miss rare events, or conditions that only appear after much longer than the average trial, is wrong. Early RCT data suggested less than 5% of people had sexual side effects on SSRIs. In fact, close to 100% do and these effects start within 30 minutes of taking the first tablet. This effect, more common than any mood benefit, was

---

32 These issues are dealt with in greater detail on samizdat.org/shipwreck/

missed because investigators were focused on mood. Drug-induced sexual dysfunction can endure forever after treatment stops. These sexual effects were even known about from healthy volunteer studies (Drug Studies) before the first clinical studies (Treatment Trials) began. How could they be missed? Dangle a primary endpoint in front of investigators' eyes.

Randomization is trumpeted as the ultimate elimination of bias. But if we designate mood effects of a drug as primary, when companies knew before the trials began sexual effects were more likely than mood benefits, and the RCT process blinds investigators to this, then RCTs must churn out the most biased form of clinical knowledge there is.

Randomization aims at managing the unknown unknowns for one of the effects of a drug, such as how it may alter mood. This is done at a cost of ignoring other effects. This gamble is worth taking for one critical piece of information—whether a poison might in certain circumstances be useful. The gamble becomes a problem if the rhetoric of RCTs gives the impression that since these drugs have been through RCTs most of what needs to be known about them is known. Proclaiming RCTs as the royal road to the truth, when they are set up to monitor only one of a drug's effects, generates an ignorance about ignorance.

There is a final twist. Controlling a drug effect with a placebo in an RCT makes less sense than might be expected. Comparing a new drug to a placebo like the original Beecher placebo would be like comparing two drugs—something that cannot be done. In a trial of an analgesic and an antibiotic for back pain, for instance, the analgesic will win. If we then only mandate the use of analgesics rather than antibiotics for back pain, out treatment will be less effective for the 10% of patients whose back pain stems from an infection. In the same way, placebos lose out to active drugs, and we are all now forced to take something that 'works'. Anything else is regarded as unethical even though it might be the best treatment for us.

In the process, the magic of medicine has been leached away. When clinicians treat individual variation as inconsequential, they practice medi-culture rather than medicine. That this might happen was not apparent in the 1960s.

Mindless Medicine

If you broke a wrist, and as part of an RCT the fracture team randomly applied a plaster cast to some limb, either a leg or an arm, the cast would beat placebo, because some casts would be on the fractured wrist. To advocate random application of a cast to a limb, on this basis, would be nuts. Practicing on the basis of RCT evidence without thinking, similarly, dumbs down care. This is increasingly how medicine is practiced.

That said, there is a notable mirror image hazard. Where there is X-ray evidence of blocked leg or coronary arteries in a patient who is in pain consistent with a blockage, surgeons confidently recommend an operation. In practice, these operations often do less to relieve pain or improve survival than getting the person to walk.

Whether the evidence comes from the social side of medicine (RCTs) or the biological side (X-rays), we need doctors who can recognize that evidence from one source rarely does away with the need for both them and their patient to make a judgment call that bears in mind we usually know much less than the surrounding rhetoric claims.

Advocates of RCTs claim they demonstrate cause and effect. Consider then the case of imipramine, the first antidepressant, launched in 1958 without an RCT in sight. Among other actions, it is a serotonin reuptake inhibitor. In later trials, it beat SSRIs in patients with melancholia (severe depression). Melancholic patients are 80 times more likely to commit suicide than mildly depressed patients. Within a year clinicians recognized that wonderful though imipramine was, it could cause an agitation and suicidality that cleared when the drug was stopped and reappeared when restarted (Challenge-Dechallenge-Rechallenge).

In an RCT of imipramine, a drug that can cause suicide, in melancholic patients, it will on average protect against suicide by reducing the risk from melancholia to a greater extent than placebo. In contrast, in the RCTs that brought SSRIs to the market, these drugs doubled the rates of suicidal acts. This was because SSRIs are weaker than imipramine and had to be tested in people with mild depression, at little risk of suicide. The low placebo suicidal act rate revealed the risk from the SSRI. It would do the same if imipramine is put into trials of mild depression. RCTs can badly mislead as regards cause and effect,

In Treatment Trials where both condition and treatment cause superficially similar difficulties, as when both bisphosphonates and osteoporosis lead to fractures, RCTs give misleading answers. The only unambiguous trials are Drug Trials in healthy volunteers where hazards stand out clearly. Companies do Drug Trials, leave the data unpublished, and use what they learn to game their subsequent Treatment Trials.

Trials can be gamed in other ways. When the SSRI antidepressants were first released, Lilly put fluoxetine and GlaxoSmithKline (GSK) put paroxetine into trials of Intermittent Brief Depressive Disorders (IBDD). IBDD patients (borderline personality disorder), are repeated self-harmers. Neither drug helped. The data remained unpublished. Despite two negative SSRI trials in this patient group, GSK undertook another paroxetine trial in IBDD.

In April 2006, defending paroxetine against accusations it could cause suicide, GSK released the following data (Table). The paroxetine Major Depressive Disorder (MDD) patients show a worrying increase in suicidal act risk.

GSK's release also contained data on the suicidal act rate in two paroxetine IBDD trials, neither of which supported using paroxetine for IBDD. Combining the MDD and IBDD data causes the risk of a suicidal act on paroxetine compared to placebo to vanish (a relative risk less than 1.0 suggests a protective effect). We can add 16 more suicidal acts to paroxetine in IBDD and still magically get an apparently protective outcome overall.

Table: Suicidal Acts in MDD & IBDD Trials

	Paroxetine	Placebo	Relative Risk
MDD Trials Acts/ Patients	11/2943	0/1671	Inf (1.3, inf)
IBDD Trials Acts/ Patients	32/147	35/151	0.9
Combined Acts/ Patients	43/3090	35/1822	0.7

This paradoxical outcome can happen in every trial of a superficially similar clinical state such as depression, pain, breast cancer, Parkinson's disease, or diabetes that are in fact different disorders. This is true of most disorders in medicine. Every time there is a mixture of more than one patient group in the trial, randomization ensures some patients will hide some treatment effects, good and bad. Standard back pains, for instance, mask the beneficial effects of an antibiotic on back pains linked to infections. This makes it possible to design RCTs that use a hazard a drug causes to hide that same hazard.

The way to overcome biases in trials is to know what we are doing. Then RCTs become a demonstration that only chance might disrupt as Fisher originally proposed.

In breast cancer trials, standard treatments show a 50% response rate. In breast cancers with a Her 2+ receptor, the drug Herceptin shows an 80% response rate. This result shows the more we understand what we are doing, the more predictable the results we get but that even in the case of Herceptin there is a lot we do not understand.

Both alcohol and SSRIs have an anxiolytic effect. To get SSRIs on the market, companies only had to show a minimal benefit on rating scales in mild nervous conditions with a high spontaneous recovery rate in two of five 6-week trials. It would be possible to get alcohol approved on this basis. After that, as part of our marketing we can do what companies typically do, which is to produce up to 50 scientific articles for every trial done, giving us 100 ghost-written publications with all hazards hidden.

A modest amount of alcohol would not give the doubling of suicidal acts found in trials with SSRIs. It would be safer in pregnancy than SSRIs. If we had difficulties stopping it after a few weeks, our doctors wouldn't tell us these difficulties come from our original disorder and that we should continue taking alcohol for life just as diabetics take insulin.

Because everyone knows what alcohol does, it is easy in this case to see the mismatch between the evidence from RCTs and the evidence from daily life. We can put the right weight on each, but few of us can do this for SSRIs, or other medicines. It would be a huge public health problem to have 10% of the population take alcohol on a close to permanent basis as we now have with SSRIs. RCTs did not show us the risk from endorsing just this for chemicals we know less about than alcohol.

Why then do RCTs now dominate healthcare? One reason is they seemed pro-consumer. Another is they justified government spending on drugs that 'work'. As Tony Hill noted, despite looking like they should cause difficulties for business, they suit companies. Both FDA and Pharma were happy to endorse a line that doctors' clinical noses are no better at sniffing out what a drug does without an RCT than their noses are at sniffing out an alteration in blood or urine without a spectrophotofluo-rimeter. The main reason they dominate, however, is because they are the gateway to a market.

DREAMS OF RATIONALITY

Lasagna published *Life Death and the Doctor* in 1968. Its publicity described him as mixing "a healthy respect for drugs with a chronic skep-ticism of some of the claims made for them. But lest he be branded a nihilist, Dr Lasagna adds: "I suppose I often overstate the case because I'm particularly likely to see the bad effects of drugs. And because I'm trying to combat the tendency of some physicians to overprescribe, the tendency for both doctors and patients to look for too much from drugs, to consider them too benign—an attitude the drug industry tends to encourage."

In 1958 at the height of the antibiotic boom, the Upjohn Pharmaceu-tical company combined tetracycline, a broad-spectrum antibiotic, with novobiocin (streptonycin) made in 1956. The combination was branded as Panalba.

In the 1950s, drug combinations created a market for brands and eliminated pharmacists as compounders of medicines. Analgesics were combined with each other. Tranquilizers like Valium were combined with analgesics, antihypertensives, and antidepressants. Antibiotic combina-tions accounted for 40% of the top 200 most popular prescription drugs.

Frowned on by academics, combinations seemed a good idea to many doctors. Academics argued it made no sense to combine a drug against one kind of infection with a drug against another unless a patient had multiple infections or an entirely unknown one. Sputum, urine, or feces should be tested for bacteria and the right antibiotic given. A combination might deliver too little of the drug needed and too much of one not needed. This is clearly true in principle but in office practice it was often convenient to cover all risks.

FDA got a new commissioner in 1965. James Goddard, a man filled with regulatory zeal and a belief in rational therapeutics. Looking at the drugs approved before 1962, whose efficacy box had never been ticked, Goddard proposed a Drug Efficacy Study Implementation (DESI) program. DESI recruited panels of academics to assess the evidence and decide which of 4000+ medicines sold by 237 companies worked. Many drugs designated as likely effective were removed because the academics did not realize that anything short of an unequivocal endorsement condemned compounds to death.

The DESI panels were against combinations. They dissed 40 antibiotic combinations, and in a further 50, suggested the combination posed risks. The data on Panalba pointed to 12-15 deaths per year that otherwise would not have happened. Both of Panalba's components were deemed effective, but FDA argued the combination had not been demonstrated to be more effective than either of its components. On December 30, 1968, it required Upjohn to remove Panalba from the market.

Upjohn could withdraw and destroy the drug immediately; stop manufacturing and marketing it but do nothing about supplies on the market; stop manufacturing but continue to market the medicines still available; produce and promote it and deploy strategies to block FDA until it was banned. Or they could opt for war.

The Panalba case has been presented in business ethics programs, across the world to Swedes, Chinese and Americans, to conservatives and socialists, to young and old. The consensus is that the responsible action is to withdraw and destroy the drug. Upjohn's decision to opt for war gets no support.

The Pharmaceutical Research and Manufacturers of America (PhRMA) and AMA claimed Panalba was a test case for "doctors in this country and the drug industry". FDA had to be prevented from making "an authoritarian official determination of what is good for medicine". FDA on the other side saw a "conflict between commercial and therapeutic goals" critical for "the future of patient care in the United States".

Goddard at this point had been replaced by Herbert Ley as FDA commissioner. Under fire from all sides on other issues, Ley, said of Panalba that the issue is:

> *Are we in this country dedicated to a rational scientific basis of antibiotic therapy or are we dedicated to contributing unnecessarily to the 1,500,000 hospital admissions annually attributed to adverse reactions to drugs?*[33]

AMA told Kefauver in 1961 they were phasing out adverts for combination products from their journals. AMA in 1969 were seeking tax exemption on its profits from drug adverts on the basis they were educational. When the DESI antibiotic panel submitted a paper to JAMA on the hazards of combinations, the journal refused to publish.

Lasagna intervened in a growing debate. He had just published a study showing antibiotics were the most commonly prescribed drugs. An antibiotic was prescribed for 60% of visits for a common cold, and chloromycetin, supposedly restricted to life-threatening infections, was dished out liberally. This appeared to play into a narrative that Lasagna himself espoused at the Kefauver Hearings, namely that modern therapeutics had become too difficult and too dangerous for today's doctor to go it alone. An academic narrative that prescribing should be done by specialists rather than generalists.

But while he would never use Panalba, and didn't believe in combinations, FDA, he argued, were overreaching. In an affidavit, he said there was

---

33 See Mintz M. "FDA and Panalba" *Science,* (August 1969), 876.

nothing in the 1962 statutes that said combinations had to be shown to be superior to their individual components. FDA were relying on the views of DESI panels, of which he had chaired one. These could not be a basis for removal. If enough individual doctors saw enough merit in Panalba to make it a blockbuster drug, who was to say they were entirely wrong.

FDA's counsel, William Goodrich, responded that Dr Lasagna's position "stands in bold contradiction to every scientific precept he has advocated publicly and to his profession." FDA's Panalba brief included Lasagna quotes about the lack of wisdom of doctors: "There is a common belief that the addition of many bits of disorganized data will somehow yield a clear picture, that the multiplication of zeros will somehow produce an important finite good."

But the later discovery that helicobacter pylori infections caused duodenal ulcers was based on just such clinical idiosyncrasies. Many doctors in the 1970s gave antibiotics for ulcers. No trials supported this. We now understand the basis for the behavior and a decade later antibiotic combinations were used to cure ulcers. It is clearly better to know the mechanism underpinning a benefit, but not prescribing until we know the mechanism is very ivory tower. Many psychotropic drugs have antibiotic properties and statins may help because they are anti-inflammatory rather than because they lower cholesterol levels.

Academics saw the average doctor as a zombie controlled by marketing. They would not concede that Panalba sales might demonstrate a benefit they knew nothing about. Lasagna laid out his position in a *Science* article on the history of drug development and regulation. "The story in regard to monitoring the quality of medicinal drugs [is one of] ignorance, ineptitude and fraud." Recognizing the fraud, and the ineptitude, he nevertheless put the greater weight on ignorance. We know less than we think we do. We know (in 1969) almost nothing about basic issues such as how drugs are metabolized in the body and how different preparations of the same drug behave compared to each other. The oddity is, the more we learn about these things, the higher the standards to which we want to hold everyone, even for prior developments.

Some saw his position as contrarian. Daniel Carpenter and Philip Hilts in their accounts of FDA's history paint a figure being dropped by those who had previously lauded him. But Nathan Kline wrote to him: "Reading the report of your testimony, I felt like shouting 'Loud Cheers.' Those of us who have both clinical and research experience certainly appear to live in a different universe from the extremists on each side. The basic irrationality of the 'absolutely scientific' position is just incomprehensible to me."

In July 1969, Nixon's Secretary of Health, Education, and Welfare, Robert Finch, intervened on behalf of Upjohn, but to no avail. Upjohn lost and Panalba was removed. Its components, tetracycline and novobiocin (Albamycin) remained. Albamycin is in use today as a treatment for MRSA infections and it later pointed the way to the fluoroquinolone antibiotics. With the removal of Panalba, doctors could still prescribe both drugs in Upjohn's original ratio or in wild and wonderful ratios of their own concoction. Panalba was a visible combination drug. Imipramine and almost all other drugs are invisible combinations. They have multiple actions that come in a fixed ratio.

In Scott Armstrong's 1977 study of business ethics using Panalba as the paradigmatic case, as noted, participants universally disapproved of Upjohn's conduct. But, put in the position of role-playing the Upjohn Board, everyone behaves as Upjohn did. Something about corporate structure makes this possible, whether the corporation is a government as in Germany, a Church as with child abuse, Health Organizations or Universities.

Company marketing is often egregious. But when prescribing is investigated after things go wrong on drugs from sulfanilamide or chloromycetin to Panalba it seems that no more than 10% of medical prescribing is appropriate. Even insulin after its introduction was pressed into rest cures and as a form of Shock Therapy. Big Corporations may stick closer to a rational path than many doctors but if things slip between the divides, because the Corporation is Big the harms are also Big. Given the money involved, this will often mean putting the management of risks to the corporation ahead of managing risks to patients.

To the Rochester Station

Lasagna spent 17 years at Hopkins without tenure. In 1969 Hopkins negotiated funds for a Chair in Clinical Pharmacology. They approached candidates, but not him. Later that year, the University of Rochester appointed him Chairman of Pharmacology with unlimited tenure. When the news broke, the *Baltimore Sun* claimed his views on controversial issues cost him his position, noting his warnings about the risks of contraceptives "before British studies showed a definite link between the pill and thromboembolic diseases."

Hopkins refused to let him take equipment he had bought on grants he secured. This, he said, was like refusing to let a tenant take the furniture they had bought for the house because the landlord or new tenant fancied it. It contrasted with how they treated others. Hopkins' lack of support, he said, "had required my going, hat in hand, to various pharmaceutical firms to raise substantial amounts of money."

Had he moved too close to the industry flame? Upjohn had certainly courted him in the year before the Panalba controversy. Senior figures in Merck, Squibb and other companies regularly sent him letters of appreciation for his input even when he painted them as inept.

A large NIH study on Upjohn's tolbutamide linked it to more cardiovascular deaths than other treatments for diabetes in 1970, a finding not found in smaller or company trials. Upjohn didn't roll over on this drug either. They lined up a series of 'independent' experts to pan the NIH study. The *Medical Tribune* turned to Lasagna. He said it was important that the NIH results not be swept under the rug. We have to accept them and work out what this means. "One possible answer to problems like this is to let physicians take risks… If medicine had insisted on definite evidence before the clinical use of antihypertensive drugs, a lot of people would have died of hypertensive complications." This was the same as his position on oral contraceptives some years before: women needed to be informed of the hazards and let decide for themselves. FDA and many academics wanted either to whitewash the risks away or ban the products.

In Rochester, Lasagna met William Wardell, a New Zealand pharmacologist, scathing of clinical trials. They wrote *Regulation and Drug Development* in which Wardell developed the idea of a Drug Lag, comparing the availability of drugs in the US and Britain. The exemplar was the beta-blockers used widely for hypertension and angina, everywhere except America. America had one, propranolol (Inderal), where some countries had ten. Inderal had been introduced in 1968 but the cardiovascular division in FDA blocked further beta-blockers for a decade until the 'Frances Kelseys,' as Wardell and Lasagna put it, moved sideways. Some FDA officials of the period boasted they had never approved a product.

Lasagna and Wardell wrote:

> *Some in FDA had served the public well by their concern about drug toxicity. The question is really a bigger one: how best to serve the public overall? All of therapeutics is based on a cost–benefit analysis and... the FDA has been too constrained by the idea the public is best protected if it primarily worries about drug toxicity. The ultimate application of this is... no drugs. Every benefit carries a risk in this world... John Locke centuries ago pointed out that the physician cannot practice agnosticism. Every clinical decision is an active one, including the decision not to treat. The bureaucrat can engage in abstract speculation, the practicing physician cannot. It is natural that the practitioner should resent a limitation of therapeutic options for himself and for his patients by regulators whose sights are too limited.*[34]

Lasagna set up Medicine in the Public Interest (MIPI) in 1974, a not-for-profit to conduct studies, perform analyses and evaluate policies on topics like generic substitution and vaccine resistance. As an independent body it could and did make representations to Congress. He set up the Center for the Study of Drug Development in 1976 on a grant from the National Science Foundation. It was soon largely funded by industry.

---

34 Lasagna L, Wardell WM, "Commentary: the FDA, politics, and the public". *JAMA* 232 (1975), 141-2.

Its most famous study claimed the cost of bringing a new drug to market in the 1980s was $1.2 billion.

He was marked as having gone over to the dark side. The changing perception worked its way through to a July 1980 Washington Drug Letter, an industry take on FDA News. Reviewing Reagan's likely healthcare platform and noting that the candidate was in favor of repealing the efficacy criterion of the 1962 regulations, it predicted (tongue in cheek) that, if Reagan were elected, Lasagna might be made director of the Bureau of Drugs.

I Have a Nightmare

In pushing drug effectiveness in 1956, Lasagna had in mind a hurdle to eliminate Snake Oils. It has proven impossible to put in place a meaningful hurdle. Where the placebo once seemed a form of hypnosis, RCTs now hypnotize clinicians into giving ever-increasing amounts of Snake Oil, because all a drug has to do to be deemed effective is to beat placebo. Snake Oil (which has analgesic properties) could do this with a judicious choice of outcome measures and a sufficiently large sample of patients.

Where doctors in 1962 for the most part prescribed short courses of one drug at a time, now, lured by the pied piper of efficacy, 40% of patients over 65 take 5 or more drugs every day. What could be wrong with taking drugs that work? The evidence is that taking 5 or more drugs shortens life spans and increases hospitalizations.

The critique of indiscriminate antibiotic prescribing in the 1960s was that treatment should be driven by diagnosis. This idea lies at the heart of the medical model. But effectiveness is a lure. Doctors now resemble farmers who quietly lace their animal feeds with antibiotics, hormones, tranquilizers, analgesics and whatever. This is not a medical model.

Effective medical treatments should be self-funding or even lead to a fall in healthcare costs. If lives are saved and people are put back to work or become more efficient at work because disability is relieved, then economies should perform better and wealth increase. But not only are healthcare costs increasing exponentially, morbidity and mortality from treatment is also and treatment induced death may now be the normative way of dying.

For four decades from 1962, the management of pregnancy was one area where skepticism about the use of drugs remained the clinical norm. By 2000, ever more drugs, especially antidepressants, were being given to pregnant women, despite mounting evidence of birth defects or behavioral disturbances in children. Industry respond that there are no RCTs showing these hazards and only RCTs can tell us what is really going on.

Drugs in pregnancy raise the question of objectivity. Does it come from the mechanical exercise that is an RCT, which claims to use chance to eliminate bias? Or does it come from using bias to eliminate chance, as has been the scientific norm? In scientific experiments from physics to biology, the norm has been to run an experiment in front of people who might have the opposite point of view, whether because of personal antagonism, another model of reality, sponsorship, or ignorance. We get objectivity by letting Catholics, Protestants, Muslims, Jews and atheists, experiment until they agree on the best way to explain the data.

In the case of pregnancy, this would mean developing pregnancy registers where every drug a woman takes gets logged along with all outcomes, physical and behavioral. We now have the capabilities to do this for pregnancy and for vaccines. The data then needs to be available for scrutiny by women, physicians, statisticians, pharmacologists, and company personnel aiming at taking a view as to whether there is likely to be a risk or not, and, if so, how great.

Perfect objectivity is a dream. We live and die in this world on the basis of the risks we take. We can dream about being rational but as Bruno Schulz, who ended up being shot arbitrarily on a Polish street by a German soldier in 1942, put it in *The Street of Crocodiles*:

> *The six days of Creation were divine and bright. But on the seventh day God broke down. On the seventh day he felt the unknown texture under his fingers and frightened he withdrew his hands from the world. Beware the seventh day.*

7: NEO-MEDICALISM

When Germany invaded Poland in 1939, the managed economies, whether of the Right or the Left, seemed to be outstripping less managed economies. The future looked like it lay not with capitalism or communism but with management, even totalitarian management.

Concerns about the shape of things to come in the West were articulated during the War by the left. Theodore Adorno and Herbert Marcuse of the Frankfurt School, who moved to America and worked for the US government, saw America, with its deployment of behavioral sciences and managerial techniques, as totalitarian as the Soviet Union.

On the right, in his 1944 *The Road to Serfdom*, a foundation stone of what became neoliberalism, Friedrich Hayek argued that in Nazi Germany, Soviet Russia and Fascist Italy central planning had shown itself inimical to science, and to the complexity of modern life. Directing countries from the top down could not lead to progress, which only came when as many individuals as possible were freed up to take risks. Neither America nor Britain, according to Hayek, had fully resisted the virus of central planning.

There was nothing in *The Road to Serfdom* about medicine or health, even though the virus of central planning first became obvious and was most evident in healthcare, leading directly to the Holocaust. Hayek's call for a return to nineteenth century economics appealed, in a way that nineteenth century medicine and its trade in proprietary medicines couldn't.

As part of the War effort, the Roosevelt government suspended the Clayton Anti-Trust Act, triggered by the emergence of Big Oil. By 1950 the US had Big Auto, Steel, Aluminum, Meat, and Tobacco. Big and its managers were in. The US also, 270 years after Petty, adopted Gross Domestic Product (GDP) as a measure of economic activity. GDP took data from manufacturing, trading, debt collection, disaster relief, and inflation. Despite warnings it could rise without a country being meaningfully better off, a rising GDP quickly became an index of economic health.

After the War, US universities competed to offer business management degrees to officers returning home with a background in military management. Concerns about a new technical managerialism quickly appeared. William H Whyte in 1956 in *The Organization Man* described an America that had become intensely collectivist with a myth of individualism. This was echoed in Vance Packard's *Hidden Persuaders*. America was transitioning from a Republic to an Empire, Gore Vidal claimed in 1959.

In contrast, in this period, the National Institutes of Health (NIH) came close to fitting Hayek's vision of a society of individuals empowered with freedom to drive progress. Hundreds of scientists visiting from rigidly hierarchical European universities were blown away by the freedom even junior researchers had to chase leads. In this heady atmosphere new techniques were deployed, new fields created, and advances in biology were remarkable. The 1956 Washington meeting, at which Lasagna starred, was typical of NIH efforts to bring people together and map ways forward unhampered by considerations of commercial confidentiality. New drug leads, new evaluative techniques, and Nobel Prizes followed.

In parallel, from 1946 to 1953, a set of Josiah Macy Conferences involving social scientists, physiologists, engineers and mathematicians created a new discipline that took its name from Norbert Wiener's 1948 book *Cybernetics*. *Cybernetics* built on mathematical and physiological work by Claude Shannon, John von Neumann, Wiener and Arturo Rosebluth. It explored the algorithms, and feedback loops, that underpin servomechanisms that were then underpinning developments in automation and computers.

Feedback loops of the kind that make thermostats work can be seen in much of biology. What is homeostasis, the critical process that keeps our physiology within tight limits, if not a feedback loop? Gregory Bateson claimed distortions in communication feedback loops could make us mentally ill by double-binding us—a hugely influential idea in 1960s antipsychiatry.

These loops even more obviously underpinned the behavioral psychology of Pavlov and B. F. Skinner and fed into a key twentieth century development, operationalism. Operationalism began before the War. P.W. Bridgman, a physicist, was one among its many promoters in a 1927 book on scientific method. Rather than debate meanings, operationalism called for a focus on defining and working with elementary units of more complex phenomena. This book was influential in physics but also psychology. It underpinned Skinner's operant conditioning, a radically new and different approach to human beings.

Margaret Mead was one of this small group. She is often cited today for her inspirational quote: "Never doubt that a small group of thoughtful, committed citizens can change the world; indeed, it's the only thing that ever does." No one knows when or about whom she said it.

Feedback loops are closed systems, reflexes. Their if X then Y operations are algorithmic, operational, and one-dimensional. They cannot work if they have internal contradictions. They can, however, be stacked one on another to create ever more detailed flowcharts onto which ever more complex functions can be mapped. If reflexes can support a great deal of human behavior, perhaps algorithms could underpin organizations.

Many were skeptical of this but by the 1960s even previous skeptics, like Denis Gabor, trumpeted: "We are now justified in considering cybernetics as deserving first priority among all the hard sciences. It may have come just in time to harden the regrettably soft social sciences and to save our free industrial society from the twin dangers of drifting into anarchy by its instabilities or stiffening into a totalitarian system." Heinz von Foerster, a physicist and cheerleader, claimed: "...we apply the competencies gained in the hard sciences to the solution of the hard problems in the soft sciences." Cybernetics "has ultimately come to stand for the science of regulation in the most general sense."[35]

Just as Lasagna rued his role in creating an RCT bandwagon, so Wiener rued the extension of cybernetics to social systems, later termed second-order cybernetics. Perhaps because he had worked on systems automating anti-aircraft weaponry, he was keenly aware the primary support to the development of cybernetics came from the military. The military were interested in more effective weapons but also in supporting industrial automation, believing this would strip ordinary people of any power to influence the political direction of the United States.

As early as 1947, in an article in Atlantic Monthly, Wiener wrote:

> *The measures taken during the war by our military agencies, in restricting the free intercourse among scientists on … projects, have gone so far that it is clear that if continued in time of peace this policy will lead to the total irresponsibility of the scientist, and ultimately to the death of science. Both of these are disastrous for our civilization and entail grave and immediate peril for the public.[36]*

While continuing to be involved in the development of cybernetics, Wiener refused to engage in research that might be put to military uses. He turned to exploring how cybernetics might have applications in health, such as enhancing the function of prostheses. In 1964 the year he died, he published *God and Golem Inc.* He warned that while algorithms can apply to lower order closed systems, they should not be applied to open situations that call for choices and responsibility. He also foresaw the perils of Full Artificial Intelligence.

Wiener's was a voice crying in the wilderness. When Peter Drucker, the doyen of management science, endorsed cybernetics, or as it was beginning to be called Systems Theory, or Operational Management, the way was open for flowcharts to underpin this new growth industry. Rather than issue directives, the new manager would create an information flow in

---

35 Kline RR, *The Cybernetic Moment* (Johns Hopkins University Press, 2015), 192.

36 See Neo-Medicalism references on samizdat.org/shipwreck/

organizations that with appraisals of individuals and benchmarking to best practices would supposedly harness the creativity of employees in a way old-style Taylorism hadn't. (If automated machines didn't replace those employees).

Some claimed cybernetic flowcharts could explain how the free market might work more efficiently than central planning systems, how social order might arise out of self-interested chaos, as Hayek proposed. Perhaps for this reason, the Soviets, who favored Taylor's *Scientific Management* as much as any capitalists, were initially wary of this new bourgeois science. An embrace of science, however, was in the DNA of the Eastern bloc and cybernetics was picked up there as well.

Where Taylorism mapped onto factory work, the new management was tailor-made for the growing service sector of the economy. After 1848 the proportion of the population working in agriculture fell from 90% to 10%. People shifted to manufacturing. After 1948 manufacturing numbers fell from 70% of the workforce to 10%, as manufacturing jobs were automated. Jobs moved to retail, tourism, hospitality, financial services, bureaucracy, computing, and management.

The new systems took time to bed in. When they did, managers realized that components of their flowcharts could be outsourced. Far from being organic, the thigh bones of the new organization need not connect to its hipbone nor the neck bone to the head bone. The organization didn't bleed if limbs were removed and relocated elsewhere. As things came apart, there was a profusion of manuals on how to keep employees onside. In lieu of a pulse, there was a turn to mission statements.

As of 1980, education and health were not part of this new sector.

One-Dimensional

The rise of Big Everything stimulated consumer activism, especially in America. Most of us, though, whether we voted Left or Right, liked Gore Vidal or preferred William F Buckley Jr., seemed comfortable with the fixed prices of cars, oil, and tobacco that bothered Estes Kefauver. We turned to consumerism to get recommendations about the safety and quality of products rather than as a revolutionary weapon.

Marx saw monopoly capitalism squeezing the middle class leaving a proletariat to square off against the capitalists in the final battle. After the War, a middle class seemed to be growing and enjoying a rising tide of material and healthcare affluence.

As wealth increased, many bought a car. Few needed cars. Most could get to work by bus or train. Local shops were close enough to walk to. As cars were bought, they changed from being a luxury to a requirement for people who lived further from work and shopped weekly in supermarkets, which stocked goods not found locally. Cities and the way we lived changed so that we needed cars. Marketers call this a distribution channel. The idea is to control it so everything sells the product. Companies now market types of cars, rather than the idea we might need one. While cars have benefits, they are also linked to changes, like climate change, so vast they seem beyond the influence of individuals.

We bought TVs, although they weren't 'needed' until the news began to break on them in the 1960s. When TVs hooked up with computers to create an informational super-highway, it was increasingly difficult for those not hooked up. Everything conspires to sell the product.

J. K. Galbraith celebrated an *Affluent Society* in 1958, which was flooding us with goods and opportunities. A decade later, in *The New Industrial State*, his tune changed as he outlined how the invisible hand of corporations shaped the distribution channels that created our wants rather than met our needs. About these corporations he later added:

> *Money gave the owner, the capitalist, the controlling power in the enterprise. So, it still does in small businesses. But in large firms the decisive power now lies with a bureaucracy that controls, but does not own, the capital. This bureaucracy is what the business schools teach*

their graduates to navigate. But bureaucratic motivation and power are outside the central subject of economics.[37]

In 1964 in *One Dimensional Man*, Herbert Marcuse saw our prior two-dimensional struggle against an Establishment being replaced by our absorption into a one-dimensional world. Medicine was soon to offer the most telling examples of both one-dimensionality and bureaucratic management, but as with Hayek and Galbraith, Marcuse looked elsewhere.

From 1800 to 1940, it was hoped science would lead to Progress and Modernity. Auschwitz and Hiroshima ushered in a post-modernity in which nothing appeared to have a stable meaning, not even science. A scientific 'follow the data' seemed to merge with business' 'follow the numbers'. Operational rather than conceptual thinking was in, instrumental rather than pure reason, when, given Auschwitz and Hiroshima, it was time to think about what we were doing rather than how we could do more of it.

The growing crisis had a 'spiritual' side. Saints and artists had cautioned against too close a link to our possessions; in the 1960s our cars, homes and material goods were becoming part of us in a new way.

Culture became an industry rather than a calling. For sponsors of art, literature, and movies the numbers of people who accessed them counted rather than the judgments of critics or what was increasingly termed an elite. If the numbers pointed to Disney rather than Shakespeare, Hollywood did Disney. There was pressure to include in television and movies the tropes shown in surveys to work rather than material forcing people to look at things in a new way. Discretion and critique were being emptied out. The media had become a business whose customers were their advertisers. Even protest music now tied us to the apparatus.

After 1800, both Right and Left accepted that running modern societies, institutions, and companies, needed an administrative apparatus, a bureaucracy. Administrative techniques, like all technique, are amoral. They

---

37 John Kenneth Galbraith, "Free Market Fraud". See: progressive.org/dispatches/john-kenneth-galbraith-free-market-fraud/

can be deployed for bad or good. The Apparatus can be perfectly logical, built on reason, and yet mad as the Nazi concentration camps showed.

These concerns fed down to college students. Through to 1960, the Left saw the alienation that comes from having your labor bought by someone else as a commodity, along with squalid urban living conditions, as a state shared by an entire class. 'We' were alienated. While African Americans and feminists maintained a 'we', disaffected college students, wanting to be authentic, began describing themselves as alienated too. Trust had been lost, especially trust in institutions. Motives were increasingly scrutinized and found to conflict. A Great Refusal took shape. The Vietnam War was protested. Civil Rights took to the streets. Women demanded freedom. Even the Vatican faced a Liberation Theology.

In 1968 unrest affected both Eastern and Western blocs. Prague was invaded. Chicago had riots. Major political figures were assassinated. After two decades of denial Germany woke up to its death camps, the role of doctors in terminating lives not worthy of life, and the fact that politicians from the 1940s were still in control.

Medicine in 1968

> *Just as despots can, it is possible to create the appearances of order in an asylum with the use of arbitrary and unlimited confinement, chains and savage treatments. But is this not the silence of the cemetery and of death? It is also possible to maintain order through the wise use of freedoms. This approach softens the often miserable existence of the alienated...*

Philippe Pinel, Treatise Sur le Manie, 1800

The turbulence of 1968 stemmed from a meeting of two torrents. One fed by an increasing sense of conformity and biomedical advances. The other by a growing openness and biomedical advances. Some saw opportunities for enhancement; others saw us diminished. Psychiatry offers a lookout point on the turbulence.

In *Madness and Civilization* (1960) and *The Birth of the Clinic* (1962) Michel Foucault hinted at a machine behind the medical model. Few heeded. By curing scourges, relieving disability, and resurrecting people from death beds, the 1950s pharmaceutical revolution had seemingly validated the medical model. This was progress incarnate. And in subjecting themselves to RCTs in 1962, the business lion seemed to lie down with the scientific lamb.

Despite their extraordinary impact, as of 1960 drugs were not the only answer to disease. These prescription-only poisons that could restore life were an option doctors could use but medicine was not yet a pharmaceutical distribution channel. Drugs had not become the fetish objects cars were. Pharma had to adapt to having doctors as an intermediate step on the road to consumption. Prescriptions meant we could not identify with our meds the way we could with our cars and later phones. Estes Kefauver's adoption of RCTs, however, was about to change that and the climate of healthcare as much as oil was changing the global climate.

After 1848, psychiatry, which introduced the medical model, specialist hospitals, and academic journals, before other branches of medicine, had retreated to its asylums. The prospects of cures for mental illness were no better in 1948. Psychiatric patients were more stigmatized than those with tuberculosis or venereal disorders, and psychiatry had almost no contact with other disciplines.

With the discovery of chlorpromazine in 1952, the outside world rushed in. Techniques as effective as chlorpromazine and penicillin can create new world orders in months, without any marketing. By 1954 German, British, Soviet, and American doctors were meeting in international conferences about this new French drug when otherwise there were restrictions on traveling between their countries.

Tranquilizing a psychosis, like curing an infection, helped restore a person to their place in the social order. Other treatments, the benzodiazepines, LSD, oral contraceptives, and plastic surgery, opened possibilities for people to change their place in that order. LSD cut to the heart of a person's identity offering psychotherapy in hours rather than years. It was pressed into use for alcoholism, homosexuality, frigidity, drug abuse and other deviant states. Like Mesmerism in the 1780s, LSD made an entire social order appear arbitrary.

Benzodiazepines act on conditioned reflexes to undo conflict avoidance and conditioned fear. They disinhibit. They are the kind of drug to help salesmen as well as women seeking to fling off the conditioning of patriarchy. Along with oral contraceptives, they fueled change.

Through to 1954 psychiatrists could do little for their patients but the field gave rise to the magisterial works of Karl Jaspers and Sigmund Freud. Chlorpromazine and its progeny dumped these works in the dustbin. Across medicine, new abilities to do with drugs and scanners seemed to eliminate thinking. No doctor newly able to help people was about to stop helping because the theory behind what they were doing wasn't fully worked out.

There was a huge increase in academic medical posts and optimism. A first Chair of Social Medicine was created in Oxford in 1943. Social meant epidemiological medicine. A majority of those appointed to academic posts in European psychiatry identified as social psychiatrists. In America, psychoanalysts were appointed, and were approached by social scientists with research proposals.

Social medicine rapidly created a mythology. In America, Henry Sigerist, a German émigré and historian of medicine, and George Rosen a physician who, unable to get into medicine in New York because of quotas for Jews, trained in Berlin in the 1930s, fingered poverty and inequality as major determinants of disease. Rosen's *History of Public Health* created the myth of Rudolf Virchow as the standard bearer of a social medicine displaced by the cuckoo of Koch's biomedicine landing in its nest. 'We' had done more for health in cleaning up food and air and with sanitation than biomedicine ever did.

This ignored the fact that the move to cities (social factors) had contaminated the food, air and water to begin with, and prior to the move those with clear rural air and food died young. It ignored social interventions like the provision of milk for children that helped spread scarlet fever and rheumatic fever. It ignored Virchow's fingering of the cell as the basis for pathology, making him central to biomedicine.

Social psychiatry joined mainstream medicine in 1948, with the inclusion of mental disorders in the *International Classification of Diseases* (ICD-6). The first edition of the *Diagnostic and Statistics Manual of Mental Disorders* (DSM-I) appeared in 1952. The ICD and DSM were part of a move to develop the metrics and procedures for the epidemiological mapping of mental disorders needed to underpin efforts at prevention.

A National Institute of Mental Health (NIMH), established in 1947, was oriented toward the behavioral sciences and epidemiology (social was a taboo word in the US). The first major project funded was a study by August Hollingshead and Friedrich Redlich showing mental disorders were more common in urban settings and lower social classes. A second undercut claims that Hutterite communities had no mental illness. And a Midtown Manhattan study showed 80% of New Yorkers had mental health issues.

Michael Shepherd, then a professor of epidemiological psychiatry, was the lead psychiatrist on ICD committees, which were largely run by Britain. Shepherd's colleagues in London's Institute of Psychiatry set up an International Pilot Study of Schizophrenia, which showed outcomes for schizophrenia were better in non-industrialized than industrialized countries. Another study showed that schizophrenia rates were higher in the US and the Soviet Union than elsewhere. When patients could be shown to attract different diagnoses depending on where their video-interview was seen, there was a push to standardize diagnostic interviews and adopt operational criteria. This was medical model medicine.

Something else was taking shape in the wings. The use of personality tests for military screening had revealed a shocking picture of neurosis and unhealthy social attitudes. This opened the prospect after the War of screening for mental factors that, in addition to leading to mental illness, might contribute to racism, fascism, and deviance. It was believed the Nazis were psychopaths, and social engineering was needed to avoid a repeat. In fact, concentration camp guards showed up as normal on US Army screening tests.

Many American psychiatrists returning from the War joined a Group for the Advancement of Psychiatry (GAP) set up by William Menninger. GAP supported psychodynamic treatments, which appealed to doctors, patients, and Hollywood. Here were keys to understand human behavior. The message from dynamically oriented psychiatrists was that no-one was perfectly adjusted, as the Midtown Manhattan study confirmed.

The idea psychiatry might have a place in rooting out racism and anti-democratic tendencies slipped into suggestions that white males who voted Republican were latently fascist, homosexual and mentally disordered. Psychiatrists claimed that Barry Goldwater was mentally unfit to be President. There was an equally strong critique of the Therapeutic State from the Right. Hollingshead, who had shown that class and poverty makes mental illness more likely, was a Goldwater Republican. Thomas Szasz claimed mental illness, was a ploy by liberals to control the population.

By this time, antipsychotic drugs were supporting falls in asylum populations. Far from splitting psychiatry into biological and social camps, their use brought institutional neuroses into view. Asylum inmates, like concentration camp survivors, were nervous about leaving. Studies with chronically psychotic patients pointed to deficits in social skills. Social Skills Training it was claimed could help treat neuroses and psychoses. This was called tertiary prevention and today is called recovery.

In between preventing illness (primary prevention) and recovery lay secondary prevention. Even if we didn't know what caused these disorders, once detected, the right treatment in the right settings should lead to the most rapid resolution, just as clean hospitals had been beneficial even before we had antibiotics. What did the right treatment look like? The War brought trauma into the frame. In addition, when officers with nervous breakdowns were given more autonomy than in traditional hospitals, they showed more improvement than was typical for mental illness. This approach, celebrated in fiction and movies, was adapted for civilian populations in therapeutic communities.

Even before the War, mental hospitals had begun to open admission wards and stays in these were generally shorter. Evidence of people rotating through the doors of psychiatric units rather than entering and never leaving, the rhetorical appeal of therapeutic communities, evidence that stress led to breakdowns, with survey data indicating that large swathes of the population were maladjusted, and the influence of psychodynamic theories, made it plausible to recast mental disorders as social disorders.

A sense society should do more for the mentally ill gave rise to a community mental health movement in the United States. On October 31,1963, the last Act Kennedy signed was a Community Mental Health Act. This created facilities for early detection and treatment as an alternative to asylums. The budget for the NIMH meanwhile increased from $300 K in 1948 to $300 M in 1967.

Preventing mental disorders required social research to identify target groups and mental germs. The first targets were the refrigerator mother in autism, the schizophrenogenic mother in psychosis, and mothers of homosexuals. Betty Friedan in *The Feminine Mystique* argued that liberation was necessary to ensure the subjugation of women didn't lead to a rising incidence of autistic children. The germs were double-bind or other distorted communication styles. The work of Erving Goffman, Thomas Scheff, Thomas Szasz, and R. D. Laing, among others, appearing in popular paperbacks, spread these ideas.

Goffman's *Asylums* in 1961 dealt with questions of identity rather than psychiatric disorder and it cast mental illness in terms of total institutionalization in overbearing societies that had shades of a concentration camp. In both, we were only likely to get a glimpse our true identities in the cracks of institutional routines. Scheff's insights on how labeling shapes the way we view ourselves had equally wide appeal.

Thomas Szasz was even more radical. *The Myth of Mental Illness* in 1961 regarded the mental health apparatus as bogus. He characterized the enthusiasm for the new drugs in terms of "Germany today, tomorrow the world." His take on the infringement of liberties in the detentions of people with psychosis powered a generation of survivor movements with a rallying call that prisons, and the police paid more attention to due process and people's rights than mental health systems.

R. D. Laing's *The Divided Self* in 1960, and *Self and Others* in 1961, made the psychoses as poetic and understandable as Freud had made the neuroses. Schizophrenia resulted from society alienating us from our true selves. Conventional medical treatment lobotomized us into an acceptance of the status quo whereas in the right hands psychotic episodes opened a window to deeper insights. Laing's willingness to accompany patients on this journey and the emergence of humanistic therapies in the hands of Abraham Maslow and Carl Rogers, which promoted psychology as a force for liberation rather than an ever more subtle oppression, colored the times.

Mental illness became a metaphor for the way we were living in Joseph Heller's *Catch 22* (1961), Anthony Burgess' *Clockwork Orange* (1962) and Ken Kesey's *One Flew Over the Cuckoo's Nest* (1962). Colonization was a common theme. Our parents colonized us. Whites colonized black consciousness. Men colonized women. The working class, which now had a level of everyday material wellbeing undreamt of by their parents, were colonized by capitalism. The oppressed were in the same boat as the mentally ill, colonized by those who rule society. And a psychotic event was a social and political event, not a medical event.

As in 1789, the social chains holding back an alienated people were conflated with the chains holding the mentally alienated. As in 1848 even medical students could feel a stint at the barricades coming on. Laing and Szasz were invited to Tokyo to speak in 1967. Their visit provoked the students at Tokyo University to occupy the department of psychiatry, forcing Hiroshi Utena from office. The students disapproved of his biological research. The occupation lasted 10 years.

Protesting students in Paris ransacked the office of Jean Delay, whose department had discovered chlorpromazine. Delay boasted that chlorpromazine had transformed the asylums into places where silence replaced shrieking. Echoing Pinel, the students responded that this was the silence of the grave. Delay, an establishment man, never recovered from the shock.

Seymour Kety, the head of Neuroscience in NIMH, was called by Congress to answer questions about psychiatric control of human behavior. He responded that:

> *The manipulation of the brain by any of the biological techniques which can be developed in the foreseeable future would involve such drastic invasions of privacy, integrity and the unalienable rights of the individual that in their application behavioral control would already have been achieved even if the electrodes carried no current and the pill were placebo.*[38]

Kety's point was that control lay in social forces rather than in biology. LSD, the benzodiazepines, and contraceptives undid behavioral control rather than imposed it. But, society banned the psychedelic drugs, as they once banned mesmerism, leaving drugs that buttress the social order, the antidepressants and antipsychotics, untouched.

Social conditions can unquestionably demoralize and alienate, may seed substance misuse and suicide, even trigger psychosis. The claims made for liberation psychiatry, however, made it inevitable mainstream psychiatry would pull back, leaving an antipsychiatry on the opposite side of a divide still in place. All of medicine shrank as a result.

An extension of psychiatric control became a self-fulfilling prophecy. Antipsychiatry legitimized the notion that all distress was continuous. So did Michael Shepherd studying primary care nervous conditions in the 1960s, who hit an iceberg of everyday nervous disorders that psychiatrists knew nothing about. Like Leo Srole who had run the Midtown Manhattan project, Shepherd failed to spot that the tools he thought might help us govern ourselves could just as readily make markets for pharmaceuticals. Psychiatrists were about to be de-institutionalized.

---

38 S Kety, "Hearings of the National Commission on Health Sciences and Society," *90th Congress, Second Session* (1968), 292.

OPERATIONAL THINKING

The arguments on either side in 1968 were value laden and passionate. The center seemed to be falling apart as it had in 1641, 1789 and 1848. The U.S. Chamber of Commerce approached Lewis Powell, one of the Supreme Court Justices, to draft a plan to save US corporations from a growing democratic threat. Powell's 1971 prescription fueled the huge increase in corporate lobbying that is such a feature of politics today.[39]

This prescription is spun as the remedy that restored corporations to good health. Power and control did seem to be restored soon after, but it is not clear that anyone on the Right or Left of politics could have had much sense as to how order was about to be conjured out of chaos. Two decades later, whether we came from the Right or Left, the idea that if we apply the best techniques to problems, we will get the best possible results was not remarkable. But in 1971, this was not on many people's radar and certainly not on Powell's.

The publication in 1980 of the 3rd Edition of the Diagnostic and Statistical Manual of Mental Disorders (DSM III) offers a paradigmatic example of a new technocratic approach, and its pitfalls.

The creation of DSM-I in 1952 marks an emergence of operational thinking in American psychiatry. The 1956 Washington Conference marks a point beyond which, despite the concerns of Freyhan, Kline and Evarts, the slide into operationalism, with its rating scales, clinical trials, and diagnostic criteria, was unavoidable.

Nevertheless DSM-II, which was introduced in 1967, was as marginal to the lives of doctors and patients as ICD 1 in 1893. Few beyond a group of homosexual doctors in the American Psychiatric Association (APA), who rallied against the coding of homosexuality as a mental disorder, were aware of DSM. APA delegated the public relations issue that homosexuality had become to Robert Spitzer, an epidemiologist from Columbia, who brokered its deletion from DSM-II. There was a brief flicker of media

---

39 Powell, Lewis F Jr, "The Lewis Powell Memo: A Corporate Blueprint to Dominate Democracy", see: greenpeace.org/usa/democracy/the-lewis-powell-memo-a-corporate-blueprint-to-dominate-democracy/

attention for an event that later entered mythology and made Spitzer's career.

Spitzer was given charge of preparing DSM III. Facing a growing divide between psychiatry and antipsychiatry, he turned to operational criteria. This involves a listing of the surface features of disorders, units, that can be checked as present or absent. If for instance we list the 9 symptoms commonly found in depression and decide we will diagnose and base depression research on anyone who has 5 or more of these 9 criteria, we should all be able to speak the same language whatever our passions and values.

An operational answer can work when distinguishing between Jews who wear phylacteries, Muslims who turn to Mecca, or Catholics who eat fish on Fridays. In ambiguous cases, though, they operate as they did when embodied in the *Malleus Maleficarum* for the detection of witches; what is seen lies in the eye of the observer.

Spitzers drafting committee saw themselves as pulling the profession back from a mission to change the world to a focus on diseases. They claimed they were adopting a neutral stance on the nature of medical disorders. Others saw a Medical Empire crossing the Rubicon with a view to dismantling a Consumer Republic.

Freud, for all his observation of patients, never described a new disorder. Along with Kraepelin, his psychiatry counterpart, he got by on roughly the same 10 categories clinicians today could get by on. DSM III coded for 163 disorders. DSM IV in 1994 for 297. This is like a turn to Ptolemaic spheres in a clinical universe that has lost its Copernican center, or like the fracturing of Protestantism after Christendom split. An initial turn to greater precision led to increasingly meaningless iterations, just as initial distinctions between good and bad cholesterol broke into multiple other fractions, or initial blood pressure or blood glucose thresholds shifted. Borges' Map of the Empire incarnate.

DSM III coded for Post-Traumatic Stress Disorder (PTSD), making it a focus for Vietnam veterans. It coded for multiple personality disorder (MPD), triggering an epidemic of MPD. The combination of PTSD and

MPD brought trauma and abuse to the fore and underpinned a Recovered Memory movement, temporarily checked in the mid-1990s by legal verdicts against therapists who had persuaded patients that even if they couldn't remember the abuse on an alien spaceship at the age of one it had happened.

The alienation and oppression of the 1960s refracted through DSM's prism became trauma and abuse. DSM swept away schizophrenogenic and refrigerator mothers, symbols of the need to return to medical roots. Abusive men replaced them. These new conditions were not medical. They labeled cultural boxes rather than provided a common focus for researchers from different backgrounds interested in trauma, genes, or hormones.

Barney Carroll from Ann Arbor created a Dexamethasone Suppression Test (DST) in 1969. This cortisol-based test distinguishes melancholia (unequivocal medical depression) from neurotic depression or mixed anxiety and depressive states, conditions that may be medical or social or existential. It did so as well as electroencephalograms (EEGs) distinguish epilepsy from functional fits. In 1976, the DST was the hottest research topic in psychiatry. Yet in 1980, the DSM criteria for Major Depressive Disorder (MDD) embraced all shades of misery from unhappiness to psychotic depression but had no mention of the DST. Nothing that cut beneath the surface of things was welcome in the DSM.

Using the new MDD criteria in clinical trials, Lilly could demonstrate that Prozac, which is ineffective in melancholia, had a marginal efficacy in 'depression'. FDA had difficulties approving it as an antidepressant, the RCT evidence was so weak. Newly adherent to bureaucratic rules about two positive trials, however, FDA ticked the approval box, allowing Lilly to market Prozac for Major Depression and build an impression it works for severe mood disorders. Had the DST featured in DSM III, designating the SSRIs as antidepressants would have been more difficult, and depression might never have come to be viewed as the greatest source of disability on the planet.

Before 1980, even though drug treatments could go wrong, and pharma and shady practices go hand in hand, most of us were pro-pharma and especially their drugs. Few mentioned Big Pharma. Michel Foucault and Ivan Illich worried about Big Medicine rather than Pharma.

A rising tide of drug consumption since 1980 has fueled claims that Pharma controlled the DSM. Scrutinizing DSM IV and 5 committees investigative journalists have unearthed evidence of links between panel members and companies with all links taken as indicating sell-outs to industry. But when it comes to generating a list of clinical features for disorders, whether every single panel member or none has links to industry makes no difference. Once the criteria are in place, like horoscopes there is no controlling what people can read into them. Like an enzyme that catalyzes a reaction, it's easier to go with them than against.

Those who are placed to take advantage can make a killing. Nothing about DSM could stop either Trauma or Pharma bandwagons, with their respective soundbites, exploiting these opportunities. Neither Spitzer nor anyone on his committees had any sense this might happen.

We are now in a universe bounded by operational criteria. There is no outside. DSM claimed to sideline beliefs about conditions, but without professional judgment there is no way to ensure that anyone who meets depression criteria, while influenzal or pregnant, will not be diagnosed with depression. Just as in the absence of discriminating judgments, there is no underpinning in reality to the algorithmic functions that are RCTs, so too with the DSM. The appeal of both operational criteria and RCTs is their apparent offer of an end run around judgment and conflict.

There was a new culture on the block by 1990. The marketing of the SSRIs and stimulants for ADHD had made biobabble part of the health-related lingo of everyday life, especially in America. Negative research results could no more eliminate these new myths than they could change a prior psychobabble.

The biobabble implied that neuroscience will in due course explain mental disorders, indeed all behavior, but to this day biological testing plays no part in mental health care. Unlike the antibiotics, the antipsychotics and antidepressants don't buttress medical models by resolving clinical states. They do, however, serve to locate disorder within us. In contrast to taking a stimulant to stay awake or a tranquilizer to sleep, when a soldier takes an SSRI, licensed for PTSD (in the absence of *any* evidence for benefits in combat troops), he relocates the disorder from the theater of combat to within himself.

The soldier will be treated by a biological psychiatrist. There were no biological psychiatrists before the soundbite was invented in 1989. 'Bio' in this sense is code for doing. It has little to do with biology. Those who 'do' dish out the same few pills to everyone in response to our numbers.

Doctors like this, increasingly called 'pharmacologists', know nothing about pharmacology or biology. They are uncomfortable with the fact anxiety can arise from physical or social sources. It needs clinical acumen to know if it stems from a cancer or a heart condition rather than the existential dread of sinners, or precarians. These doctors know little about the biology underpinning temperaments; that when anxious, introverts become obsessive and phobic while extraverts become ADHDy or borderline. These differences are biologically based; scores on introversion-extraversion scales, for instance, predict how much anesthetic is needed to put someone to sleep. They don't know Pavlov demonstrated a century ago that trauma could lead to nervous breakdowns in dogs some of whom responded to stimulants, and others to sedatives, depending on their temperament. Everyone now gets an SSRI.

RCTs assume an average man and make no accommodation to the possibility that other differences between us might be as great as ethnic or sexual differences. Because RCTs accommodate more readily to apparently specific DSM disease entities, difficult children, some of whom might have been helped with a stimulant and others with a sedative, become cases of ADHD (stimulant responders) or juvenile bipolar disorder (sedative responders). The labels eliminate interest in further enquiry, in favor of doing. The continuity with prior medical diagnoses is superficial. These one-dimensional labels are not medical.

Different temperaments also respond differently to trauma. Just as postmortems may show what people can live with rather than what they die from, so a clinical history will often reveal considerable trauma with little consequence. Extraverted patients, however, are exquisitely sensitive to the expectations of therapists, and an unwary therapist, or one ideologically committed to the central role of trauma in mental health, can quickly make such patients relive rather than just remember a trauma that never happened.

Abuse unquestionably happens and many have vested interests in not seeing the alienation their power visits on the rest of us. Questions of abuse and trauma now fuel the politics of identity (chapter 10). Clinical practice, however, needs judgment calls as to whether a traumatic event in an individual case has in fact had significant outcomes.

There Is No Alternative… to Neoliberalism?

Far from DSM III solving our belief and value problems, an unanchored technical process is itself a belief system. Across medicine, the focus is now on the superficial numbers for blood pressure, peak flow, or bone density readings (chapters 9 and 11), with little interest in teasing out environmental and genetic inputs to superficially similar conditions or to individual cases. The figures lead to a doing rather than a thinking.

Objecting is almost impossible. Marcuse called for more philosophy to combat one-dimensionality, but medicine now has more philosophy in the form of bioethics than ever before with no effect.

Even to those for whom the superficiality of the apparatus is clearly value based, there seems little option but to suspend disbelief in the stage act. Apparent efficiency wins out over—what? It is difficult to specify what the alternative might be. As a key neoliberal phrase of the 1980s put it "there is no alternative." The Iron Cage has snapped shut.

Spitzer and others writing about operational criteria in the 1970s made no reference to outside forces but the turn to operational criteria in medicine coincided with an advance of operational thinking in economics, which brought a focus on money rather than what it represented. The roots of this 'monetarism' can be traced to Hayek and the 'Vienna School' of the 1930s, Clark Warburton in the 1940s and Milton Friedman in the Chicago School of Economics in the 1950s.

Monetarists argued that managing the economy should hinge on a monetary thermostat rather than political judgment. *Pecunia non olet* (money doesn't smell). Socialists and capitalists might have irreconcilable values but controlling the money supply would be good for both. Algorithms have neither a right nor a left side.

The Allende government in Chile in 1970 famously adopted computers to crunch economic data. This was not management by algorithm. It was still treating the country, the way a doctor would treat a patient—if something isn't working, change course. A few years after the Pinochet coup, Chile became the site of a first ever cybernetic management of a country with the supply of money given a thermostat function in running an economy. This made superficial sense in the 1970s with rampant inflation but controlling the money supply regardless of the state of the country was simplistic. Chile didn't do well, nor did Britain a short while later, but neither could seemingly change course.

Monetarism has since been rebadged as neo-liberalism. It is not clear who coined this term, and it remains undefined other than operationally. The sense is Western governments since the 1980s have managed liberalism. In this new dispensation, just as raised blood pressure figures or depression scores trigger interventions, money supply or inflation targets dictate responses, in which judgment plays no more part than it does in the computer systems underpinning the financial markets, which carry out a million transactions a second.

Government has been replaced by governance. Leaders by managers, for whom it is as impossible to abandon meaningless even harmful figures, such as those for GDP, as it is for a doctor to engage with a patient without any measuring instruments. This unwillingness to listen to and engage with judgments underpins the all-encompassing generalization from economic data to government found in neo-liberalism in contrast to liberalism. Neo-medicalism has similarly generalized from the limited area of our lives diseases once occupied to the totality of our behavior.

In 1976 Michael Jensen and William Meckling pushed thermostats into the management of corporations. Where corporate executives once used their discretion in the application of flowcharts, managers now had to be bound by an 'ethical responsibility' to maximize shareholder value, even if that meant outsourcing components of the firm, and laying off workers. This justifies using profits to buy back shares rather than invest in new production. This generates inequality rather than wealth.

The obligation to maximize share-holder value underpinned a growing scope to play the numbers, as part of what is now called financialization.[40] This was increasingly fertile ground for hedge funds, making them over time powerful enough to shape the behavior of countries. If judgment is suspended, numbers become a one-way street.

There is a parallel pharmaceuticalization in medicine. A dopamine antagonizing antipsychotic marketed as a mood-stabilizer (without any good evidence) may be given to someone who is diagnosed bipolar, a now fashionable diagnosis. This treatment causes a loss of focus and ability to concentrate, that will produce a-meets-criteria-for-ADHD state on a rating scale, prompting the addition of a stimulant, a drug with just the opposite effects on the dopamine system. The stimulant in turn may produce depressive features and a growing cascade of prescription drugs. Clinical practice of this kind can be and is increasingly done remotely. The doctor may never meet us. He may operate from rating scales emailed to us. As the consumption of drugs chasing the tail of the drug before increases, life expectancy falls.

Soon after DSM III was published, the Berlin Wall came down. East and West embraced technocracy. Talk of an end to history replaced both the noisy medical and political struggles of the 1960s. There is no evidence Lewis Powell had any sense this was about to happen or that his contribution made any difference. He may simply have introduced a useful fig leaf—many now see corporate lobbying as the kind of thing that needs to be put right. This diverts attention from what we are doing to ourselves.

Few dismiss Powell in this way but the idea that any medical grandee in 1971, full of sound and fury, thundering about the need to roll back antipsychiatry and homeopathy, foresaw what was coming is ludicrous.

---

40 Like neo-liberalism, a word with no accepted definition.

Twenty years later, Milton Friedman, one of the founding fathers of monetarism, writing about healthcare, clearly couldn't see even what was then happening, stating that: "The intellectuals may have learnt the words but they do not yet have the tune… On both sides of the Atlantic, it is only a little overstated to say that we preach individualism and competitive capitalism, and practice socialism."[41]

In helping produce greater health (and therefore wealth) doctors, loosely speaking, occupied the role of capitalists in 1968. The emerging patient movements were socialists, in the sense of seeking a seat at the table where issues of production are decided. A neo-medicalism has since produced a Silent 1990s and 2000s. This doesn't mean that capitalism triumphed over socialism. Both the medical model, which produced real advances in health, and patient values, which in any universe are central to healthcare, were replaced by something else that has enabled pharma-ceuticalization (chapters 9 and 11). Capitalism and socialism have been similarly subverted by management (bureaucracy) and financialization, neither of which are productive. The socialist mission to harness capitalist forces of production is dead. Only those with opportunities to extract rent gain from this situation.

Our need now is to harness technical processes and to distinguish between technocratic expertise and merit. In this no-one has a more important role than the drug wrecked among us who are forced to be entrepreneurial (risk-taking) and to adopt a medical model.

We commonly hear about Cyberspace and Cyborgs, but not now about Cybernetics. Cyber- misleadingly links these words to computers. Cyber comes from the Greek Kubernetes, the helmsman or pilot of a ship. This became the Latin Gubernator, which gave us government, and governance, a word that suggests we the people have a role in government. In practice it means anything but. Governance now allows political appointees to wash their hands of responsibility.

---

41 Friedman M, *Preface to The Road to Serfdom* (1994).

8: ACCESS TO MEDICINES

In March 1963, Estes Kefauver set political hare running when he contacted Bill Haddad, about a story in his breakfast paper. America had declared a war on generic drugs with Colombia its target. The Colombians were trying to get life-saving tetracycline antibiotics in generic form. President Lleras Camargo had an offer from John Nolan, head of McKesson and Robbins, to supply the medication at a cent a capsule to campesinos and slum dwellers, compared to the 53 cents charged for the branded product. But McKesson were being blocked by brand name companies. As Kefauver put it:

> *the main issue is simply the desire of some major American drug companies to continue to sell drugs in Latin America at exorbitant markups, a willingness of some other American companies to sell at more modest although still satisfactory markups and certain alleged concerted efforts on the part of the former to prevent the latter from doing so.*[42]

In an election year, subpoenas but would be too hot. Could Bill get the media involved? Haddad engaged the *New York Herald Tribune*.

On August 10, 1963, Kefauver died of a heart attack. Haddad visited Colombia, where the president confirmed the story. Company people, often the unsung heroes, handed Haddad files pointing to a brand cartel

---

42 Childs M, "Kefauver's Last Fight", *New York Post*, (September 24, 1963)

complete with kickbacks, rebates to ensure business as usual, regular strategy meetings with US advisers, and disinformation campaigns. Colombian doctors were told quality products could not be produced at low prices. Pharmacists were told generics would bankrupt them. Medical journals wrote critical editorials. And someone contaminated the low-cost drugs. The branded industry insisted their only concerns lay with patent infringements, although lower cost could adversely affect US balance of payments. They were reluctant to disclose their records for fear of compromising US foreign policy. The story took five years to play out.

Haddad meanwhile ran for Congress in 1964 in New York's 19th district. After finding the Brooklyn Navy Yard stored drugs for the military and the President, bought as generics at one fifth of the prices New York hospitals paid for the branded versions, he campaigned on exorbitant drug prices. New York State filed a civil suit against pharmaceutical companies and Haddad traveled the country urging other States to join in. In Florida he was given a secret FBI file showing he was being tailed. He lost the election.

On February 5, 1969, Cyanamid, Pfizer, Upjohn, Bristol-Myers, and Squib settled the Columbia case for $200 Million, then the biggest anti-trust settlement. The cost-of-drugs genie was out of the bottle. Supporters of Medicare claimed drug costs might be the straw to break the camel's back. Opponents of Medicare painted cost containment as socializing medicine. Rational medicine for some was rationing for others.

Healthcare costs rose 6% in the 1960s, but drug prices, industry claimed, fell as a proportion of that rise by 0.1%. Fifty years later branded drugs still take 10% of healthcare budgets leaving companies grinning, and politicians confused. If drugs work as we are told, they should take 20% or more of a falling healthcare budget instead of 10% of an escalating one.

By 1960 there were over 4000 pharmaceutical brands mostly prescription-only. A succession of anti-substitution laws meant pharmacists had to hand over exactly what the doctor wrote. The aim of these laws was to reduce counterfeiting. But they put a premium on the sentiments of doctors as Arthur Sackler and others realized. The net result was that 94%

of dispensing was for brand name drugs in what was a $10 billion business. Drug brands for most doctors conjured up Merck's Diuril and Tryptizol, Mercedes drugs. The idea that all that might be on offer was the brand, Coca Cola drugs, was not on anyone's radar.

Up to 1950, US chemical manufacturers, later called generic companies, were small family companies who supplied raw materials to larger houses. In the 1950s, some of these companies were portrayed as fly-by-night operations but Good Manufacturing Practices sorted out most abuses.

Haddad wrote to the Industrial Medical Association (IMA), a pharmaceutical trade organization, in 1965 asking what the basis was for claiming a difference between generic and branded drugs. Clark Bridges, the Chairman replied, "your letter requesting information on the effectiveness of brand name drugs vs. generic drugs indicates the need for some basic understanding of this subject. We suggest that you consult any physician or pharmacist and have him explain this situation to you."[43]

Industry were confident physicians and pharmacists would sing from a song sheet over a decade in the making. The chorus line centered on bio-equivalence. Not all versions of a drug were the same, it was claimed. In a small number of celebrated examples an important difference between brand and generic had shown up.

But pharmacists were getting restless. It was close to impossible to stock all 4000+ brands, many of which pharmacists regarded as junk. Besides, many pharmacists figured they knew more about equivalence than doctors. Some pharmacists favored repealing the anti-substitution laws. Others didn't. Facing escalating healthcare costs, the Nixon administration didn't feel able to reign in consumer interest in price competition.

Kentucky passed a substitution law in 1972. New York was key to what would happen next. Haddad had a position in a New York State Assembly Office of Legislative Oversight and Analysis. Based in the World Trade Center, armed with subpoena powers to extract documents, he built support for generic substitution. It became clear that for military

---

43 Clark Bridges, IMA Managing Director (March 12, 1965).

purposes, FDA had been testing generic drugs for equivalence for years and had a list of interchangeable drugs. Haddad got hold of this list, and teed up *Newsweek*, *60 Minutes*, the *New York Post*, the *Herald Tribune*, and other media outlets. On April 28 1977 he produced a list of 1,250 brand name drugs and their equivalents, and a cloak and dagger story as to how the list had come to light. There was no going back. New York passed a 'Haddad Bill,' as industry called it, which came into force on April 1, 1978. A year later 49 States had repealed their anti-substitution laws.

Industry geared up for war. Following the Kentucky law change, an article castigating the move to generic prescribing appeared in *Drug Therapy* entitled "The Generic vs Brand Name Substitution Controversy: A Mad Tea Party," authored by Louis Lasagna.

Joseph Sargent, president of New York State Physicians Union, wrote to the editor of Labor News saying the case for generics was shot through with inaccuracies and misstatements. Neither FDA nor New York State, he noted, were offering to be legally responsible for adverse reactions on generics, whereas brand name houses were legally responsible for both the safety and efficacy of their drugs. He attached a Lasagna article "Generic Substitution; Trick or Treat?" which argued generics were inadequate and not significantly cheaper than branded compounds.

Yet another Lasagna article in *Drug Therapy* in May 1978, "The New York State Generic Substitution Law: an exercise in surrealism," began with the phrase "It is entirely appropriate that April Fools' Day 1978 is the date of implementation of New York State's Public Health Law ... to encourage generic substitution." Therapeutic equivalence, bioequivalence, and medical interchangeability were not the same thing, he said. A pharmacist might know if drugs were bioequivalent but only a doctor knew if they were therapeutically equivalent.

In September 1978, Patricia Coyne of *Private Practice* reported on a debate between *Private Practice*'s Francis Davis MD and Haddad, telling her readers that in these battles "the conservative free-enterprise coalition have learnt that its liberal consumerism opponents don't play fair." For them, the end justifies the means. They know the industry is wicked and small firms virtuous. Don't be fooled by Haddad, she warned. He can be reasonable in debate but off the record he is a hatemonger. He claims the federal government has failed miserably to protect the States and the consumer from the last of the Robber Barons—the prescription drug industry. He is horrified that, several months after New York's new law, doctors haven't switched over to generics and claims Congress is still a pushover for the drug industry. She ended with a swipe; Haddad claimed his crusade was inspired by Kefauver whose heart was broken by the branded industry, but everyone knew Kefauver was an alcoholic.

In the October edition of *Private Practice*, Coyne reported on a National Consumer Alliance's Conference on Generic Drugs. In *Fear and Loathing and Generic Drugs*, she noted with delight that Stanley Steingut, the New York politico, held up a copy of *Private Practice* and branded it industry propaganda. Even the Ku Klux Klan or the Weathermen, she claimed, would be hard put to outdo the consumerists for sheer suspicion and hostility. Brands drive genericists wild. They are intent on removing choice. To their chagrin, she claimed, people and doctors don't support them. For the believers, this can't be the fault of consumerist philosophy. The fault must lie with companies and this fuels their hatred. If the branded industry could be brought to its knees, medicine would fare better.

A series of adverts in *Private Practice,* under the brand "Medicine and Politics Don't Mix", promoted doctors who "don't want to bargain with your health." The adverts suggested, "you trust the doctor who prescribed it [your medicine], shouldn't you be able to trust the company who made it as well." The drug companies "keep the brand in mind because they have you in mind." The politicians are "out to save money on medicine even if it kills you.... Soon the law could say your doctor can't prescribe the medicine he thinks is best for you."

Oklahoma Congressman Mickey Edwards claimed the generic argument was like a football scout saying to the team coach he could no longer sign O. J. Simpson, because FDA had decided any footballer was the generic equivalent of O. J. Did O. J.'s touchdowns only happen, the mystified coach responds, because he had a good publicity department?

The main industry ploy was to introduce branded generics, drugs that had gone off patent but which with a brand name could be pitched at a higher price than an anonymous generic. New York's physicians turned to branded generics, which were made in factories making generics of the same drug, packaged differently. Haddad was not impressed.

An Empire State Chamber of Commerce press release in 1979 headed 'Wild Bill Rides Again' crowed; "the prize for our "now we've heard everything" award belongs to William F. Haddad. Having steamrollered a generic substitution drug bill to law on April 1 he is now engaged in a frenetic running gun battle to deny reputable manufacturers of "brand name" drugs the chance to serve the new market his bill has created, backing these up with their own names, reputations, and financial liability.

Echoing a 1940 advert from E R Squibb & Son, the press release claimed; "the priceless ingredient of a product is the character and integrity of its maker. We think Mr. Haddad is playing with dynamite and he had better give a little thought to where it is leading him."

Blaming the 1960s

Congressional Hearings on medicines littered the 1970s. On January 4,1970 Gaylord Nelson's Hearings on the safety of oral contraceptives was triggered by Barbara Seaman's 1969 book *The Doctors' Case Against the Pill*. Not a single woman presented. Faced with angry feminists, Nelson at one point asked the "girls" to keep quiet, unwittingly adding to pharma's growing consumer revolt. This was further stoked by later hearings on tranquilizers and their marketing to women.

Lasagna had been saying for years the pill caused thrombosis. A 1968 British study confirmed a link between contraceptives and thrombosis. The British considered making patient information available but rejected it as compromising the doctor-patient relationship and banned high-dose estrogen pills instead.

FDA's endorsement of the pill was the fundamental dictum shaping its use, American experts said. If FDA considered it safe, women had no way to gainsay this. FDA leant toward providing patient information, via package inserts. AMA opposed this. In February 1972, FDA introduced a close-to-unintelligible first insert. When AMA objected, the insert's inclusion was left to medical discretion.

In January 1978, Jimmy Carter in his State of the Union address promised an Act to protect the drug consumer without hitting industry's research capability or interfering with the doctor- patient relationship. On March 17, his administration introduced Ted Kennedy's Drug Regulation Reform Act. This aimed at getting valuable drugs to market as quickly as possible, making available the data underpinning their approval, instituting post marketing surveillance of drugs, making patient inserts routine, fostering competition among manufacturers, ending drug promotion, and advertising abuses, and establishing a national center for Clinical Pharmacology.

Haddad's National Consumers Alliance saw consumers as overprescribed, overcharged, and underprotected. It welcomed the inserts, post-marketing surveillance, the possibility of independent review of drug trial data, and an independent clinical pharmacology center that might test medicines on young and old, which pharma rarely did. But it was unhappy with proposals to relax safety and efficacy testing for breakthrough drugs and the failure to tackle the difference in price between trade and generic drugs.

The Pharmaceutical Manufacturers Association didn't agree their members exerted too much influence on physicians. They saw doctors as too cautious in prescribing new life-saving drugs. They branded FDA over-protective, citing Wardell and Lasagna's Drug Lag and approval times for drugs that were twice as long in America as in Europe.

They noted that there had been a 95% increase in the price of all consumer items between 1960 and 1977 and a 144% increase in wages, but only a 12% increase in drug price. Profits had been maintained, they said, only because of a switch from small to large companies. Why the mania to eliminate brand names in an area where quality differences are vital? Their members now made generic drugs to a much higher standard than fly-by-night companies.

Lasagna testified to increasing alarm at the disastrous effects [of regulation] on drug research and development. The bill contains "Nice words including on the need to deregulate but in fact it increases regulations." The difficulty is not a matter of regulations, it's one of attitude. FDA behavior is not law based. It's a culture and no law will change this. FDA are detective, prosecutor, judge, jury, and appeal court for drug approval. The public had been given an insight, he said, on the lunacy FDA was capable of when it banned saccharine on the slenderest of data but did nothing about tobacco.

In close to a reversal of his 1962 position, he said there was no way to make valid risk-benefit assessments. And no way to assess relative efficacy. Relative efficacy and risk-benefit assessments could only be done at the patient level. They should not enter regulatory decisions. He claimed doctors didn't need raw data and this requirement would accelerate the flight of US companies elsewhere. As regards increasing the consumer presence on FDA panels, why not consumers from disease-oriented groups who want access to drugs rather than consumers trying to restrict access.

Speculation mounted Kennedy would run against Carter in 1980, with healthcare an issue. His Bill died in Senate in September 1979 for lack of administration support.

Orphan Drugs

While outlining Drug Lags, Lasagna flagged up an Orphan Drugs issue. Unless a drug was likely to be used by 200,000 people, companies claimed they could not make a return on their development costs, which now included a need for clinical trials, regulatory delay, and a shorter effective patent life. There was no room for a company to be public spirited and bring a drug on the market to serve a clear need. Drugs such as carnitine, EDTA, dopamine, and 5-HTP, therefore, became orphans: no one was willing to adopt them. We risked the same fate for new multiple sclerosis, epilepsy, and cancer treatments.

There the issue sat until Abbey Meyer, a self-described Connecticut housewife, picked it up. The story Meyer told in *Orphan Drugs: A Global Crusade* began in 1968 with the birth of her son, David. When he was a few years old he began to show signs of what her doctor called tics. As his difficulties grew, her concerns grew. Then in a Sunday newspaper she read about Tourette Syndrome. This led to clinical appointments. The standard drug, haloperidol, turned David into a zombie. He was enrolled in a trial of a new drug, pimozide, which was better, but supplies were cut off in 1976 when McNeil pharmaceuticals opted not to develop it. Her doctor used the term orphan drug.

Chasing the idea of orphan drugs, Meyer came across Marjorie Guthrie, wife of Woody Guthrie whose Huntington's disease led her to campaign for orphan diseases. A group of women got together, including Muriel Seligman from Los Angeles, whose son Adam had Tourette's. Seligman approached her Congressman, Henry Waxman, who convened a hearing in June 1980 inviting pharmaceutical companies. No-one showed apart from a few families with rare diseases and a *Los Angeles Times* reporter.

Following an *LA Times* article, Meyer was contacted by Jack Klugman who ran Quincy MD, a TV medical series. Klugman created an episode that had a boy testify at a Congressional Hearing in emotional terms about the damage caused by lack of treatment. The show, *Seldom Silent, Never Heard*, ran in March 1981. Thousands of letters flooded in. Waxman convened a follow up hearing at which Quincy testified. There was standing room only. The *Wall Street Journal* laughed at the idea Congress would listen to an actor. But Nancy Kassebaum (R. Kansas) introduced a bill in the Senate, which Waxman took to the House. It passed in December 1982 and was signed into law by Ronald Reagan in January 1983, allowing accelerated access and a longer period of monopoly for orphan drugs.

Meyer and others then formed the National Organization for Rare Diseases (NORD) and catalogued over 6000 conditions that might qualify. She met Haddad, who in 1980 became Executive Director of a new organization, the Generic Pharmaceutical Industry of America (GPIA). Pushing an Act to regularize the position of generic drugs, Haddad said that if branded companies didn't bring orphan drugs to the market, generic companies would.

Haddad provided funds for an office for NORD in Danbury Connecticut. When the landlord heard about NORD, he asked whether patients with the just named AIDS might visit the premises. Meyer had no answer. The landlord told her she would have to go elsewhere, but after a 'meal' with one of Meyer's supporters he made a substantial donation. AZT was the first drug approved under Orphan Drug provisions, with almost all other drugs for AIDS and its associated infections approved in the same way.

Haddad introduced Meyer to Agnes Varis, the owner of AgVar, a generic company. Varis was connected to everyone in the generic industry and the Democratic Party. At this stage rare diseases were fronted by ALS, multiple sclerosis (MS) and hemophilia. A drug called copaxone had shown benefit for MS, but Meyer couldn't persuade a branded company to pick it up. It had been discovered in the Weizmann Institute in Israel. Varis strong-armed Teva, a small Israeli generic company, to pick it up. It was approved under the Orphan Drugs Act and became a blockbuster, earning Teva over $1 billion per year.

While *Orphan Drugs* is a compelling read, as of 2016, branded drugs were a $1,275 billion-dollar industry, half of whose profits ($638 billion) came from drugs brought to market in the standard way while the other half ($637 billion) were orphans. These included AbbVie's Humira, the most profitable drug ever, Merck's Vioxx, Lilly's Cialis, Astra's Crestor, Bristol Myers Squibb's Abilify, Botox, and many best-selling drugs.

While it is possible to close some loopholes that lead from orphans to blockbusters, the precedent of allowing high prices for drugs that will supposedly only ever occupy niche markets has laid a niche-busting business model for personalized medicines. If genetic tests ever permit a tailoring of medicines to specific patient groups, the orphan argument will apply. Without mentioning Waxman, the *Wall Street Journal* began trumpeting the lifeline the Orphan Drugs Act had thrown the pharmaceutical industry

Patent Wars

After the collapse of the Drug Regulation Reform Act in 1979, Pharma lobbied for a Patent Term Extension Act, arguing that bureaucracy had reduced effective patent life from 17 to 7.5 years and was producing a drug lag, and fewer drugs. While companies had avoided collapse and managed to hold prices steady when all other prices were rising, politicians needed to act before America's pharmaceutical industry went the way of its automobile industry. Granting patent extension of 7 years would return patent life to what Thomas Jefferson intended. The argument had wide support.

The rollback of anti-substitution laws had created a fledgling generic industry. But the expected wholesale switch from costly branded drugs to low-cost generics hadn't happened. Generics had less than 10% of market share with little sign of change. Kennedy's Act contained proposals to facilitate the licensing of generic drugs. Its collapse left generic companies in limbo. The move to patent extension threatened to kill them.

The companies banded together in 1980 to form GPIA, with Haddad its CEO and Alfred Engelberg as legal counsel. Engelberg's parents fled Germany in 1938 and he was born a year later. He attended law school at night in 1961 and worked by day in the patent office. The work there was done by up to a thousand examiners, half of whom were students like him, who simply looked for 'prior art'. He then moved to the Justice Department, defending the US Government when they infringed patents, as they regularly and legally did. He joined a Manhattan law firm and in 1974 slipped into defending Primo Pharmaceuticals charged with infringing the patent on Upjohn's tolbutamide. To his surprise, Upjohn were keen to settle and to pay to delay anyone else becoming aware of this. Engelberg got a name in generic circles.

Henry Waxman and Al Gore fronted the opposition to the Patent Term Extension Act, backed by Engelberg and Haddad. Gore's response to pro-extension industry arguments was there was no evidence for falling profits, reduced research spending, or fewer effective drugs. Jefferson had sanctioned patents as a reward for disclosing an invention. Patents helped raise capital and were designed to benefit the community rather guarantee a fixed period for commercial exploitation.

The power of the pharmaceutical industry, Engelberg argued, lay not in patents but in its ability to monopolize markets through brands and the ability to persuade doctors there were important differences between two drops of water. Roche's Librium and Valium were close to identical drugs but had been targeted by Arthur Sackler at subtly different markets. When Librium went off patent, even though it was 16 times the price of the generic competition, it still accounted for over 90% of its market niche and hadn't interfered with Valium becoming the biggest selling drug in the world.

Industry had an even tighter lock on the market than this, Congress was told. The first patent application on Valium was filed in 1959, after which a series of others were filed until the final patent was granted in 1968. The 17 years of patent protection only began trickling through the hourglass after this. Haddad branded strategies for patent prolongation as "evergreening".

Industry and the Reagan government contrasted Washington delay with private company efficiency. Where did FDA delay begin and end, Gore asked? Post-thalidomide, even if there were no FDA, no prudent businessman would bring a drug to market without animal tests and clinical trials. It made business sense to cover the legal liabilities and explore markets at the same time under the cover of patent protection. The only delay FDA could be blamed for was the time spent scrutinizing the paperwork. User fees could overcome that.

Industry's Patent Restoration Act passed in the Senate. It needed a two-thirds majority in the House of Representatives. It failed by 5 votes.

Waxman took the initiative. He introduced a Drug Price Competition and Patent Term Restoration Act. The goal was to lower drug prices by fostering competition while providing incentives for innovation. A key issue was whether a generic company could develop a generic to present to FDA without infringing the branded patent. Passage of the bill required a deal. In a series of meetings over 10 days, Haddad and Engelberg for GPIA and lawyers for government and industry traded a baseline 5-year period of exclusivity from the time of marketing for access to prepare an application and acceptance that with equivalence testing the generic chemical would be regarded as kosher. It also became easier for generic companies to challenge patents. Finally, a medicine is a chemical plus information. As regards the information, the generic companies would adopt the branded label.

This pragmatism drew fire from both leading branded companies and Public Citizen. But it made sense to let a branded company make a market and tackle initial safety issues. Relationships were central to the deal. The Act needed a sponsor in the Senate. Mylan Pushkar, owner of Mylan, the only Republican among the generic company owners, lined up Orrin Hatch (R Utah). Hatch and Haddad bonded. The bill passed just as Congress recessed for the 1984 presidential election.

Changing Roles

Challenged by a case in which Leonard Arthur, an English pediatrician, had been acquitted of murder, having issued instructions "for nursing care only" on the birth of a healthy baby with Down's syndrome, in 1982 Lasagna wrote *Murder Most Foul*. English medicine, he said, had lost its moral compass. He mentioned his son Christopher had Down's syndrome, which limited him in some ways, but also endowed him with a congenital inability to hate.

Arthur Sackler wrote to him:

> *I have so much to thank you for. Whenever I read one of your papers, get together with you in a scientific meeting, even in the simplest interchange, I come away enriched…You do manage to constantly probe issues which, whether recognized or submerged, are central to so much of our thinking and decision-making.*

Sackler wrote an editorial on *Murder Most Foul* in *Medical Tribune*. He then invited Lasagna to become dean of the new Sackler School of Medicine at Tufts in Boston. Lasagna moved to Boston in 1984 and the Center for the Study of Drug Development moved with him. Sackler died from a heart attack in 1987.

Haddad meanwhile became executive Vice-President of DeLorean Motor Cars (DMC). John DeLorean prided himself on making deals and saw himself as a future president. Both men agreed the company was not just about making money. It was about making ethical cars in locations that needed jobs, like Belfast and the Bronx, made by people whom others said couldn't or wouldn't work. It was great branding, but DeLorean ended up in jail.

After Hatch-Waxman, Haddad became the CEO of Danbury (later Schein) Pharmaceuticals. Here too, he had a vision of a business that would promote a public good—access to medicines. The owners didn't share the vision: a business was for making money.

Whether it was for making money or promoting the public good, there was an obvious strategy for a generic company: target the patents of the best-selling branded compounds. The use of beta-blockers as anti-hy-pertensives had provided a cornerstone for Lasagna to make a drug-lag argument. Except for propranolol (Inderal) which had come on the US market in 1968, the US had none of these drugs while Europe was full of them. Under huge pressure, FDA licensed a series of beta-blockers and by the mid-1980s three of the ten best-selling drugs were beta-blockers.

Knowing the beta-blocker patents were granted by students, Engelberg checked them out. They were indistinguishable from each other structurally and functionally. There was no novelty. He quit his Manhattan law firm and set up joint ventures with Schein and other companies to target patents, the deal being he got a share of the profits if the challenge succeeded.

He challenged cyclobenzaprine, sold by Merck as Flexeril for back pain. This was very similar to Merck's antidepressant amitriptyline. The patent was unenforceable because Merck had withheld information about the similarity to amitriptyline. For two and half years after generic cyclo-benzaprine launched, Engelberg got a cheque for $6.25 million every quarter. A patent challenge on buspirone gave him $38 million. He retired and became a philanthropist. Other lawyers flocked to the action. A significant proportion of the generic industry ended up owned by lawyers, who often only had to file challenges to get 'paid to delay'.

The Price of Drugs

Healthcare reform was part of the Clinton presidential platform in 1992. Drug costs were central to this. After the election Donna Shalala, the newly appointed Health and Human Services Secretary, held hearings at which branded and generic industries were asked why prescription drug prices were so much higher in America than elsewhere?

The generic industry was in some trouble at this point. Hatch-Waxman had included a period of exclusivity for a company that filed first after the patent on a branded product expired. Mylan claimed it kept being pipped at the post. It hired a private investigator, who targeted the trash of Charles Chang, an FDA official, and found evidence that Par Pharmaceuticals had been bribing Chang and other officials. The spreading net caught Bolar Pharmaceuticals who had submitted branded diazoxide for bio-equivalence testing of its generic version. Executives from the company went to jail. A generic drug scandal featured in the press, leading to Congressional Hearings, marked by disenchantment that the good guys had turned out to be as greedy as others more than by evidence of substantial wrongdoing. Dee Fensterer, the lead for GPIA at this point, was credited with steering the new industry through choppy waters.

In 1992 responding to Donna Shalala's questions about drug costs, Robert Allnutt, vice-president of PhRMA agreed it was unsatisfactory that 70 million Americans were without prescription drug coverage. PhRMA believed all prescription drugs should come with a benefit to help cover costs. Within a managed competition system, prices could be kept down. Companies would be willing to do this on an industry wide basis, if the justice department didn't regard it as monopoly behavior. He also noted that price increases had slowed dramatically and were often higher in Europe for new drugs. Price controls, he concluded, would bias drug development toward low risk, low benefit products.

Dee Fensterer responded that there were two different industries. A generic fiercely competitive industry, and the branded industry. The branded beta-blocker Inderal cost $37 for 100 tablets in 1988, while generic propranolol cost $4. Inderal cost $57 in 1992, while propranolol cost $1.84. Rebates and perverse incentives were part of the problem. Medicaid incentives favored brands.

Generics were taking close to 45% of the 1992 market in pharmaceuticals, despite the generic scandal. Twenty years later they were taking 85% of the US market, and the global generic market was worth $260 billion. But drug costs were still taking 10% of the healthcare budget. The branded industry, meanwhile, a $20 billion industry in 1984 had grown to a $1,275 billion industry worldwide, $400 billion in the United States.

Direct to Consumer Advertising (DTCA) had helped this growth. In May 1983, the Boots Pharmaceutical Company, discoverer of an analgesic, ibuprofen, ran a television advert in Florida noting their brand of ibuprofen was cheaper than others. This was information consumer associations had said they wanted. The Federal Trade Commission (FTC) told Boots to take it down. There followed two years of debate over DTCA. Lasagna argued companies would find DTCA bothersome, but many patients might welcome the relief from the paternalism of FDA. On the back of the precedent of providing contraceptive information to consumers, FTC agreed to DTCA. Little happened until 1997 when Schering began broadcasting adverts for their branded generic Claritin, after which DTCA took off.

In the meantime, the generic industry was consolidating. Some of its leading members, such as Teva, had become members of PhRMA. Traveling in the opposite direction, Novartis's Sandoz and Pfizer's Greenstone were among the top 5 leading generic companies.

Another player also emerged. The first pharmacy benefits management (PBM) company was set up in 1968 to negotiate with health insurers, drug companies and pharmacies on prices. With generic discounts on branded products, the potential for PBMs grew. PBMs originally promoted low-cost generics but later helped branded companies with new high-cost drugs. The branded companies bought and then divested themselves of PBMs, after which PBMs bought pharmacy chains and required patients to collect their drugs from PBM pharmacies. Backroom deals were done involving rebates and spreads. The costlier the drug a PBM endorsed, the greater it made on rebates. PBMs raked in billions in profits while drug prices escalated.

In the 2016 presidential election, both branded and generic drug prices were an issue. Breathtaking spikes in the prices of generic drugs led Trump and Clinton to promise an end to company gouging. The furor centered on Mylan's Epipen and Turing Pharma's Daraprim.

Daraprim (pyrimethamine) was licensed by FDA in 1952. As of 2010, it was primarily used to treat toxoplasmosis in patients with AIDS and secondarily for malaria. Owned by GSK, it retailed at $1 a pill in 2010 when sold to Core Pharma, which in turn was bought by Impax. The price rose to $13.50. When Turing bought it, the price jumped to $750.

Daraprim was not unique. Several older drugs were bought by unknown pharmaceutical companies, who hiked prices by 100% to 5000% to support future research. These companies, owned by hedge funds, had no research plans. The gamble worked because Medicare and Medicaid became cash cows when the Bush administration blocked their ability to negotiate on price. The hedge funds made money unless, like Turing, a brash executive, Martin Shkreli, and a 5000% hike tripped them up.

ACCIDENT OR MURDER?

On February 4, 1970, with the French government still shaking after the 1968 revolution, sixteen miners died, and others were maimed in an explosion at a mine in Lens. The mine owners pitched the event as an accident. It didn't help their case that Northern France had a history of mine disasters, including in 1906 the worst ever in Europe. This is the reason we have insurance, the owners said.

The miners asked the Marxist philosopher Jean-Paul Sartre to present their case. There are no accidents, Sartre claimed. The owners knew there would be a certain number of deaths each year and factored this into their costs. There had been five the year before. Injured workers thought their job was risky and if injured they were just unlucky. They were mistaken, Sartre said. It was murder.

Calling the deaths murder made them an event. A pivotal moment for the Left. But despite a lack of trust in the government, French society didn't follow Sartre down this route. The crushing of the Prague Spring in 1968 made it seem unlikely the miners would have been treated any differently in Eastern Europe. When Sartre was buried in 1980, French Marxism was buried with him.

Michel Foucault, who had emerged in France as offering an alternative to Marxism, branded Sartre as a nineteenth century Liberal, a believer in contracts and the Rule of Law. The twentieth century, Foucault claimed, required a turn from economics to seeing power as the key issue. He and Francois Ewald pitched an 1898 Worker's Compensation Law as marking the advent of the Providential State. Where Liberal Society was based on contracts, the 1898 Law, they said, marked a wider distribution of power. It pointed to a Third Way, neither Left nor Right, that sought stakeholder consensus around what the science showed.

As Sartre was buried, the idea America might face an overwhelming plague and its people wonder which of their sins had led to this visitation would have seemed fanciful. But like Banquo's ghost, reports emerged in 1980 of patients dying of a rare infection, Pneumocystis Carini. This was followed in 1981 by reports of deaths from a rare skin disorder, Kaposi's sarcoma. The patients were white homosexual men. Twelve articles in 1982 described other deaths from rare conditions. The 12 publications mushroomed to 2,700 scientific articles by 1986 in addition to acres of newsprint and hours of TV coverage devoted to the new plague. Those dying were immune deficient. They had Acquired Immune-Deficiency Syndrome (AIDS). The homosexual link fueled speculation about promiscuous and perverse sex, despite reports of a similar disorder in drug users, and then hemophiliacs, and women, and finally in babies born to women with the disorder.

The idea a virus might cause AIDS appeared in 1982. If it was a virus, it was different to anything previously encountered. Retroviruses had been discovered in the 1960s but were thought to be commensals we can live with. In 1983 Robert Gallo claimed a retrovirus caused AIDS. As with germs in the 1880s, the idea of a virus dampened some fears by pointing to ways we might avoid it, while spreading the fear anyone could catch it.

When Luc Montagnier, a French virologist, pinpointed a different virus, a dispute between two white men playing out in the media helped spread awareness. The US Government celebrated and patented Gallo's achievement but Montagnier was right. An antibody test to the Montagnier virus was developed and in 1986 the new virus was named Human Immuno-Deficiency Virus (HIV). While this kindled hope for a future treatment, the lack of a treatment meant a positive test was close to a death sentence.

In 1960 Jerome Horwitz a cancer researcher from Michigan had designed azidothymidine, later called zidovudine, AZT for short, as a possible anticancer agent. It didn't work. Burroughs-Wellcome acquired the drug and tested it for anti-viral properties. It didn't work. In 1985 the National Cancer Institute called for reverse transcriptase inhibitors to tackle a retrovirus. AZT did this in test tubes. Given clinically, it increased T-cell counts, the cells depleted by the virus in AIDS patients.

Wellcome submitted a New Drug Application to FDA in July 1985 aimed at showing increased T Cell counts in patients given AZT. They reported the finding in the *Lancet* in March 1986. A larger study stopped early in September 1986 as there was apparently a clinical benefit in addition to improved white cell counts. AZT was approved in 1987, two years after first submission, the first Orphan Drug. Wellcome, whose share-price was booming, launched it with a price tag of $8-10,000, for a compound on which they had done almost no work, and which was a quarter of a century old.

AZT was debatably beneficial, definitely toxic, and with a tendency to produce resistance. Against a background of dampened hopes, conspiracy theories flourished. Some blamed the virus on the CIA. Peter Duesberg, an eminent virologist, claimed it was a hoax. Buyers' Clubs, later celebrated in Hollywood movies, were set up to import drugs from Mexico. The authorities agreed to previously inconceivable public health measures, such as supplying clean needles to intravenous drug users. Even the Vatican accepted a role for condoms.

Establishment experts, however, appeared to be withholding treatments in the interests of purist research. For sufferers this was close to sadistic. In 1987 Larry Kramer established an AIDS Coalition to Unleash Power (ACT-UP) in New York. Related groups formed in San Francisco and around the country, comprised of people who compared themselves to troops in a War being led by academic generals and bureaucrats as out of touch as any British generals in World War I. Armchair ideas about how RCTs should work, these activists felt, were not appropriate in a life-and-death battlefield situation.

ACT-UP took to the streets with theater, demonstrations, and publicity-grabbing headlines. Holocausts, they reminded people, happened because of inaction and there was a genocidal inaction here. These deaths were not accidents. They were murder. Human need, suffering and death, seemed to count for little to FDA compared to the importance of orderly process and well-maintained policies.

In the trials for AZT and other compounds, patients began to break the blind and share the medication around. In the case of another compound, ddC, activists found a way to make it in bathtubs. The volunteers didn't agree they had donated their bodies to science. In their view key decisions, including those of trial design, must remain with the person whose life was on the line. Manuals were produced on how manage doctors and experts.

This activism made it clear that professionalism or expertise can only function where there isn't an opposing community. In the face of a community, authority loses its footing. This was a replay of the history of trade unionism. And of drug discovery. AIDS activists viewed FDA as boxed into the position *vis-à-vis* new treatments that Evarts and Kline (chapter 6) had predicted in 1956: "You're going to freeze yourself into one moderately successful drug to treat AIDS."

On October 11, 1988, demonstrating outside FDA's headquarters, the activists were invited in. Well versed in trial methods and regulatory codes by this point, their message was 'we can do business', but we have to change RCTs from a gold-standard tick-box for bureaucrats to something that works for people whose lives are on the line. FDA's brief, they argued, was not just to keep people safe but to promote health. Few wanted to fuel Republican style deregulation, but AIDS Activists and Republicans found themselves on one side of a fence with traditional consumer activists and liberals on the other.

In 1988 Lasagna chaired a Presidential Committee to look at access to AIDS and cancer drugs. This followed his call in 1982:

> *The time is ripe to proclaim and implement a new mission for the FDA—to speed the public's access to important new drugs. No change in the law is needed to do this—simply acceptance that past approaches have not served the public well enough.*[44]

He found himself facing a consumer group who "must have read everything I ever wrote and quoted whatever served their purpose. It was quite an experience." A group, who were proud of looking bizarre and given to dramatics like dangling a watch in front of the committee. They advocated everything he had been suggesting for decades, especially the right to take risks. The activists found him sympathetic. Treatments for AIDs, perhaps coincidentally, made more progress in the decade that followed than the treatment of mental illness has made in seven decades.

Over time, the Activists and Experts converged. Both sides agreed that conflicting study results showed how hype could shape perceptions. While agreeing there was some merit in individuals foregoing their rights to further a wider public benefit, activists argued that on ethical and pragmatic grounds, entry into trials had to be voluntary. Trials would work better if compassionate approval let some patients access the drugs without having to enter a trial. This would ensure the integrity of trials that took

---

44 Lasagna L. "Will all new drugs become orphans?" *Clinical Pharmacology & Therapeutics 31* (1982), 285-9.

place. There was also a call to take patients as they were, which included treating their opportunistic infections rather than deny them all treatment other than the trial compound.

These debates revealed that both experts and activists expected trials to settle issues and be authoritative. Both wanted to be told what treatment to recommend. Unless we understand the biology, however, trials can do little other than steer people away from junk treatments. The search for certainty risks disillusion and recrimination. When AZT failed to meet hopes, every rise in Wellcome's share-price led to outrage, every company donation to activists became an effort to co-opt.

Little of the science was happening in companies. Most of it was in NIH. The hierarchy at the top of science didn't seem accidental to the activists, or that scientists kept advocating more of the same. There was a move to take the research back from NIH. A County Community Consortium in San Francisco and a Community Research Initiative in New York ran their own studies. Based on these studies, in 1989 FDA approved pentamidine for PCP infections. This was a first ever license for community-based research. This success ironically may have helped turn some Family Medicine clinics into clinical trial mills through which from 1990 onwards pharma marched a lot of shoddy drugs.

FDA culture however was changed by these controversies. It endorsed compassionate use and accelerated approval without an Act of Congress. Reviewing developments, the National Research Council (NRC) stated that every aspect of the process by which new drugs are identified, evaluated, regulated, and allocated had been tested by the exigencies of this epidemic. The NRC didn't address the question of whether it was appropriate for trials to be part of the regulatory system. The activist view was that it would have been easier for doctors and patients to organize good trials after a drug became available than it was to do so before approval. The activist view is arguably the correct place for clinical trials in medicine.

Struggles in ACT UP had white males focused on curing AIDS on one side. For this faction a seat at the regulatory table was critical. On the other side were activists, including many women, who wanted to reform healthcare in general. This group wanted to boycott the establishment. This echoed the split between socialists for whom a seat at the table is important and communists.

It was estimated 400,000 people in the US were HIV positive in 1994 and 4 million worldwide. Just at the point activists had begun to accept trials had a role in winnowing out bright ideas and test-tube wonders, and the search for effective solutions would be a long haul, an answer came. It did not come from clinical trials.

Progress in mapping the HIV virus suggested combining drugs that intervened at more than one spot in the virus's mechanics. A range of drugs including protease inhibitors, reverse transcriptase inhibitors, integrase inhibitors and others, came on the market in 1996. None were any better than AZT. Each were approved separately on the basis of modest blood test results. But, it quickly became clear that combining 3 drugs together from at least two groups produced an almost Lazarus-like effect. Highly Active Anti-Retroviral Therapy (HAART) was consolidated into one tablet combinations—Triple Therapy. Trials weren't needed to convince anyone. Terminally ill people came back to life in days on Triple Therapy, almost like rehydrating cholera patients.

Triple Therapy came with a $15,000 per annum price tag and it would have to be taken for life. There were estimates that 8000 people were dying a day in Southern Africa, none of whom could afford this price. Pressure built to review prices.

Companies talked about branded generics at $1200 per annum and blocked efforts to introduce lower cost generic drugs. In February 1998, industry took Nelson Mandela to court, saying his government's attempts to make affordable medicines available violated the South African constitution and World Trade Agreements. There was public outrage.

In May 2000, the US government filed a complaint with the World Trade Organization (WTO) against Brazil for compulsorily licensing AIDS medicines so indigenous companies could make them. US government representatives claimed it was pointless making treatment available at reduced costs because Africans and Latinos were so uneducated they would never be able to make it work. In failing they would create treatment resistance that would harm Americans. Even the *Wall Street Journal* asked, "Can the pharmaceutical industry inflict more damage upon its ailing public image?"

The WTO complaint fell apart in the wake of an anthrax scare in the weeks after 9/11, when the Bush Government publicly considered compulsorily licensing Bayer's Cipro, making everyone aware that US administrations routinely infringed patents.

David Langdon, a Peace Corp activist, took the obvious step and contacted Bill Haddad. Haddad contacted Agnes Varis, who directed him to Yusuf Hamied, the owner of Cipla, an Indian generics company. An Access to Medicines campaign began. Haddad and a group of activists flew to London to meet Hamied who agreed to help bust a cartel. Gaining access to a meeting between EU and African leaders, Hamied pitched triple therapy at a price of $900. There were no takers. He then offered triple therapy at $354, less than a dollar a day. He threw in nevirapine for free, a treatment that inhibited transmission between pregnant women and their offspring. This price made it impossible for international donor programs not to mount an effort to ensure that everyone who needed treatment could have it. A few years later the price of triple therapy had dropped to $100 a year.

These events made clear the pharmaceutical industry operate a pay us what we want, or you will die business model. The ratio between the price offered by branded companies for Triple Therapy and the price Hamied offered was the same ratio separating branded and McKesson's offer to Colombia forty years before.

Coda

Michel Foucault had been one of the first to argue we needed to look closely at medicine and not just assume it was a story of progress. When Russian tanks rolled into Prague in 1968, they undermined Sartre and made Foucault famous.

After 1968, with its growing affluence and flourishing sciences, the West seemed to be pulling ever further ahead of the Eastern bloc. "If you don't think the Free Market is a good system, just ask yourself whether you would get better drugs in Eastern Europe" was a regular battle cry. (Czechoslovakia and Hungary in the 1960s produced many of the drugs that fed Western pharmaceutical companies).

A growing mismatch in Eastern Europe between what people wanted and were told they wanted led to uprisings in Hungary and Poland and the crushing of socialism with a human face in Prague. After 1968, the Czechs with *Charter 77* and Poles with *Solidarnosc* created 'dissent' to tackle a new kind of dictatorship. Classical dictatorship had been imposed by a minority, was temporary, and usurped the rule of law. The new dictatorship governed in the name of the majority, looked permanent, and depended on law and process.

This dictatorship, Vaclav Havel said, depended on an act of hypnosis enabled by that part of us that wants to allocate responsibility to a system rather than assume it ourselves. We will mouth slogans and embrace rituals that bind us into something we can hide behind, if this lets us get on with life. While at one level we know functionaries, claiming to have our interests at heart, deal in numbers and not people, and there is no safety net beneath us, paradoxically we seem to trust the authorities even more in the era of Big Brother. They will pull things out the fire if we end up being asked to get on a train travelling East.

The new dissidents resisted being labelled a political opposition. Their call was to avoid compromising with the lie. They took a stand on the value of lives as people chose to live them. They saw a West seduced by consumer goods into its own false consciousness. What inner prompting or outer circumstance turns some into dissidents is unclear, but in the 1980s Eastern dissent grew in strength.

ACT UP was a comparable dissident campaign that took a stand on the value of enabling people to live the lives they wanted to live. It branded AIDS deaths as murder not accidents.

Eastern dissent burst into flame in 1989. The Berlin Wall came down. Vaclav Havel and Lech Walesa became their countries leaders. The Soviet Union disintegrated. In 1992 Francis Fukayama's *End of History* claimed we were witnessing the universalization of Western liberal democracy. Chicago had become the spiritual home of neoliberalism and in 1994 the University of Chicago Press reissued Hayek's *The Road to Serfdom.*

Foucault didn't live to see the Velvet or ACT-UP revolutions. He died from AIDS in 1984. His father, Paul, was a doctor. The son's deconstruction of medicine would not have seemed accidental to a Freudian, especially given his name—Paul Michel Foucault. Nor would his death from AIDS. The fact that Luc Montagnier, the discoverer of the AIDS virus, had been taught by Paul Foucault would seem closer to an accident (random), even though French medical circles were small enough for this link to be possible.

There is as good a case for calling Foucault an early neo-liberal as there was for calling Sartre an old-style liberal. He saw a possible Third Way through technocracy but didn't live to see the financialization and pharmaceuticalization of the 1990s that technology facilitated.

When Triple Therapy began saving lives in 1996, it apparently fulfilled Western promise. But the AIDS epidemic, cutting across the trajectory of a newly emerging passionless one-dimensional, odor-free medicine, was like Banquo's ghost turning up at a feast to mark the start of a new and uncomfortable reign. Triple Therapy was a pharmaceutical sideshow. The market in medicines by then was about anti-hypertensives, antidepressants, hypoglycemics, bisphosphonates and other risk managing drugs. Drug profits have since climbed 20-fold, with cocktail treatment the norm and life expectancy falling.

Yusuf Hamied kickstarted the Indian and Chinese generic industries. Uncontrolled by regulators, these may have caused more deaths than they have prevented. The branded industry has also moved production facilities to developing countries, where there is no oversight of their products. AIDS was a 1968 moment; a moment where apparent liberation was a harbinger of ever deeper enmeshment in an apparatus.

Reviewing the freedom his countrymen in 2015 had to live the lives they chose to live, Havel regarded their position as worse than it had been in 1989. Campaigning for access to lifesaving medicines has become a ticket to polypharmacy, drugs of lower quality, and an earlier death. Accident?

9: BIG RISK AND PHARMACEUTICALIZATION

Before 1800 the word accident was applied in two ways. Arms and legs were accidents in the sense of incidental rather than essential to being a human. They were also Acts of God; something that had no explanation, such as when it rains fish, or a cow jumps over a fence and lands on a passing car. In showing certain events recur predictably, statistics transform recurrent events into risks. These events and power interact. As patients or workers, we live in a world of risks we should avoid and for which we are responsible. Owners or managers, however, handle accidents for which they can't be held responsible.

Risk is recent. As of 1970, the word risk featured in the titles or abstracts of 200 academic articles. By 1990 it was 20,000. As Freud sank from view, a new realization that no one is 'rational' produced new risk perception and risk communication industries. This rediscovery of everyday irrationality put a premium on getting to grips with the dynamics of the popular mind on issues like dioxins, nuclear power, and drug wrecks. A newly emerging set of health services turned away from healthcare to the management of health risks.

Risk Prevention

When Josephine Baker created preventive medicine, aimed at building resilience in individuals and reducing contributory causes of disease, she met resistance from many physicians.

In 1981 Geoffrey Rose, a London physician, claimed infant and maternal healthcare had succeeded by focusing on children and mothers when well to prevent them getting ill. The traditional medical focus on disease, he claimed, was wrong. Just as getting everyone to wear a seat belt can save more lives than getting joyriders only to wear seat belts, so focusing on a population, most of whom are at minimal risk, would save more lives than focusing on high risk or diseased individuals. To eliminate heart attacks, medicine must treat all elevations of blood pressure.

Rose fingered salt as the cause of hypertension. When he tried in Wales to reduce dietary salt, it made no difference. His idea of treating entire populations, however, fascinated public health departments, even though medicating people who are well crucially differs from preventing them from smoking or using salt. Few worried at the prospect of 'poisoning' hundreds of people to prevent a cardiac death, even if overall mortality rose.

Risk Prevention, later badged as Health Promotion, invited us to manage risks lying within us rather than in our environment. While there was some promotion of healthy lifestyles, doctors didn't argue with a preventive medicine that meant dishing out more pills not less. A promise of cost savings swung governments and insurers behind mandatory screening and withholding information about the harms of treatment in case anyone might be dissuaded from treatment. As with vaccines, the population risks seemed to lie in non-treatment.

Since Hippocrates, medicine had focused on acute life-threatening crises from infections, trauma, epilepsy, and obstetrics along with a few chronic disorders like leprosy, or arthritis. After Rose, the focus switched to what became Chronic Disease Management—even though few of those being managed have anything medically wrong with them. They have mild thinning of their bones, a wheeze, minimal elevations of blood pressure, blood sugars, or lipids, or nerves. These risk states make Pharma its money rather than medical diseases for which, apart from HAART for AIDS, Solvaldi for hepatitis and Gleevec for leukemia, we have no better treatments than we had in 1980.

The new focus made Lasagna look as much like a nineteenth century liberal as Sartre. Meeting organizers scrambling to explain the new concept of risk to audiences asked him to lecture, missing his endorsement of risk taking rather than risk avoiding, his view that risk benefit assessments could not be undertaken, and that deaths as a result of FDA inaction were closer to murder than accidents.

A few years before, in 1976, the pharmaceutical industry had told Congress their share prices were about to collapse even though:

> *Human beings have within reach the capacity to control or prevent human disease… there do not appear to be any impenetrable, incomprehensible diseases. This in itself represents a major advance for biomedical science, and it is a change that has occurred only in the last twenty-five years.*[45]

Share prices will stay up, if there is no competition and an industry can charge whatever it wants. But the branded industry was facing competition from generic drugs, and orphan drugs had not yet thrown it a lifeline. The other way to maintain share price is to 'grow' the market. With antihypertensives, hypoglycemics, and drugs for osteoporosis and lipid lowering, Rose's argument could be used to portray the population as having several 'diseases' at the same time and in perpetuity.

The US drugs market was worth just over $20 billion in 1984. Five years later Glaxo's antacid, Zantac, became the first blockbuster drug—a drug grossing $1 billion per annum. A decade later Pfizer's lipid lowering Lipitor was grossing $13 billion per annum. By then more money was being spent in the US on marketing the risks of cholesterol than on research on dementia, autism, arthritis, multiple sclerosis, sickle cell anemia and other traditional medical disorders combined. Company share prices held up.

---

45 *President's Biomedical Research Panel*, (April 1976).

Patients in 1980 were typically on one medicine only; seven is now the norm for anyone over 60. Anyone put on an antibiotic is likely to already be on some combination of antihypertensives, statins, bisphosphonates, hypoglycemics and psychotropics. Medicine, traditionally skeptical of vitamins, dietary fads, and fashions whipped up to counter notional risks had a Damascene conversion to Risk Prevention. This was key to transforming healthcare into health services.

Risk Management

Numbers create risk. The data from rating scales, peak flow meters, cholesterol levels and bone density scans, set up new risk markets. As with all measurements from the first weighing scales in the 1870s, these measures provide data from one aspect of life. This data captures our attention. A focus on the data from stopwatches in athletics for instance can be put to constructive use. A focus on the data from rating scales for ADHD or peak flow rates also hypnotizes us and is likely to put us at the mercy of suggestions that the numbers point to risks drugs can manage. The data conjure up Lipitor, Fosamax, or Januvia nervosa disorders, the way weighing scale data conjures up anorexia nervosa.

Around 1960, companies began to market depression (melancholia), hypertension (process hypertension) and Type 1 diabetes. These are real and sometimes lethal disorders. Merck's Diuril for hypertension and Tryptizol for depression saved lives. Distinguished physicians wrote books on depression and hypertension and their treatments. Companies distributed these for educational purposes, along with teaching aids, rating scales, and blood-pressure monitoring devices. The risks of treatment were spelt out.

This set a template for selling pills by selling disorders. By 2000, thousands of ghostwritten publications were being pumped out to sell osteoporosis, social anxiety disorder, erectile dysfunction, and restless legs syndrome. Diuril was a benign treatment for the malignant hypertension that killed Franklin Roosevelt. Restless legs, however, already had a good treatment, but was marketed to sell dopamine-agonists like ropinirole which are capable of inducing compulsive gambling, sexual perversions and other impulsive behaviors.

In 1960 clinical judgment aimed at distinguishing a process hypertension that might become malignant from a benign even helpful ageing related blood pressure increase. The goal was to treat the one where the benefits of medication might outweigh the risks, while managing the other conservatively. After 1981, there was a shift to medicating all elevations of blood pressure, reductions in respiratory flow or loss of bone density. Where physicians once tried to establish the cause of a patient's blood pressure rise, or fall in their respiratory flow, the new focus was simply on treating numbers. This focus inhibits a recognition that a 70-year-old woman's fatigue might stem from her antihypertensive, hypoglycemic or bisphosphonate rather than her age. Without diagnostic discrimination, treatment can become a disorder that mandates further treatment.

Before 1981 physicians focused on avoidable triggers to reduce the likelihood of an asthma attack but there is little interest now in pinpointing triggers. Many epilepsies can be managed without medication through judicious food intake, avoiding fatigue, and recognizing stressors, but few get told this now. In the 1980s companies making H-2 antagonists for gastric acid, like the blockbuster Zantac, blocked efforts to establish that *h. pylori* infections might cause ulcers that antibiotics could cure.

As a result of this sea-change, forty years after their share price was ostensibly about to collapse, while companies still claimed to be keeping drug prices at 10% of overall health expenditures, the 2016 US drug bill was $400 billion. Total healthcare spend had risen to $4 trillion, 18% of GDP. Rather than delivering care, a large proportion of the extra $3.6 trillion funds a distribution channel that ensures what industry terms unmet needs get met.

Some years ago, I slipped in the shower on a Friday and fractured my shoulder. A surgeon advised a plate to avoid losing the function of my arm. The operation was done that day and I was back at work on Monday. A service this effective could be provided for free from the savings on sick leave and payments for locums. It benefits me and my community.

Shortly afterwards, a letter invited me to have my bones screened. In most health services, everyone of a certain age who has a fracture gets a similar letter. A sizeable proportion of those screened are told they have some bone thinning (osteopenia) and are invited to avoid risks by taking a bone thickening drug. This is bankrupting us.

Osteopenia (bone thinning) is a non-illness, manufactured to bring consumers to products they would otherwise never buy, in this case the bone thickening bisphosphonate drugs. These drugs emerged in the 1980s, with the statins to lower cholesterol levels and other drugs, whose marketing centers on generating perceptions that treating the risk of a fracture, heart attack, or suicide is the same as treating a fracture, heart attack or mental illness.

Company claims that drug increases in bone densities offer the same benefits as the plate in my shoulder led to screening programs, facilitated by free bone scanners provided by companies. Rates of long bone fractures rose. Auditors were hired to monitor adherence to screening. Then managers were hired to sort out failing programs. As developments took shape, the data behind company claims for these drugs became inaccessible, the medical articles about the drugs ghost-written, and guidelines emerged that almost forced doctors to prescribe bisphosphonates (chapter 11). Emergency departments were faced with dramatic rarely seen before spiral fractures of long bones. These were used to support more screening and treatment, even though they are caused by bisphosphonates.

Talk of drug treatments for osteoporosis leads many to lose confidence in their body which, in turn, reduces physical activity, and increases the risk of fractures. Bisphosphonates are also associated with other costly treatment-induced disorders. This health 'care' makes people less productive.

Money spent on screeners, auditors and managers mean we employ a pharmaceutical sales force. In so doing, along with the costs of treating drug-induced injuries, we enable companies to claim the cost of new high-cost drugs remains a constant fraction of overall budgets. Pointing to hospital costs that remain one third of health spend, companies imply more medicines will keep people out of hospital and costs down even as treatment-induced disabilities become a leading cause of admission and prolonged stays. Replacing a hip is costly but hip replacements are restricted to people in need and the gain in productivity on getting us back to work could allow us to deliver replacements for free. The funds that might do this, instead, get diverted to feed the osteopenic cuckoos in the medical nest.

Treating these new conditions does not save lives or reduce disability. These 'treatments' are, however, more gratifying for doctors than classic medical treatments. Blood pressures fall on an antihypertensive, and cholesterol on a statin, more reliably than a heart attack, stroke or cancer responds to treatment. The outcomes on risk prevention drugs are quality outcomes, in a Big Mac sense of quality, namely that we get the same hamburger every time. This makes the new health services seductive, and doctors measurably better, but leaves anyone receiving services meaning-fully worse off.

The measurability of treatment gives a rationale to reimburse doctors for screening and for ensuring a proportion of those screened get treated for their cholesterol or glucose levels or bone densities or for anxiety. The upshot is that where we once went to a doctor for care when we had some-thing obviously wrong, services now come to us suggesting screening for this and that. In the process, they give us 'medical' conditions we never knew we had. A health service industry has replaced healthcare.

This is not harmless. We put ourselves at risk of being labelled pre-diabetic, or hyper-lipidemic. An unwillingness to take a statin will be entered in our medical record and will affect our insurance premiums. Unhappiness at some side-effect may be labelled a lack of insight or mental disorder.

When Crusoe set sail for the New World in 1660, health was domi-nated by handbooks like the *Tacuinum Sanitatis*. These came illustrated with beautiful images of scenes from daily life designed to tell people, depending on their constitutional types, which foods to eat at which times of the year. This risk prevention made Theriac Europe's best-selling drug for a millennium and introduced Rx (short for Recipe—take and mix; Theriac had 80 components) into medicine. The medical model delivered us from this. Now, though, ever more of us take a modern equivalent to Theriac, unaware how dangerous Eye of Novartis and Toe of Pfizer can be.

The hypertension, lipidemia, osteopenia and depression we now hear about sound real and biological but aren't. Melancholia is a real disease but the lowering of serotonin, used to justify SSRI use, is a marketing myth. This myth has co-opted everyone from psychologists to the complementary health market, whose publications encourage us to eat foods or engage in activities to enhance our serotonin levels, confirming antidepressant validity in the process. The same happens with nutraceuticals (foods) used to lower cholesterol levels or blood pressure. The distribution channel has been captured when even those who hate you sell your products for you and do so for free.

Politics have also been captured. Intervening on behalf of the public's health was once the badge of progressive politics. But by the 1980s everyone, whether on the Left or Right, following the apparent evidence had little option but to focus on changing individuals rather than the environment or society. Scientific impersonality meshed with bureaucratic impersonality. Conscientiously keeping to procedures is one way of behaving ethically, but it doesn't generate trust, isn't always moral, and can lead to a Holocaust.

Risk-Benefit

The Reagan and Thatcher governments, portrayed as bent on privatization and deregulation under the banner of neo-liberalism, are widely blamed for killing a democracy struggling to be born in the 1970s. While these claims badge a change, it was risk-benefit analyses rather than deregulation that did for medical democracy.

In the 1930s the US Army Corps of Engineers introduced cost-benefit analysis for major projects, aimed at transforming a hodge-podge of largely self-serving assumptions into something more 'objective' by sprinkling the fairy dust of quantification on them. This was of a piece with the GDP metric simultaneously introduced by Roosevelt's government. Cost-benefit analyses are rhetorically potent rather than objective. So potent that Johnson with Medicare, Reagan as Governor of California, and Nixon all subjected public projects to cost-benefit analyses, to give the appearances of removing partisan judgments from the process.

In the wake of Ralph Nader's 1965 *Unsafe at any Speed*, there were calls to regulate the automobile industry. The chemical industries also faced Clean Air and Toxic Substances Acts. Both motor and chemical industries mobilized. Their weapon was cost-benefit analysis. It was easy to cost regulations and translate these costs into jobs lost, increases to inflation, taxes on consumers and a stifling of innovation. Industry sponsored cost-benefit analyses delayed the removal of lead from gasoline, and stalled efforts to remove vinyl chloride, dioxin, PCPs and other chemicals beyond safe lower limits.

Risk-benefit analyses of drugs turn cost-benefit analyses inside out. In 1978 Lasagna said that FDA proposals to undertake risk-benefit analyses of drug applications could not be done. Stepping through a Looking Glass, however, industry conjured health economics out of thin air to demonstrate how much treatment benefits would save the economy. It was easy to estimate these benefits where estimating the benefits from seat belts or airbags had been impossible. The onus was left to patients or doctors to cost any risks of treatment.

The mantra that RCTs deliver the best, indeed the only reliable information on medicines, had taken hold by 1990. With cost-benefit analyses in other industries, industry won because the studies showing lives and productivity lost were drowned out by industry studies. In medicine, industry ran all the studies.

The benefits of drugs are changes on rating scales or cholesterol levels rather than lives saved or people restored to work. There are few drugs apart from Triple Therapy for which we could think about making a valid risk-benefit analysis. There are a growing number of drugs claiming a favorable risk-benefit balance, where more people die on treatment than on placebo. As regards harms, aside from industry's favored harm of not getting treatment, RCTs are not designed to detect them. Where they happen, ghostwriters make them vanish.

Once, industry realized regulators could do little against a claim that a drug's risk-benefit profile remained favorable, until a company removed it from the market, a drug was safe, even if it caused heart attacks, diabetes, suicide, gambling or promiscuity.

These risk-benefit analyses are as notional as Pascal's wager on God—if there is a chance he exists it makes sense to believe in him. Or the analyses that underpinned colonialism that favor the benefits presumed to have been bought to benighted people. Or those that put a greater value on the sacraments delivered by priests than the abuse also delivered. Risk-benefit was a juggernaut that flattened regulators and the media and will do so until a fall in life expectancies becomes impossible to ignore.

In this mirror image world, an effectiveness mandate is gold. The precautionary principle works for pharma because nuking rather than balancing risks is easier. In other industries regulators aim at safety. No one in the Securities Exchange Commission, or airline regulation advises on efficacy. The concern is to make investing and travel safe. Road safety makes sense; road efficacy doesn't. The effectiveness criterion, however, makes junk drugs more valuable to pharma than life-saving ones.

In this Alice in Wonderland market, patients injured by a drug or doctors concerned about marketing find other patients and doctors view them as an enemy of the people. Patients on antidepressants hear the message "it may be wiser not to treat" morph into "your illness is trivial." Doctors giving a statin hear their good intentions questioned. Both mobilize without prompting from Pharma. If RCTs deny the risks, the only rational course of action for patients and doctors is to defend the drug and brand attacks as anti-medical and irrational.

If we adhere to the guidelines for managing all risks, however, we exponentially increase the risk of killing or maiming people, as five medicines or more per day reduces life expectancy and increases hospitalization rates. We now live in a Medical Sheffield, where we get ill and die prematurely because the poisoning from our medicines blots out the sun and contaminates the air.

The beta-blockers were discovered by James Black in the 1960s and have been cited since as one of the greatest contributions ever to cardiology. FDA were castigated for being slow to license them. In 1997, however, a major study showed that while they were reliably antihypertensive, they did nothing to save lives. As one commentator put it, "It's tough when patients take a pill, see their numbers improve, and think their health has improved."[46]

Having lobbied for beta blockers in the 70s, Lasagna was later alone in promoting a 1982 study in which a family doctor, Sanjeebit Jachuk, looked at the effect of a beta-blocker on blood pressure in 75 patients. In every case, the doctor, witnessing the fall in blood pressure, was satisfied with the outcome. In half the cases the patient was satisfied, perhaps because their doctor was. In 74 of the cases, however, a key relative was unhappy at seeing a man now worried about his health and symptomatic from his treatment. Treating a disease may save a life. Treating a risk adds a drop of ink to an identity that may never clear.[47]

Whether the focus is on prostate risks based on a deeply flawed test or counteracting the effect of poor diets or sedentary living, the New Medical State is not about treating diseases. It's about identities and burdening us with risks bundled up in branded disorders that encompass ever more of our lives. On a management level, it's about meeting targets. In the effort to meet targets, trust is lost. When I snap a bone badly enough to need plating, and let a surgeon mutilate me confident this is what she would have done for herself, things can go wrong but it's a risk we both take and trust (social capital) likely grows from the outcome. If I feel fine but get talked into an osteoporosis drug that compromises my daily functioning, and might leave me unable to walk properly again, by someone I sense would never take these drugs herself, trust is corroded, and healing compromised.

---

46 Epstein D, "When Evidence says No but Doctors say Yes", *The Atlantic* (February 22, 2017).

47 Mangin D, "NAPCRG Lecture" See: tapermd.com/videos/

Risk Politics

Just as a turn to operational criteria coincided with the rise of monetarism, the turn to risk prevention coincided with a rise of risk politics. Ulrich Beck, a German sociologist, Francois Ewald, Foucault's successor, and Zygmunt Bauman, a sociologist driven out of Poland in 1968, reflected the new politics.

In 1986 Beck claimed we now live in Risk Societies. The creation of the Atomic Bomb and the widespread use of DDT meant the greatest threats to both nature and us now came from us rather than nature. With the advent of fertility control and the ability to save lives, the lives of women and men were no longer dictated by traditional roles. We had arrived at an End of Nature, and an End of Tradition. Our futures lay in our own hands. While our powers to intervene in the world were ever greater and could make it safer, we could also bring about ever greater unintended disasters. Disease comes from nature, drug wrecks from man. Beck doesn't mention drug wrecks.

Ewald also put risk center stage in 1987 in *L'Etat Providence* (the Providential State). Risk was a property of populations and managing it with insurance, private or public, was an act of solidarity. When around 1900 countries adopted workers' and health insurance, they moved from a liberal to a communitarian world, whose challenges require capitalists and workers to work together. Unnoticed by Ewald, our management of drug wrecks is steadily becoming less communitarian.

In *Liquid Modernity*, Zygmunt Bauman focused on identity. Like figures from a Leonard Cohen song, we were becoming visitors who settled in careers or relationships for a while rather than committed to them, trading some security for freedom. In *Modernity and the Holocaust*, he reframed the Holocaust not as an aberration from but as an expression of modernity, a triumph of process over content, of bureaucracy over meaning. There was consternation when he said Max Weber predicted the Holocaust. Bauman would likely be less surprised by *Shipwreck*.

All was changing. The management of heart attacks and strokes cannot be industrialized or subjected to quality criteria, in the way screening services for osteopenia, hypertension or cholesterol levels can. Where traditional medicine was aimed at patients, risk prevention opened the way to a new medical service sector.

The changes could be seen on the front pages of newspapers. Except for a few dramatic events epitomizing progress, such as the first heart transplants, health had rarely been front page news before 1980. After that, a trickle of stories increased to a stream, and then a flood. The stories split between risk containing breakthroughs (that never materialized), and new risks to worry about such as cancer from saccharine. Risk and its prevention brought health to a place once occupied by religion. Where once we avoided occasions of sin, the true path was now to avoid risks.

It also placed the new service industry at the center of politics. A new breed of metro-politicians, especially notional progressives like Blair and Clinton, told us we should no longer look to public authorities to keep us safe. The greatest threats now came not from epidemics but from raised cholesterol, diabetes, and other aspects of our lifestyles. We needed to choose wisely and be responsible for the outcomes of our decisions.

Despite this language of choice, and although we know we shouldn't smoke or drink to excess and should mind our diets, doctors increasingly enquire about our smoking, alcohol, dietary and other habits. They insist it is our duty to vaccinate our children and lower our cholesterol or sugar levels with medicines.

The trumpeting of choice and responsibility has become increasingly coercive. Our choices, supposed to reflect our involvement in the new world order, in practice entail an acceptance of rule by bureaucratic process and management. Once shaped by commandments from above, and then by laws, our behavior is now shaped by guidelines that put us in the position of the mental patient who has a choice to stay informally or be detained.

As Annemarie Mol described in *The Logic of Care*, when pregnant in 1990 guidelines recommended amniocentesis for women in their 30s. The procedure is hazardous. Lying on a bed, Mol's small talk "I hope it goes well" to the radiographer met a "well, it's your choice" response.

Just as the emergence of germs in 1880 supported new livelihoods in plumbing and food hygiene, the emergence of risk provided a *raison d'être* for a new managerial class with a focus on audit trails. Both germs and risk call on 'consumers' to become more responsible. And just as with extreme cleanliness, risk monitoring from PSA tests to baby monitors can lead to more problems than it solves.

The guideline mandated statins, bisphosphonates and other chemicals of risk prevention are hazardous. The man-made framework in which they come, a framework of ghostwritten articles, lack of access to trial data, involuntary screening, supervised by managers, present us with a new kind of risk. There are no insurance policies designed to cover us in the event of wrecks that result from lies and fictions. No policies cover a world where the doctor who keeps to the guidelines might be the most dangerous.

Along with nuclear weapons, drug wrecks are a quintessential man-made risk. But there is no mention of them in risk discourse, other than how to ensure people don't see prescribed drugs or vaccines as risky. If you are drug wrecked today, there is no solidarity. If you pitch up on some island, you'll be left there.

Big Risk, Big Pharma

The health insurance industry and public intervention in healthcare (Big Risk) were born from efforts to prevent industrial and other injuries.

Around 1990, the Human Genome Project and claims we could become better than well on SSRI antidepressants made it impossible for Big Risk not to engage with the drugs tumbling out for what seemed like medical disorders. If the drugs saved lives, they would have been of great value. If not, Big Risk should have been the market force to check Big Pharma.

Now, we have more admissions for falls on antihypertensives or hypo-glycemic episodes on diabetic treatments, than we have from diabetes or hypertension. There are more suicides on antidepressants than there would be without them. The likeliest cause of strokes stems not just from anti-coagulants or anti-platelet drugs but, if on them, we are likely to be on 8 or 9 other drugs also. Treatment induced death is becoming a modal cause of death, even if it rarely features on death certificates. Treatment induced disability, given the number of medicines people now take, has to be our greatest source of disability.

It should be in Big Risk's interest to map the epidemiology of drug wrecks to eliminate them, but this isn't happening. Instead, statins, bisphosphonates, antidepressants and other medicines are guideline mandated, and doctors can find themselves out of a job if they don't prescribe for someone with minimal bone thinning, a mildly elevated lipid level or slightly raised depression score. If they are going to lose a job for not prescribing, it doesn't pay to recognize the warning signs of a drug wreck.

It should be in Big Risk's interest to stop Big Pharma from taking out separate patents on isomeric drugs as similar as two drops of water, as the anti-convulsant sodium valproate and semi-sodium valproate, the reflux drugs omeprazole (Prilosec) and esomeprazole (Nexium), the anti-psychotics risperidone (Risperdal) and paliperidone (Invega) and charging far more for the 'new' drugs. Refusing to reimburse would do it.

It should be impossible for Big Pharma to ghostwrite 90+% of the literature for on-patent drugs and sequester the data from clinical trials. Refusing to reimburse treatments without access to the data would stop this. A market that worked would hold Pharma to account for a flood of medicines whose informational component is as adulterated as London's lead painted sweets of the 1850s.

This market is failing on a massive scale. Some may argue this failure is not a surprise, this is capitalism. The real surprise lies in how the failure came about.

In the 1950s, epidemiology (social medicine) was on a roll, linking smoking to cancer and DDT to chronic poisoning. With their proliferation in the 1960s, RCTs were billed as a new potent weapon and a means to contain the pharmaceutical industry. Social medicine in the 1950s was not hostile to biology. RCTs, though, could show that however compelling the biological rationale for a treatment might be, such as unblocking coronary arteries, if the treatment data doesn't stack up, it doesn't stack up, whatever the biology says.

In the 1990s, RCTs underpinned a new movement that was given a local habitation in the Cochrane Collaboration and a name, Evidence Based Medicine (EBM).

Archie Cochrane was a minor figure in British social medicine compared with Tony Hill and Michael Shepherd. He came complete with wartime experience, a left-wing background, and a commitment to the NHS. His 1972 book *Effectiveness and Efficiency*, of little interest at the time, argued that RCTs might contribute to a better functioning health system. Cochrane noted that while rising wealth made for better health, more doctors made for greater mortality. Medical experts, for instance, were certain the then new coronary care units had to produce better outcomes for heart attacks than care at home, but an RCT showed they didn't. For Cochrane, RCTs were about challenging medical arrogance and stopping high-cost therapies grabbing the money in healthcare. We would be better off if we put our money into geriatric or rehabilitation facilities, which enabled our natural recuperative powers to bring about recoveries.

Cochrane died in 1989. In 1989 David Sackett and Gordon Guyatt in McMaster University in Canada coined the term Evidence Based Medicine (EBM). A movement took shape in 1992 when Iain Chalmers set up the Cochrane Collaboration. Chalmers argued most of what passed as evidence in medicine were review articles by medical authorities that selectively cited studies favoring the reviewer's point of view. We needed a collaborative effort to collect all the evidence, winnow it to avoid multiple publications of the same study being seen as separate studies, and present the results in systematic reviews.

Cochrane used RCTs as a weapon to get a more equitable health service. For the advocates of EBM, however, RCTs had become the highest form of evidence and were value neutral. No one needed to worry about what kind of health service we should have. If doctors stuck to the evidence, the health service would take care of itself. This was operational thinking par excellence. Keeping to the rules rather than thinking. RCTs shape shifted from a means to debunk claims to being the fuel of therapeutic bandwagons.

From the get-go, EBM enthusiasts were more skeptical of biomedicine than social medicine had been. The new movement, however, was welcomed by most doctors as pharmaceutical marketing seemed more potent than ever. Protest groups like No Free Lunch were appearing. A mission viewed by many as containing the pharmaceutical industry seemed to make EBM a natural ally for Big Risk. In practice, EBM now stands in the way of realizing any efforts to prevent, treat, or mitigate the consequences of drug wrecks.

This has happened because EBM sees RCTs as a primary value. Nothing can be let counter this perception. When collating the evidence, EBM includes ghostwritten publications. It tolerates a denial of access to data when it had put itself in a powerful position to bring Pharma to the table by restricting its reviews to trials whose data was accessible. When challenged on this, EBM claims a primary interest in efficacy rather than safety, and for this it doesn't need the data. Focusing on efficacy, however, is to focus on something held out as an answer to risks. The promise of a means to manage danger is a potent lure to take a pill. The development of EBM has led to the statistical outputs of RCTs being called data and to this data now seeming more real than the increasingly invisible people from whom the outputs came.

In the mid-1980s, against a background of prescribing irrationality exposed in every crisis linked to a drug disaster, there had been a push to create Evidence based Guidance to support clinical judgment. Guideline committees formed. Industry set up its own guideline panels. And disbanded them, when companies realized their control of clinical trials meant they controlled even independent guidelines. Just as with RCTs in the 1960s, in the 1990s Pharma encouraged physicians to practice EBM.

The imprimatur of EBM and the Cochrane Collaboration helped Pharma further by solidifying what was initially seen as guidance into guidelines. Allied to the measurability of cholesterol levels, bone densities and peak flow rates, insurance and health service managers could now track what consumers *should* be having. He who pays the piper could now call the tune as in a proper business. Gandhi's "he who would do a great evil must first of all persuade himself he is doing a great good" applied in spades to EBM.

Louis Lasagna and Michael Shepherd were central to the development of social medicine and RCTs. They met for the last time in 1992 at the 50ᵗʰ American Psychosomatic Society meeting in New York. Lasagna was chairing. Shepherd speaking on The Placebo, drew distinctions between The Powerful Placebo of the 1950s and the clinical trial placebo, which, by definition, everything on the market beats. After the lecture, Lasagna asked for questions. There were none. Lasagna commented on the silence:

There are 3 possible explanations. First you were all asleep and there-fore you heard nothing. Secondly it was so bad that since this speaker has come 3,000 miles you didn't want to embarrass him. Third it is genuinely so original and new that you don't quite know what to make of it. I'll leave you to decide which it was.[48]

At dinner, Lasagna told Shepherd placebos were as eclipsed within American medicine as LSD. Few could grasp the issues he had raised. Both agreed that when it comes to treating an individual patient or evaluating what is going on, drug responses in trials tell us nothing. A judgement needs to be made on the patient. As Lasagna put it:

Evidence Based Medicine has become synonymous with randomized placebo-controlled clinical trials even though such trials invariably fail to tell the physician what he or she wants to know which is which drug is best for Mr Jones or Ms Smith—not what happens to a non-existent average person.

The days when a drug company would go to skilled and sophis-ticated psychiatrists and give them a supply of a new drug and ask them to try it on some different patients seem gone forever. Is this a cause for celebration or depression? In contrast to my role in the

---

48 Shephard and Lasagna Interviews, see: samizdathealth.org/shipwreck/

1950s, which was to try to convince people to do RCTs, now I find myself telling people that it's not the only way to the truth.

When asked in 1995 about what was then a new craze for Evidence Based Medicine, Shepherd responded that if we went down this route:

We would also, of course, never make any advances because all advances depend on guesses which we call hypotheses—most of which are wrong but some of which are right. In terms of the logic of the scientific process the evidence comes after the hypothesis. You must begin with a guess.

I knew Cochrane but [Evidence Based Medicine] is pushing the thing to an absurd extreme. Of course, it's true that the whole discipline is cluttered up with procedures for which the evidence is meagre at best and there is a case for trying to make quite certain that is minimized... but [the risk is you] eventually stifle everything else.

Medicine used to involve a judicious taking of risks, taking a poison (pill) or agreeing to a mutilation (surgery), following a consultation with a doctor. Risk management, which is central to the logic of a health service, aims at covering risks to the service.

This bureaucratic culture has encompassed everything. Nursery staff now faced with a 3-year-old's birthday cake brought in from home will cut it up and send the pieces home with children in party bags so parents can take responsibility for feeding someone else's cake to their child. Bureaucracies substitute procedures for trust.

In contrast, as one family doctor recently put it in a debate about liability insurance:

[Medicine is] high risk and my job is to manage that risk. If I sent everyone to hospital on a "you can't be too careful basis" the hospitals would be full by lunchtime. If managing risk we are wrong at some point—that's not negligence.[49]

---

49 Peter Holden, BMA medico-legal committee. See: http://bma.org.uk/news-views-analysis (April 23 2016).

Medical liability insurance, like travel insurance and health insurance, was once about enabling people. But liability and health insurance have become inimical to a medicine that involves mutilation and poisoning. The idea of bringing good out of the use of a poison sounds more like magic than science. It doesn't compute for insurers.

Vaccines are the domain in which the choices of doctors and patients have been most clearly replaced by those of bureaucrats. Here the bureaucrat acts as physician to a population. If the entire population is going to be treated, myths like herd immunity, and denial that vaccines can have adverse effects are important. So, while the evidence grows that flu vaccines have caused narcolepsy, or that shingles, dengue and HPV vaccines trigger auto-immune reactions, research is poured into overcoming vaccine hesitancy rather than predicting who might react adversely.

Medicines are not vaccines but, endorsed by guidelines, the bureaucratic apparatus responsible for their delivery denies their harms also. It would now be easy to capture all the effects of drugs in pregnancy or of vaccines in registries, but this isn't done.

In the 1980s, a balance in drug development tipped from producing effective poisons to marketing panaceas. A balance within prevention also tipped. Where the collection of real data had allowed us to create insurance schemes and prevention programs that enabled health, we have stepped back to a horoscope medicine, consulting cholesterol and bone density entrails that provide no basis for picking out people whom treatment might benefit.

While insurance began with Big Data, and there is now a growth in Big Data industries from Google to Facebook, it is not yet clear whether these companies will mesh with our interests or those of the apparatus. The internet initially appeared to empower us, but enslavement now looks more likely (chapter 10). These last decades have seen a growth of Corporate Dinosaurs, when what we need are warm-blooded creatures who can live on their wits.

Medicine Today; Tomorrow the World

There was no mention of pharmaceuticals at the formation of the World Health Organization (WHO) in 1946. In 1977 WHO caused a stir when it produced an Essential Drugs list that had 186 drugs from 25 different categories. This list was a product of the times. In 1971 *Médecins sans Frontiers* (MSF) (Doctors Without Borders) formed, and in 1981 Health Action International (HAI), with other groups following. All committed to access to essential medicines. Some drugs, they said, are public goods rather than commodities. The branded pharmaceutical companies and leading governments pushed back. An Essential Drugs list, they claimed, condemned poorer countries to older and (by implication) inferior drugs.

Long before the Access to Medicines movement succeeded with Triple Therapy, WHO had been neutered. Previously an international co-operation, it was folded into a global health bureaucracy, run by the World Bank. In 1992 the World Bank commissioned the Harvard Center for Population and Development Studies to look at the Global Burden of Disease. This aimed at raising the global profile of non-communicable diseases, for which we needed 1990s rather than 1950s drugs. Astonishingly, in 1996 this research revealed depression to be the second greatest source of disability on earth. It has since become the greatest source of disability. This is not medical model medicine.

The Harvard Department of Social Medicine became a Department of Global Health and Social Medicine in 2008. Global Mental Health (GMH) and Public Mental Health (PMH) linked to Harvard and the London School of Hygiene and Tropical Medicine also arrived. Claiming it is important to ensure that places like Gambia and Burkina Faso eliminate the kinds of abuses that led to the mentally ill being chained to bedposts in attics or outhouses in 1840s Britain, GMH has rolled out educational programs telling the rest of the world how to have Western disorders. Some of its advocates identified the lack of access survivors of the 2004 Tsunami had to the latest on patent Western psychotropics as equivalent to the lack of access to AIDS medicines a decade earlier.

Global Public Health and Public Mental Health come badged as Soft Healing in contrast to the Hard Healing of traditional medicine. Soft healing supposedly aims at prevention and at populations and is delivered through economic incentives, surveillance, media, advocacy, school and worksite programs to nudge people to better health. It explores the management of vaccine resistance. It tilts its lance against the windmills of income inequality. It screens but has no sense that identifying disorders in children, once aimed at improving parenting skills, is now a conduit to early drug prescribing. It doesn't screen for death or disability from medicines or vaccines.

As mainstream medicine turned to Risk Prevention in the 1980s, Wellness programs took off. Mental health turned to Wellbeing programs, after a 1996 article by Felicia Huppert claimed improving Wellbeing would prevent mental disorders. In the name of Wellness and Wellbeing, there have been calls to tackle income inequality, marriage breakdown, and discrimination against transgender individuals along with calls to roll out cognitive behavior therapy to stop low-grade depression compromising workers' functioning. Society, we are told, should offer opportunities for self-expression, social usefulness, and the attainment of satisfactions.

Corporations rapidly became the biggest consumers of Wellbeing and Wellness 'products' for their staff, from mindfulness to the latest Apps to monitor a growing array of personal metrics. As of 2018 more than 50 million Americans were engaged with work-based Wellness programs or in private clinics. For many these had replaced family medicine.

Britain's Chief Medical Officer, Sally Davies, slated Wellness programs in 2014 as asking policy makers and funders to take a leap of faith these programs work, despite poor quality research and almost no evidence for efficacy. She faced a backlash. Public mental health doesn't fit into biomedical reductionism. The issues are too important to be held to a high evidential standard. Besides as Geoffrey Rose argued even miniscule effects on an individual level can have large population effects.

Davies had no more success than Canute at stemming an incoming tide. By 2020, ideas about replacing GDP, as an indicator of a country's wealth, with measures that included wellbeing and wellness were being taken seriously. The pitfalls in operationalism become strikingly apparent at this point, in that measures of wellness or quality of life are almost identical to depression rating scales. This sets up a sales pitch for improving the wealth of the country by mass treatment with the latest psychotropic drug.

Between 1981 and 2020, bodies like WHO and CDC, as well as regulators in America and Europe, were increasingly funded by pharma. Some see this funding as the top-down braces holding up the neoliberal trousers. *Shipwreck* argues that value-free numbers are alarmingly seductive. These constitute the system and hold it in place. The bribery deflects scrutiny.

10: FOOTPRINT IN THE SAND

The trajectory of Western medicine from 1800 hinged on developments in our understanding of extraordinary complexities at the interface of biology and society. Success impacted on our life expectancies, and our identities.

Before then Europe had seen Cathar, Waldensian, Lollard, and Hussite movements, and religious revivals, with many convinced the End of Time was near. Concerns about Satan and all his works led to witch-hunts and an Office of the Inquisition. Identities were at stake in these crises; would we be among the dammed or the saved? Luther's 1517 proclamation split Christian identities, leading to savage wars and a rise of national identities.

Charles I's decapitation marked a point at which a hierarchy fractured. *Hieros* refers to a primacy of the moral or sacred in society and a need for justice and benevolence. Till then, the discretion of a monarch underpinned justice and the care of others, making hierarchy another word for top-down government. In the new world, something else was needed.

Supported by the role of techniques in triggering science, Descartes, Locke, and Kant filled the void with the ideal of an autonomous subject reasoning in a detached way about our place in the universe. This individual wouldn't take the word of the Ruler as gospel. In this dispensation, the requirements of justice and benevolence led to constitutional government, universal human rights, an independent judiciary, the development of contracts and later welfare systems.

A Romantic reaction insisted this vision fell short of what was needed. The decapitation of Louis XVI points to the molten lava that swirled beneath the thin crust of liberal civilization. A detached approach, the romantics said, was taking us into a world of instruments, procedures, and bureaucracy. We must supplement philosophy and science with something else. Some turned to Nature, others to Art, some to the People, others to forces rolling through history that religion had harnessed but technocracy seemed less able to address.

Techniques and procedures embody an intelligible element, an algorithm. Everything that functions from bacteria and viruses to thermostats and computers must have an intelligible basis. Is there more to humanity than a collection of intelligible elements? In caricature form, science and technocracy says no. Marxism and psychoanalysis were in this sense romantic. Semi-religions reborn in a scientific age. Their technical aspects gave the appearance of science, but the materialism of dialectical materialism and the libido of psychoanalysis were mystical concepts rather than entities with a precise meaning.

As Charles' and Louis' heads came off, medical colors began to replace religious colors. Contagion which had encompassed the spread of social deviance, such as homosexuality and drug abuse, would be restricted to infectious conditions. In the 1860s, ideas about how biology might lead to social degeneracy facilitated the first descriptions of schizophrenia, colored Lombroso's *L'Uomo Deliquente*, the first study of psychopaths, and underpinned racism and eugenics. In the 1920s, the establishment of departments of health were an early marker for bureaucratic totalitarianism.

By 1960 health was poised to replace religion in shaping our identities. Authenticity had become the keyword which, rather than having a spiritual reference, increasingly meant being psychologically adjusted and now means physically adjusted. As the health universe embraced all of life, we gained bodies we were responsible for. As life became a commodity, we looked for the warranty we came with. As health services replaced healthcare, pressure grew on us as consumers to establish and manage our identities where before our selves had stemmed from the communities in which we lived.

The Tyranny of Numbers

Periodic starvation has been culturally sanctioned for millennia, and the 2016 Nobel Prize for medicine endorsed the idea that fasting may be good for us. In the 1870s when fasting was still religiously sanctioned, a new condition, anorexia nervosa was described. It affected women more than men. It increased in frequency in the twentieth century, exponentially in the 1960s, throwing up variants such as bulimia nervosa, where weight is controlled by purging and vomiting. Its prevalence in Western settings, grounded speculation on the changing roles of women in the West, the role of child abuse, and trauma.

None of these theories explain anorexia nervosa any better than its link to weighing scales. It emerged with the first weighing scales for people. It became more frequent when the life insurance industry linked weight to health, and public weighing scales began to carry ideal weight norms pinned to them, with beauty linked to these norms. It mushroomed in the 1960s as weighing scales migrated into homes. As weighing scales spread, it spread.

Scales, like stopwatches or any measuring instrument, offer a tool through which we can attempt to control an aspect of our identities. Measurement becomes maladaptive, even life-threatening, if we measure one aspect of our lives intensely and neglect all else. Just as social conditions and constitutional differences interact with microbes to produce infections, social conditions and temperaments interacting with measurement can infect our identities.

In the 1840s, a thinning of bone density linked to rare fractures was labelled osteoporosis. In the 1980s, the advent of bone scanners and their dissemination by companies marketing bisphosphonates created a socially rather than a clinically defined condition. The new diagnosis happens decades earlier than the traditional one, with even teenage girls now aware of it. It leads to maladaptive behaviors, such as increased inactivity. Rather than a poison that brings about benefits, bisphosphonate drugs make serious fractures more rather than less likely, a not surprising consequence of abnormally thickening bones.

In Type II diabetes, a premium on monitoring blood glucose levels by machinery can lead to a loss of the ability to read our own bodies. This combined with aggressive treatment to keep sugar levels within narrow bands has increased the incidence of low sugar episodes. We are told we must achieve tight control of raised sugar levels or risk losing our eyesight or feet, rare in Type II diabetes. We are not told that hypoglycemic episodes can cause dementia. By doing as we are told, we help doctors meet targets set by health service providers. They have stopped helping us lead the lives we want to live.

Measurement linked disorders will become more common in an era of Health Apps geared to map our heart and brain waves, and fluctuations in our moods and attitudes. Every variation from the average can be portrayed as risky. Even without a marketing overlay, these Apps will cause difficulties for many. The Marketers, poised in the wings, are aware that measuring throws up data for which, "because you're worth it," their drug or technique can be an answer. Apps are more likely to create dis-ease than liberate us from disease: likely to be the drop of ink that clouds an identity.

The Tyrannies of Beauty and Brains

Hair loss in men can be immensely distressing. It often begins when appearances are most important. The distress stems in part from the premium our culture puts on the superficial. Internet forums for men grappling with hair loss reveal bitterness, misogyny, and confusion at a vanity the sufferer never expected. The affected obsessively self-monitor. Their obsessions are neither delusions, nor obsessive-compulsive, but can be equally debilitating.

The distress may be aggravated by sensory changes when the rate of hair loss is greatest. Accounts talk of the crisis passing, when a reduced rate of loss allows the conflict to slip out of awareness. Strategies to take control, such as shaving hair off, help some.

New options such as treatment with finasteride (Propecia) or transplants have emerged. While these restore hair, part of the benefit may stem from a restoration of agency. This availability of treatments has probably helped reconfigure hair loss as a disorder. When is it appropriate to support a turn to finasteride or transplants and when not? Finasteride is not harmless: it can cause permanent sexual dysfunction. It needs as much wisdom to know when to use it, as it does to know when nose-straightening, breast augmentation or reduction, or vulvoplasty may help. Yesterday's wisdom may not be todays. Viagra, for instance, swept aside a clinical wisdom that once stressed the need to grapple with the psychodynamics of impotence.

Propecia and Viagra mark a new enhancement domain, where we have to negotiate identities. Can we distinguish a medical use of stimulants for hyperactivity, or HRT for menopausal symptoms, from the use of these drugs in efforts to keep up with others? Medicine and surgery traditionally restored us to our place in the social order. Plastic surgery, HRT, and stimulants enable competition for places in the social order.

Our increasingly unequal world has put a premium on education. Tiger parents now push children to tick the boxes that will ensure entry to degree courses to ensure their future. University students increasingly take psychotropic drugs that, like glasses for short-sightedness, they perceive as managing glitches holding them back from being themselves.

This is an intensification of the 'gardening' process Western nations turned to in the 1930s.

Should the management of dis-eases like these and the treatment of disease be funded in the same way? What does healthy aging now mean?

The Tyranny of Identity

A diagnosis of a terminal condition can plunge us into a mismatch between our hopes and plans and the exigencies of our situation, an identity crisis. Facing chemotherapy, identity issues shape the choice of whether to opt for quality of life or a brief extension of life. Before 1990, clinicians dealt with these concerns, but now, even in palliative care, they default to antidepressants.

For most of the twentieth century it was accepted that adolescents became semi-psychotic as they struggled to find their place in the world. The traction Erving Goffman, and R. D. Laing had in the 1960s hinged on a growing importance of identity. These agonies, once seen as important, are likely now to lead to a psychotropic drug prescription.

If identity issues became overwhelming, we could once escape. A century ago, Archibald Belaney moved from England to Canada and became Grey Owl. Television brought an interest in things Native American and Grey Owl featured as an exemplar of the Native way of life and its emphasis on conservation. When it was discovered, after his death, he was English, he was regarded as a fraud. Ethnic Dysphoria Disorder, a recently invented term, is not an historical curiosity. Rachel Dolezal's claim to be African American worked for years but came unstuck in 2015. She too was regarded as a Fake.

Many religious vocations have likely been driven by similar needs. The sense of being a fraud, or the felt risk of being outed as a fraud, are tied to identity issues with many successful women afraid of exposure as imposters.

These issues now come to their clearest focus in gender politics. While several states we might now call transgender date back centuries and some filled a social niche, before 1970 gender was a grammatical notion. The modern story began in the 1950s with new technical possibilities. Pierre Deniker, of chlorpromazine fame, describing one of the first cases in 1955 predicted the new media would put a trans-sexual option on the radar for an increasing number of people at odds with themselves or their situation.

Just as with the sensory input in hair loss, a physiological input may drive a desire for radical change. But whether biologically or socially driven, in transgender cases the level of distress in being at odds with what feels like a truer identity compares with the distress faced by people with obsessions or psychoses. Getting involved in a gender reassignment program may help some in part because of the element of control it offers.

The force-field around gender is dynamic. Early transgender programs soon faced new non-binary states. Where the bulk of those involved initially were older men, by 2010 most cases involved rapid onset gender dysphoria among young women. This had cult-like features reminiscent of the Children of God and Moonies of the 1960s. Young people with any self-doubts faced pressure to decide about their identity immediately, paying no heed to non-believers, branded as transphobic.

Regulatory bodies began claiming transgender states are no more a disease than homosexuality. But rather than leaving people alone to be who they are, the regulators required clinicians to treat these dis-eases with hormones, especially if anyone threatened suicide. Doctors were told that requests to delay puberty with hormone-antagonists, like leuprolide, which have shocking side effects, should be undertaken without question.

This is the 1960s turned inside out. The labels are the condition. The issues are so complex and fast moving that nothing can ever be shown to work, yet mandatory guidelines for conditions that need judicious input, emerged. Anyone raising questions about transgender states, even gay activists concerned about latent homophobia, risked No Platforming.

Apotemnophilia is a limit version of trans-states. Individuals with this feel they will be more themselves without an arm or a leg. The idea that abnormal bodily sensations might underpin this was recognized in the 1890s. Following amputation, some report feeling better. The Internet now enables those affected to find and support each other, but it equally risks seducing some into thinking their dis-ease stems from this source. Without a realization that dis-ease may stem from existential discontent or abnormal physical sensations and states in between, some of us risk surgery we might regret.

The Forgotten Man has a core discontent that for centuries, perhaps millennia, has led to a turn to religion and politics. It's difficult to draw a line between what health-identity sites on the Internet do now and what religious sects and political movements have done for centuries. Will a consumption of body modifiers slake this thirst for something else?

Autistic Spectrum Disorders (ASD) is another happening. Autism is a serious medical disorder that emerged in the twentieth century. ASD diagnoses exploded after 1990. Some parents seek a diagnosis for social advantage. Others checking criteria on the internet tick enough boxes to make a diagnosis. Presented to a health professional these may confirm a diagnosis of ASD, as professionalism has been so hollowed out practitioners are unable to counter horoscopes like this. Meanwhile, 'neurodiversity' became fashionable enough to feature in situation comedies about lovable nerds (and their transparents).

As the wars between Protestants and Catholics, or Sunni and Shia show, struggles around identity can be vicious. Battlelines are now drawn between those who celebrate and those unwilling to celebrate gender diversity. Some neurodiverse individuals berate the parents of autistic children for drawing attention to the real disabilities of their children. This is a modern Gnosticism. An identification as Christian without buying into a Crucifixion.

Powered by a search for identity, the speed with which transgender and neurodiverse stories have unfolded suggests a religious revival of yesteryear. Untouched by drug, device and therapy markets, these conditions force us to confront the fact that we cannot simply blame Pharma for our difficulty in knowing whether to turn to politics, religion, or health.

Direct to Identity Adverts

Our search for identity drives the marketing of drugs from Prozac to Viagra. This is seen in drug adverts, which like pornography might throw up options we have not considered but basically work on our pre-existing desires.

Humira was the best-selling drug in the world in 2018. Linked to a monoclonal antibody, it was one of the first biologic drugs. This novel mechanism justified an eye-watering price when it came on the market in 2003 for severe rheumatoid arthritis, a state rare enough to enable its development as an Orphan Drug. It became a best-seller by pushing the envelope to psoriasis and other conditions. This happened even though it causes an acquired immune deficiency syndrome that, like AIDS, can leave us at risk of opportunistic histoplasmosis, tuberculosis, other infections, and unusual cancers. The company knew about these hazards while running adverts featuring women inhibited from wearing bathing suits or backless dresses by minor psoriatic blemishes at the base of a hairline.

Other high-cost biologics have since been marketed for skin conditions. The marketing is almost entirely about identity; the physiological effects of the drug are close to irrelevant. It trades on the insights of Erving Goffman on illness and identity, in a way that equally effective non-drug treatments for acne and psoriasis never did. Panels of patients with genital psoriasis are convened to advise marketers on how to encourage us to grasp control by identifying as psoriatic (or bipolar, or osteoporotic).

Taking Valium in the 1970s was pleasant but a sign of weakness. Taking Prozac in the 1990s was less pleasant but it told others we were in control. We now embrace the asylum as our new home. When 1950s drugs emptied the asylums, recoveries were put down to drug-induced cures. Out of the asylum, some of us recovered in a different sense—we no longer defined ourselves by our disorder. Modern marketing outdoes the witches in Macbeth by holding out the promise of cures from barely effective medicines to our ears, while breaking it to our hope by making it impossible for us to recover in either the first or the second sense.

Life without a condition is becoming rare. Antipsychiatry branded psychoses as political rather than medical events. Now both medicine and antimedicine embrace dis-ease as a health rather than a political issue. Even the drug-free are affected. The marketing of drugs for sexual functioning change our expectations about clitoral sensitivity and erections, and in the process redefines the experience of lovemaking. Apps fine-tuned to our emotional states will aggravate this.

The alienation of the Forgotten Man does not stem from companies extracting value from our biologies as capitalism extracted value from land or labor. Companies are not scouring our biology ever more thoroughly. It is our dis-ease that is being mined. Trading on life's burdens, we are offered sacramental means of salvation. Our selves have become a brand we have to manage. Astonishingly, parties labelling themselves progressive push this most.

In the Line of Fire

In war, soldiers in fugue states may end up densely amnesic, with symptoms but without abnormalities on testing, or, as Beecher found, feeling less pain than expected from serious injuries. These phenomena led some doctors into psychiatry after World War II and others into family medicine where they face requests to certify sick-leave or prescribe medication often without a clear basis.

Even among psychiatrists, who prescribe SSRIs almost regardless of diagnosis, there is a bias toward seeing these phenomena as mental. The patients are diagnosed as somatising, or emotionally unstable, codes for hysteria.

In the 1990s, the concept of Medically Unexplained Symptoms (MUS) emerged. MUS show up in a third of family medicine and half of secondary care presentations. Peripheral neuropathies and gynecological symptoms are particularly common along with back pains, headaches, abdominal pain, and fatigue. Women present more often than men, even discounting their greater overall use of healthcare.

It was hoped MUS might capture a middle ground and enable physicians and patients faced with symptoms to acknowledge uncertainty. Physicians, however, default into viewing MUS as somatization, and patients default into anger at a medical system that can't diagnose them or hints their condition is psychological.

The delicate art of clinical medicine that took shape between 1800 and 1950 enabled some physicians to keep a door open to uncertainty. Adopting the medical model, they viewed what presented in clinical settings in a particular way even though this approach did not lead to immediate answers. We, who came to them for help, may have been able to let them do this because there was less expectation that a ready answer was at hand and both they and we were less constrained by tests.

Clinical medicine is now in a precarious position. Through to 1960 clinicians continued to observe subtle abnormalities of the kind that had been the hallmark of medicine. But clinical observation is drying up, with a turn to doing, aggravated by an increasing array of tests, Freud's message that words in clinics don't mean what they might appear to mean, and company abilities to block publication of treatment effects (chapter 11).

If we take symptoms involving our skin, senses, gut, or muscles to a doctor today, s/he will know little more about these systems than we knew one hundred years ago. Many patients with burning feet, strange sensations around their body, food intolerance, or pain syndromes have MUS. Given our increasing exposure to chemicals and pharmaceuticals, whose effects are largely unexplored, these complaints could be a gateway to new discoveries. The War indicated that part of the clinical art lies in recognizing the contribution of context to the expression of symptoms. Whatever it was about the 1950s context, it was possible for doctors then to put new occupational injuries on the map and recognize the role of toxins and medicines in causing birth defects and adverse events. If these are not being explored now, we should look to the context in which physicians operate.

This should be but is not a golden age of clinical medicine. It is not possible to publish cases linking a new condition to a current treatment. New phenomena like asexuality, or permanent sexual dysfunction following treatment with antibiotics, isotretinoin, or finasteride are missed or dismissed. People presenting with numb genitals, following which they lose libido, or sensory and emotional numbing that leads to depersonalization, suggest there is more of us in our bodies and less in our "minds/brains" than our current cognitive-centricity concedes. But these leads to Who or What we are do not fit with current marketing or service plans.

Hyper-reality

In 1961 Erving Goffman brought identity center-stage. In *Gender Advertisements* (1976) he anticipated the major features of Direct-to-Consumer Advertising of medicines. This now $6 billion industry focuses primarily on women and risk states. Goffman framed adverts as hyper-ritualization, something borrowed from daily life which exaggerated becomes more real than reality. A fetish.

Hyper-reality is central to Brands and Identities. While there was a ritual to taking a 1960s drug, drug effects were anchored in a flesh and blood world. Treatment could go wrong. By 1990 branded drugs had stepped back from this world and become sacraments or fetish objects. Nothing could go wrong. Up to the 1960s, our selves arose in part from communities where others knew our strengths and weaknesses and from where we came. By 1990 we had identities, that like brands, cannot permit internal contradictions. We exist in an already saved state, unless held back by some treatable chemical or psychic glitch.

In 1980, DSM III flung an operational bridge across the divide between the biological and social sides of medicine. Like many management processes, operational criteria give the appearance rather than the substance of solutions. Before 1980 two opposing camps struggled for the soul of medicine. There are two camps now but both are unidimensional, operational criteria adherent.

Like adverts, operationalism has become more real than reality as the Trauma DSM brought into being demonstrates. The 1980 criteria for Post-traumatic stress disorder (PTSD) stated the trauma should be exceptional and compromise most people's function. The push to establish the new disorder came from morally conflicted US veterans. It did not come from Holocaust survivors, the Vietnamese, the Irish, or others savaged by invaders.

Let loose from the committee room, Trauma became a badge of identity. It fanned the flames of a concern with sexual abuse during childhood. For some it became the cause of every psychiatric disorder from schizophrenia to anxiety. The bandwagon was temporarily checked in the mid-1990s by a series of legal verdicts against therapists for recovering memories of abuse that hadn't happened.

Trauma recovered momentum with a study on Adverse Childhood Experiences (ACEs) published in 1998 in the *American Journal of Preventive Medicine*, showing that children experiencing physical, sexual, or emotional abuse or neglect, or witnessing domestic violence, substance abuse, relationship break-up, familial mental illness or incarceration of a family member, were more likely to have nervous disorders, high risk behaviors including alcohol and drug abuse, and health conditions from diabetes to heart attacks. The more events, the more likely later conditions.

Acute trauma following a disaster is as much a medical emergency as acute lead poisoning. Both can be managed imperfectly. Both chronic lead poisoning and chronic adversity knock points off an IQ, lead to delinquency and future health conditions, but neither has a reliable treatment. The largely American literature on both avoids referring to race or class, but experiences such as having a parent imprisoned, like chronic lead poisoning, speak strongly to race and poverty. Being brought up in fractured homes can create a loss of agency that leaves us less well placed to manage our selves afterwards, and at risk of perpetuating a cycle. Findings like this call for collective actions to rejuvenate slums, provide community supports, lift families out of poverty, and to identify and support children at risk. They do not call for trauma-informed therapy.

We need to distinguish between specific toxicity and generic inequality or adversity. A judgment is needed as to whether the difficulties this person, with a history of adversity, has stem from adversity or not. Funneling people with ACEs into programs where they meet therapists who believe trauma is everything, whose practice cannot be gainsaid, now that they can point to evidence that a host of minor adversities can cause problems, is not a recipe for success. Despite the Recovered Memory story, these programs have little appreciation that the coping styles of some of us involve abilities to provide what a caregiver seems to want. If they want memories of trauma, we can convincingly relive things that never happened.

Chelating lead to remove it from the body is necessary in acute lead poisoning. Chelating lead chronically lodged in bones and other organs can do more harm than good. Chelating chronic trauma can become the trauma it seeks to cure.

The failure to exercise clinical judgment in these areas has turned negative or strong emotions, micro-aggression and bullying into mental health issues. These important dis-eases need remedies; social or clinical that is the question.

Biology has become a calling card of traumatology. Cortisol levels are supposedly raised in ACE patients. Elevations of this stress hormone can be loosely linked to heart attacks, diabetes and other conditions. But this cortisol is as much part of a biobabble as serotonin. There is a failure to appreciate that biology varies among individuals and that social class and hierarchies are built into our biologies. While the resulting variations may bring a disadvantage in certain settings, intervening in variation is not the same as correcting an abnormality.

The Dexamethasone Suppression Test (DST) in contrast pointed to an abnormality of cortisol in patients with melancholia but not neurotic depression. It picked out patients likely to respond to tricyclic antide-pressants and not SSRIs. Cortisol levels otherwise show huge variations. EEGs, similarly, show inter-individual variations in brain-wave patterns that could be studied endlessly. Like the DST, though, it is the ability of EEG patterns to reveal an abnormality that responds to anticonvulsants that makes them clinically useful. The EEG was too established to be eclipsed by the changing culture around 1980. The eclipse of the DST in 1980 offers a symbol for the changes this chapter covers.

We are increasingly able to map bodily variations from brain activity to cholesterol fractions, patterns of bone density or ACEs. The goal of Health Service Cartographers is a complete map of the Risk Empire. A map like this has nothing to do with HealthCare for which the goal of a diagnostic test was to capture a variation malignant enough to warrant intervening with a poison. How long will it take for our new Risk Maps to get discarded along with Borges' Map of the Empire?

Footprint in the Sand

Freud claimed hysteria was caused by sexual abuse in 1893. Soon after, he recast patient claims from evidence of real events into fantasies stemming from an infantile sexuality. Bringing our fantasy life into view was a breakthrough, and clearly most of our fantasies are not based on real events.

Two real events, however, shaped Freud's new analysis. One was a treatment induced injury suffered by Emma Eckstein, a patient whom Freud referred to Wilhelm Fliess, a surgeon who claimed to be able to control masturbation by removing part of the nasal turbinate bone. The operation left Eckstein with repeated nasal hemorrhages. Freud argued she produced these to get attention.

A prior event primed this explanation. At the time, he asked people in therapy to freely associate. While doing so, one woman, Friday, by his account turned to embrace him. He framed her impulse as a reflection of her desire for her father. Just like finding a footprint in the sand, bumping into rather than just passing by someone, can consternate. Freud retreated from the moment into words. Many wonderful words and astute observations but essentially speculation rather than science. His use of libido had no more anchor in reality than serotonin a century later. He kickstarted a psychobabble.

Drug wrecks, from the phocomelia of thalidomide to the spiral fractures caused by bisphosphonates, are now our greatest source of disease and mortality. Badly traumatized, those affected may be unable to raise concerns with their 'abuser'. Trauma focused therapists, who routinely denounce biomedicine and supposed chemical imbalance in tones Christians reserve for Satan, never engage with this. They never attempt to tackle a power that silences us and them.

Psychotropic drugs are especially pernicious. Treatment induced hallucinations or suicidality can lead to legal detention in hospital. where the treatment that is our illness is forced upon us. Psychologists, nurses, and others rather than confront prescribers, side-step conflict by claiming they reject the medical model. But it's not possible to claim a drug might cause suicidality, aggression or dependence without a medical model. Drug wrecks are the best evidence for the medical model. In the case of drug wrecks, we are not up against biomedicine but against the branding that fetishes a drug, makes it hyper-real, a sacrament, a fantasy. But who can deal with fantasies now?

We have moved from the Oedipus Complex to the Oedipus Effect. From a world that recognized fantasy and reality could clash to one where the prophecy of the oracle becomes self-fulfilling. "This boy will kill his father" leads to behaviors that ineluctably bring about the horror they were designed to avoid.

Before Freud, trauma produced real and specific wounds, whose edges could be felt. After Freud, the assessment of trauma could not be distinguished from the interpretation of träume (dreams). Reality and fantasy blurred. Now we have a babble of trauma imbalances and chemical imbalances with neither having a footing in considered judgment.

Freud's encounter with Friday prefigured the idea of boundary violations. A therapist should not take advantage of us, should not use a position of power to get us to do what he wants. With the erasure of the boundary between dis-ease and disease, the identities of both prescribers and therapists have been disordered and both, increasingly promiscuously, take advantage of us.

The Forgotten Woman

In the 1980s a concern about abusive clergy emerged in Ireland. It led to the fall of the Irish Government and triggered a crisis that engulfed the Catholic Church worldwide. The crisis came to a head during a visit by Jose Mario Bergoglio to Chile in 2018. Facing anger about the Church's failure to confront child abuse, he effectively responded: if you have faith you believe in us [the clergy] but for us to believe in you [the abused] we need proof. The powerful are innocent until proven guilty. The powerless have anecdotes but not evidence.

Substitute prescribers for clergy and drug wrecked for abused and we have *Shipwreck's* central point. A doctor or a therapist confronted now by a patient raising adverse treatment effects recoils like a Freud, or a Pope, facing a footprint in the sand. Bumping into others risks a loss of control and might change an identity.

Sexual abuse is now reported because there has been a loss of deference to former pillars of society. But although drug companies are not popular, our fear of challenging them has grown. Despite increasing talk of bullying and micro-aggression, no-one mentions how nasty doctors get when adverse effects are raised. Powerlessness compromises agency.

The Irish struggling with English power found their efforts portrayed as feminine emotionality in contrast to the masculine rationality of John Bull. Combatting power and its colonizing effects became central to Irish identity. But colonization is not a medical disease. Combatting power is a political matter.

Combatting power should not mean combatting science. Science is visionary. It harnesses techniques but is not technical. It works when shared not when sequestered.

The algorithms we are up against are not science. Operationalism is an ideology not part of science. But the intelligible elements, algorithmic processes, we the people have now put in place with which to govern ourselves can be capitalized and become crushingly powerful, as Google and Facebook show.

In contrast, what had been valuable but is now suspect is judgment and discretion. Marx was one of the first to note this. While his primary framing was in terms of workers being alienated from their labor, Wall Street picked up on his point that alienation was capitalizable. What from 1860 to 1960 looked like an alienation of workers from the work of their hands, now looks more like an atomization of all of us and a loss of the solidarity that comes from bumping into each other. We no longer meet our doctor, our bank manager, the chef, the owner of the Inn. We are not recognized by anyone. As our systems fill with intelligible components, they become increasingly lifeless.

There will be no birth of freedom if government of the people, by the people and for the people means following rules even rules notionally generated by us the people (governance). Freedom will only come with leadership by us, for us.

A footprint in the sand can't be managed by an algorithm or discourse analysis. It faces us with a judgment call and an embrace of risks.

11: SHADOW GOVERNMENT

In *The Theory of the Business Enterprise* (1904), Thorstein Veblen outlined a latent conflict in any science-based business—the divergence between business practicalities and further possibilities company scientists might envisage. Once on the market, businessmen want to maximize sales of the product, where scientists gravitate toward new challenges. A business that wants to make money must keep its scientists in check.

In the 1950s, the benefits of a drug on blood pressure or nerves had to be Evident to a doctor. In the case of evident adverse effects, doctors, nurses and others were less inhibited in declaring that, if someone turned blue after taking a drug and their hue returned to normal when the drug stopped, the drug had caused it. These evident effects led to more potent drugs than the ones developed since and to everything we know about drug wrecks.

The evidence in Evidence Based Medicine (EBM) means just the opposite. A medicine is a chemical plus the information on how to use it safely. It is as difficult to make chemicals that will save lives as it ever was but easy now to make chemicals that will make money. The key lies in the information. After 1980, drugs could come to market without anyone seeing an evident benefit, licensed on the basis of a statistical change in a marginal effect. As of 1990, thanks to clinical trials evident adverse effects became anecdotes and it can now take decades to recognize them where it once took months.

By introducing RCTs as a gateway to the market, Estes Kefauver helped made Pharma Big. The expense of running trials squeezed out smaller players. The advent of Big Pharma did not involve a switch to a more rapacious industry, or domination by greedier capitalists, any more than Henry Ford was more rapacious than other auto manufacturers when he turned to assembly lines. The change came from turning to clinical trial assembly lines.

Managed Drug Discovery

In 1962 everyone assumed the flood tide of new drugs would continue. A flood of managers began to replace the physicians and scientists previously running the industry. The managers called in a new breed of management consultants to secure success.

Through to 1970, companies prospected for drugs the way they looked for oil—by drilling in likely spots. Scientists in both pharma and academia undertook blue-skies research and new compounds rained on them. Drug development was like staking out the American West.

With the coming of the consultants, Pharma's mission changed to one of meeting clinical targets specified in five-year programs. If that meant discarding intriguing leads, like LSD, so be it. As the share price came to depend on a scrutiny of pipelines and business plans by analysts, the nature of the enterprise changed from being entrepreneurial to being corporate. Research drilling was no longer an option. Nor was the best but least plannable way to find new drugs, which is to watch closely for side-effects in people on treatment.

In the 1970s, a second wave of drug development stemming from advances in biology was made possible by the serendipitous drug discoveries of the 1950s. Out of the new biology came James Black's beta-blockers for hypertension, and H-2 antagonists for ulcers, the first blockbuster drugs, and Arvid Carlsson's SSRI antidepressants. A marriage of science and business briefly seemed possible.

Based on the beta-blockers, H-2 antagonists, and SSRIs, around 1980 Pharma put capital-intensive drug development schemes in place to screen the receptor profile of thousands of compounds per day. This approach seemed as certain a home run, as the later prospect of new drugs based on Human Genome Research. But the breakthroughs didn't follow. In response, companies began to outsource research to nimbler start up biotech outfits, keeping some in-house for credibility and tax purposes. Companies became market intensive rather than research intensive.

These industry changes coincided with four other developments. Government funding for clinical research in the US and Europe evaporated. There was continued funding for basic science, but RCT funding didn't seem a priority as industry was trapped into funding trials to get approval for drugs, and RCTs were supposedly impervious to bias.

University training in medicine and related sciences expanded. Through to 1970, Pharma had been beholden to a handful of magisterial clinical academics, like Lasagna, any of whom could make or break a drug. After 1970, companies could approach the next generation of academics who were open to the seduction of being made into opinion leaders and more likely to accommodate to company interests than the grandees. These newbies had little to do other than be notional investigators. Companies supplied off-the-peg RCT protocols developed by the previous generation of academics.

During the War, the US Government funded 75% of all research in the United States. This increased in the 1950s and 1960s and was distributed to ever more universities. Perceptions grew that science-based businesses were the industries of the future. Universities began to think about patents, and industries began to invest in university research. The science-based post-war growth of Germany and Japan had put them in a position to compete with America. Claiming US research needed incentives, Senators Birch Bayh and Robert Dole in 1979 introduced a Universities and Small Business Patents Procedures Act. This created biotech and start-up companies able to pick up drug development just as pharmaceutical companies were looking to outsource what had been their core function.

A final factor hinged on access to RCT data. Early trials were conducted in a single university or hospital. As of 1970 they became multi-centered, and then multinational. This was not because the drugs were better. Just the opposite. Less effective drugs require larger trials to show statistically significant benefits. This proliferation of sites meant investigators no longer knew the patients or supervised the process. Clinicians who previously held the data for a whole study, at best now only had the data from their own site. Company personnel shuttling between sites lodged the data 'centrally'. Rather than data, the rest of us have statistical outputs from carefully constructed sets of figures.

Investigators requesting access to the data found the information was now proprietary. Without accessible data, these trials had the appearance but not the substance of science. The way was open to transforming trials from a means of weeding out ineffective treatments into a means to sell ineffective treatments. Industry control of the data from 'their' trials meant statistical outputs could be selectively used in articles to sell diseases on which a drug had some effect and to counteract publicity about treatment hazards. The apparent involvement of companies in science allowed governments a warm glow when encouraging academics to partner with industry.

For companies, business is war. The purpose of trials is to gain a beachhead in the market, not to answer scientific questions. The only trials that count are ones that turn up a positive result that can be published in a reputable journal under the names of leading academics. This is the process companies have industrialized, from which they expect quality and timely publications that optimize their ability to sell the product or counter negative publicity.

Outsourcing RCTs

As part of a re-engineering of drug development, running clinical trials was outsourced to clinical research organizations (CROs). Quintiles appeared in 1982, followed by Parexel and Covance. By 2010, the CRO business was worth $30 billion. Few clinicians noticed the transition from science to business.

CROs compete for business on price, access to patients and timely completion of studies. Clinicians are paid per patient, with most patients recruited by advertisement rather than through clinical care. There is little concern about whether recruits have the disorder being researched. As early as 1996, Richard Borison and Bruce Diamond from the Medical College of Georgia were jailed for recruiting non-existent patients. Trials had been approved by independent institutional review boards, but after 1980 CRO's set up privatized review systems. As the business grew and competition for patients increased, CROs moved trials out of hospitals to primary care and then to Eastern Europe, Asia, Africa, and American foster homes, jails, and lodging houses. They are now going virtual.

In clinical trials, people and their medical records are the raw data. Companies don't own this but claiming copyright on the thousands of pages of trial paperwork is enough. Where once academics interrogated the data, CROs now cumulate adverse events from trial paperwork, missing some events and coding the rest. These tables of coded events are the closest academics get to the data. The denial of access is an exercise of *force majeure* without scientific, legal, or moral support. The result is called EBM. It is not data-based medicine.

In the proprietary medicine era, hucksters could trumpet new treatments for cancer or whatever without making any data available. Neither hucksters nor the practitioners of alternative therapies got asked to medical meetings precisely because of this. Yet making claims on the basis of statistical outputs but without data is what academics speaking for companies now do.

At first there were only occasional company trials, scattered among articles in peripheral journals. Many assumed that academics presenting company RCTs had access to the data. When it became clear they didn't, doctors took refuge in the thought that regulators like FDA had seen all the data. They haven't. Now most RCTs reported in leading journals, and at conferences are company trials. The velvet glove of scientific appearances is welcomed. The iron fist of refusal to part with data is ignored.

Outsourcing Communications

Medical writing has been a steady business since 1900. All drug companies had in house medical writing divisions through to 1970. After that, just as companies outsourced their trials, so too with medical writing. By 2000, hundreds of writing agencies were competing for contracts on price per article, stature of the academic 'authors', and access to prestigious journals. Many of the original agencies have since become subsidiaries of public relations companies, which are in turn branches of global advertising companies such as WPP, Omnicon, and Interpublic. The journals are primarily owned by Elsevier, who shares board members with the major pharmaceutical companies.

By 2000, Axis Healthcare Communications offered to "brand the science". Envision Pharma recognized, "data generated from clinical trials are the most powerful marketing tools available to a pharmaceutical company." The PR firm, GYMR, claimed:

> *We know how to take the language of science and medicine and transform it into the more understandable language of health. We advise clients of the best dissemination strategy for their news and make sure that the message they deliver is compelling, documented and contributes to other national dialogues in a real and meaningful way.*

Current Medical Directions delivered:

> *scientifically accurate information strategically developed for specific target audiences… [We] write up studies, review articles, abstracts, journal supplements, product monographs, expert commentaries and textbook chapters, conduct meta-analyses, organize journal supplements, satellite symposia, and consensus conferences as well as advisory boards for clients.[50]*

The ghostwriters have PhDs. The work offers an opportunity to work from home, often on a different continent to the study. Ghosts have codes of practice. They ensure submissions meet a journal's requirement

---

50 All quotes from Healy D, *Pharmageddon* (California University Press, 2012)

for conflict-of-interest statements and authorship declarations in a way academics often fail to do. They see themselves as resisting the overt promotion that marketing departments favor, while ensuring an article in line with a business rather than an academic timetable.

In the 1940s ghosted articles appeared in lower grade journals. By the 1980s, the editors of prestigious journals like *BMJ* and *JAMA* regularly attended medical writer meetings and encouraged ghosts to contact editorial desks to find out if their topic was of interest. In the 1990s, as RCTs became the currency of academic medicine, leading journals realized their influence depended on the publication of key RCTs. Given ghosts produce articles that tick all quality boxes, avoid the excesses of the marketers, and turn around a product in a timely fashion, with a paper trail that makes for accountability, why would editors not co-operate?

By 2000, the odds were that the named authors on articles in *New England Journal of Medicine* (NEJM) or the *Lancet* would know little about a published study. The ghost was often the person best placed to answer questions arising from a publication. As a result, at academic meetings poster presentations of a study's results might be tended by confident women whom passing physicians assumed were post-doctoral researchers linked to the study.

Distinguished biomedical scientists might once have authored 400 articles by their 60s. Today marketing copy describes opinion leaders as people whose views we can trust because they have 1000 articles to their name. When choosing names for an authorship line, companies put most store on the potential of names as advocates for the study. For trials run in India or Africa, the authorship line may be entirely Western.

In the 1950s, ghosted articles were a small part of the literature. Today, over 90% of articles on patented compounds are written by ghosts. No independent research balances these company articles. An antidepressant will have articles festooned with statistical outputs on its use for anxiety, panic disorder, depression, dysthymia, obsessive-compulsive disorder, for children, the elderly, and women, and on trivial features where it beats its competitors, but none exploring its hazards.

THE DISTRIBUTION CHANNEL

Around 1962, operations like tonsillectomy were viewed in the US and Europe as optional. In contrast, interventions for heart attacks, cancer and hip fractures were essential. Expecting essential treatments to comprise the bulk of care, in a 1970s series of studies on hospital bed usage in Vermont, Maine, and New Hampshire, Jack Wennberg found admissions for essential procedures were relatively constant from hospital to hospital but only accounted for 15% of admissions.

Preference sensitive procedures, such as hysterectomies, tonsillectomies, prostatectomies, spinal fusions, appendectomies, gall-bladder surgery, mammography, PSA screening, and elective coronary artery stenting, accounted for 25%. The preferences were those of specialists, not generalists or patients and there were large variations between hospitals.

Supply sensitive care for congestive heart failure, diabetes, chronic pulmonary conditions, gastroenteritis, cellulitis, kidney infections, bronchitis, asthma, and angina, took up 60% of admissions. Rates depended on bed numbers. The death rates were highest in areas with the most beds. More care was a mixed blessing.

A finding that organized care had better outcomes than many prestigious medical centers was music to the ears of Health Maintenance Organizations (HMOs). In the face of cost pressures in the 1980s, the Reagan government claimed allowing HMOs, previously non-profit, to become for-profit would push costs down. Prior to 1985, fee for service provided 96% of the US health service market. A decade later it was less than 50%, as employers switched to prepaid group schemes.

In 1989 Congress funded an Agency for Healthcare Research and Quality (AHRQ), with a brief to map variation, track outcomes, and see where value for money lay. On the back of the failed Clinton healthcare plan and protests by spinal surgeons, in 1995 Congress slashed funding to AHRQ. The idea of attempting to establish what worked and fit best with patient values reappeared in the Affordable Care Act in 2010 but sank from sight.

Britain elected a Labour government in 1997. A Quality Outcomes Framework (QOF) was put in place. Family doctors would be paid for all patients investigated across a range of respiratory, cardiovascular, metabolic, and other indices. And treated. The aim was to reduce variation from health inequalities. British socialists were paying doctors to give more services, while American republicans withdrew funding from efforts to reduce services. Life expectancy is now falling in both countries.

As the number of RCTs grew, there was a push in the 1980s for evidence-based guidance. This push appealed to Wennberg's evidence for medical variation. Guidelines would reduce variation, eliminate rogue clinicians, and surgical operations of debatable value, as well as contain the pharmaceutical industry.

Many countries set up national guideline bodies, of which Britain's National Institute of Clinical Excellence (NICE) is among the best known. These standards of care cover more than the use of medicines but pivot on prescription only arrangements, primarily because there is a greater body of 'higher quality' evidence (RCTs) for drugs than for anything else. Based on the best evidence, independent guidelines invariably have the latest high cost, and often least effective drugs, on top with more effective and cheaper drugs down the hierarchy. The guidelines are the shadow government of healthcare. They leave little middle ground between company medicine and complementary medicine. NICE Guidelines were formally made the benchmark for British health services in 2002. This marks a stage in the transformation of healthcare into health services.

In the mid-1990s, the first studies undertaken to demonstrate an expected improvement in guideline driven health found no benefit. Efforts to pinpoint why things had not turned out as expected focused on conflicts of interest. Ethicists and others castigated academics involved in guidelines for ever having taken payments from industry for lectures, research, or consulting. Transparency would solve the problem. The academics fought back. They hadn't changed their views for payments. They were following the data.

The idea markets might bring public virtue out of private vice cut no ice with critics. Nor the idea that science is the ultimate free market, where an invisible hand consistently produces progress, whether by playing on our desire to solve puzzles or on our self-interest. It only does so however if others can access the data. If there is Cisparency.

Transparency is important, but less so in sciences based on data than in disciplines based on argument like law or ethics. In physics, an author's views of what the data mean is almost irrelevant to other physicists who simply want the data. The rhetoric of clinical trials suggests the same ethos, but without access to the people in a trial, therapeutics is just not scientific. Claims cannot be contested. Experts with or without links to companies are forced to sing from the same song sheet, as much in New York as in North Korea. Our difficulties are compounded by the fact that scientists still operate with the credibility vicars once had. Blaming this on experts getting paid for their time misses the mark.

Britain's NICE Guideline apparatus appeared to get to grips with transparency issues. Medical input was counter-balanced by input from patients and stakeholders such as clinical psychologists and social workers in the case of mental illness guidelines. As NICE was drawing up guidelines for childhood depression in 2004, New York State lodged a fraud action against GlaxoSmithKline (GSK). The fraud lay in publishing a ghostwritten article on Study 329, comparing paroxetine to placebo in depressed children, that claimed paroxetine was effective and safe. This lawsuit (chapter 12) brought ghostwriting, hidden studies, and hidden data into wider view, and made clear that the raw data of company trials might be seriously at odds with the published statistical outputs.

The NICE childhood depression guideline team wrote an editorial "Depressing Research" in June 2004 asking, between the lines, whether it was possible to base guidelines on a ghostwritten literature without access to trial data. Reform briefly seemed possible but was snuffed out as thoroughly as the Prague Spring in 1968. To this day, no senior person from NICE or any politician, on the Left or Right from any country will share a platform with anyone who might state the obvious—that guidelines are largely based on junk.

In 2008, another opportunity for reform emerged. On the back of the Study 329 revelations, Senator Charles Grassley (R) began chasing links between academics and industry. Emory University's Chief of Psychiatry, Charles Nemeroff, who earned millions of dollars from companies, emerged as a poster boy for conflict of interest. Grassley's efforts in 2010 led to a Sunshine Act being incorporated into The Affordable Care Act. But the Sunshine Act focuses on the people who game the rules, rather than on the rules of the game. It requires companies to make public their payments to doctors not their trial data. It does nothing for those wrecked by treatments. After a brief hiccup, the careers of Nemeroff and others fingered by Grassley continued onwards and upwards.

While these dramas were playing out, the experience of most Western physicians was like that of Rip van Winkle; they fell asleep in the 1970s in a Medical Republic and woke two decades later in a Pharmaceutical Empire, with no sense of how to restore the Republic.

FROM PROGRESS TO PROCESS

The service sector of the economy began growing in the 1950s. Health and education seemed to occupy a different domain.

The first canaries in US, Canadian, British, and French universities registered a change in the atmosphere in the 1980s. The changes were ascribed to neoliberalism or a privatization of public knowledge. The idea of a university, which valued the engagement of its 'fellows' with the big issues, was changing. Academic worth would be rated on the number of publications staff had in leading journals instead. Just as operational criteria side-lined judgments about what depressive illnesses are, so judgments about the merits of ideas, or even having ideas, were side-lined.

College brands became important. There was a switch from challenging students to giving them educational products, on the grounds the students would complain if fed anything other than material that would help them tick the boxes leading to qualification. Risk management consultants moved in to advise on everything from the need for trigger warnings on courses about nursery rhymes, to monitoring students for risks posed by radicalization or mental health. PR departments took over the management of campus events and questions about the mission of the campus.

Traditionally faculties and administrations had worked together to govern universities. The administration shape-shifted into a management with executive-style pay-packets. The replacement of academic wisdom by risk management meant the power and size of the bureaucracy had to expand. This was paid for by tuition fee increases and savings from filling teaching posts with underpaid, non-tenured staff, mostly women, who could be expected to keep to diktats. The talk was of governance which translates as keeping to a flowchart rather than setting a direction.

Management requires a turn to process, which is invariably risk-averse, compliance driven, and rights indifferent. It was extraordinary that this might happen in universities, where the belief in Progress that created modernity hinged on a belief in what people in universities do.

Perhaps progress itself was to blame. Notwithstanding the Holocaust, the successes of the 1950s were so astonishing that continuing evolution seemed assured. This boils down to a belief luck will be on our side. If the dice always roll our way, drawing development maps, as management consultants advised Pharma in the 1960s, is not unreasonable.

If what we have, however, is a set of lucky throws rather than a stable system, or if progress has been replaced by a rhetoric of progress, then rigid adherence to the maps is ideological. When an ideology runs into difficulties, something more than operational thinking is needed but ideologies double down. As things fall apart, we look for the people responsible rather at the system, and the milieu turns hostile.

In resisting what was happening, academics defended a supposedly vanishing intellectual commons against neo-liberalism. They did so in articles and books on which they held copyright, unaware the traditional university was liberalism incarnate, and they were private property owners and celebrities—individuals whose livelihood depended on their reputation. The visceral reaction to neo-liberalism points to an academic identity crisis.

Despite the rhetoric of getting the best out of everyone, university management turned to supermarket check-out or airline check-in delivery models with basic functions undertaken by frontline staff in heavily circumscribed jobs supervised by a person allowed a limited amount of discretion (professionals). The Map designers escape blame when things go wrong as long as the Map continues to be viewed as more real than anything else.

Healthcare has been as central as universities to our ideas of progress. Soon after 1980, the new tide of process began lapping up against the seawall of healthcare. It was initially welcomed. Pretty well everyone embraced the idea of auditing performance against standards and seeing what could be improved (quality improvement). There was little sense of the tsunami to come. Nor of the twist that locks the Iron Cage of process in place in healthcare more securely than elsewhere.

Once the Reagan government turned to HMOs, the new companies capitalized rapidly. They employed managers, who unlike professionals are not licensed or accountable. These promised an embrace of standards of care, which would eliminate variation, improve quality, and drive down costs. Instead, disenchanted Americans now figure their payments fund the salaries of people employed to restrict their access to care rather than improve it.

In Britain's single payer system, comparable processes, put in place to 'bring services closer to local people', led to an increase from 1000 managers to 26,000 between 1985 and 1995. Health-spend which in 1985 took 3% of the British budget has climbed past 10% and is now chasing the 20% US figure. Concerns grew about a diversion of money from frontline care into decorating managers' offices, and frontline time into ticking boxes rather than caring. Patient and staff complaints about being done to rather than listened to, about organizational deafness, and pseudo-innovations bedecked with ever changing names like clinical governance, grew.

The role of the 1962 FDA Amendments in giving health services their shape comes through here. By mandating an industrial production of RCTs, Congress changed medicine in unforeseeable ways. Before guidelines emerged, the delicate art of medicine hinged on the interactions between a doctor and patient. Funders had little option but to defer to the doctor expecting that doctors as a profession, rogue practitioners or surgeons addicted to spinal fusions aside, would give funders and patients a reasonable deal (having taken a comfortable slice for themselves). But with guidelines, business rules—he who pays the piper calls the tune—could apply. Protests that the standards are based on junk would sound fantastic. Doctors became technicians contracted to guideline adherence. Previously decent people who became managers often turned nasty.

The growing ability of computers to capture patient details let group practices, clinics or hospitals transform their clientele into populations. These could be screened with targets set to ensure that 80% or more patients with raised cholesterol ended up on statins. Physician variation could also be tracked. This would not have had the same impact without independent standards. These standards exposed clinics and practices to the threat of legal action if certain treatment approaches were not followed. Clinical discretion and the relationships between doctors and patients became problematic rather than the celebrated heart of medicine.

The similar outcomes for staff and patients in the state-run UK and private US systems point to common factors such as a benchmarking against standards of care. Making the UK system private, or the US single-payer, would trap their new managers in the same bind.

Management view guidelines like a weather forecast. Doctors had been better than the rest of us at telling the local weather, but we expect expert forecasts on average to beat local lore. Of course, as the guideline makers put it, the best bet was to marry expert forecasts with local knowledge. When there is a clash, however, the expert forecast will always trump the local view (legally), especially in an organization standardizing services over widely dispersed locales. The fact that depending on weather forecasts kills our ability to read the indicators all around us as to how today's weather is likely to turn out is just too bad.

In the 1950s, a new epidemiology showed the chronic effects of DDT, vinyl chloride, sulfates and PCBs were at odds with the experiments run in industrial hygiene laboratories that gave these compounds a clean bill of health. The laboratory data dealt with the acute, average, and unilinear effects of these chemicals, while chronic effects were accumulating dangerously in us and other species. RCTs now give chemicals a clean bill of health based on their average and immediate effects, while chronic effects poison ever more of us. Managers now require doctors to dust us with the latest DDTs and dioxins, assured by the best science this is perfectly safe.

This scenario would arise even if RCTs were done by angels. It is in practice compounded by pharma gaming health systems to deliver new and more expensive rather than more effective and safer treatments.

If a patient dies now, perhaps suicide while on an antidepressant, the service review of the death will check all encounters against benchmarks and guidelines. Noting the presence of depression and prescription of an antidepressant, it will likely give the organization a clean bill of health. Any family expecting a review to find the cause of death will end up mystified. For a service to pinpoint a drug as a cause of death, it would have to have a box in the flowchart for treatment as a cause of death and services in place to minimize this hazard. A box like this would require an acknowledgement of the fraud built into the guidelines. Such as acknowledgement is above the paygrade of managers or politicians. The closed systems that health services have become cannot entertain this possibility.

Guidelines are as amoral as thermostats. The "good" doctor or nurse keeps to them, as workers in munitions factories do, or those in the German extermination apparatus did. In the face of bigger picture failures, health systems are as closed as the concentration camp system was when it refused German military requests for transport vehicles for the Eastern front. Closed systems follow procedures rather than act intelligently or morally and in the face of difficulties do even more of the same.

By 2000, deteriorating outcomes linked to increasingly unsatisfactory encounters between patients, physicians and bureaucrats made for escalating discontent among clinicians and patients. Health service providers and insurers, especially in America, appeared to be engaged in efforts to prevent medicine and were even more reviled than Big Pharma. But by 2000, there was no-one to articulate this discontent. AMA had ceased to be a force. Consumer facing groups such as the Boston Women's Collaborative or Wikipedia were hoist on the evidence-based petard clinicians hung from.

There are national and system consequences from spending ever more on treatments that cannot save lives or return us to work or decent functioning. Treatments that increase sick leave, disability, impair functioning at work, force older people into care and put them at risk of premature death and a poorer quality of life.

For example, in 1980 osteoporosis was a rare condition. But a new set of bisphosphonate drugs set up flowcharts that mandated osteoporosis clinics, and screening programs and created osteopenia, a new condition. Now up to one third of women over 50 think they are at risk of bone disease. Services fund staff, clinics, screening, and ever more managers to ensure flowchart adherence as audits point to increasing fracture rates. This, rather than new treatments that save lives and reduce costs, is the new health service norm.

We could likely pay Pharma as much as we now pay them for only 20% of their drugs and still save money if companies stopped marketing non-conditions. The savings would come from eliminating screening, from not having to treat drug wrecks, from reducing managerial costs and from better staff and patient morale. Across mental health, diabetes, cardio-vascular, and other programs, we end up with drug options now because discretion cannot be evaluated through RCTs and doesn't make it into the standards. This is not something an apparatus can deal with. Flowcharts have no-one at home. Where physicians once ordered and patients bought, drug companies now sell to health service companies with no input from patients or doctors.

Pharmaceutical companies do well from this without appearing to rule the universe. Just like automobile manufacturers, they control a distribution channel. Just as vast amounts of money get spent on transport budgets, urban infrastructure and the like, with comparatively little going on cars, but all contribute to car sales, so it is with drugs and health services.

MURDER OR ACCIDENT?

America's Institute of Medicine published *To Err is Human* in 1989, a report on deaths from preventable medical errors. Whether from operating on the wrong limb, transfusion errors, drug mix-ups, falls, burns, pressure sores, deaths from restraint, or other reasons, these were then heading toward 50,000 per year costing over $20 billion. *To Err* blamed the lack of a system, fragmented care, variations in medical care, and a culture that had difficulty owning up to harms. (Some reviewers noted that injuries short of death are good for medical business).

There is darker side to preventable deaths symbolized by Harold Shipman and the Sackler brothers. A family doctor in Britain, Shipman was arrested for murder in 1998. He was a prolific serial killer, who killed several hundred patients with prescribed opioids. After conviction, he committed suicide in jail with no-one any wiser as to why he killed. Medicine is stuffed as full of dodgy doctors, many who murder, as the Catholic Church has had pedophile priests. Like the Church, rather than tackle the issue, medical systems worldwide have passed these doctors on to others.

In response to Shipman's killing spree, British medicine's regulatory apparatus had to be seen to act. Better training was the answer. Mandatory courses that take staff away from becoming better carers by seeing people, delivered by managers from scripts that portray caring as coming from the top down rather than bottom up, were put in place along with appraisals. The System would foster a safety culture; this could not be left to the people in it. A clinical governance Trojan Horse gave an impression of clinician empowerment.

Rather than patients or staff feeling safer, trust evaporated. Shipman had been assiduous at ticking the boxes of procedure. The new tick boxes, while safeguarding the System, make a future Shipman more rather than less likely. No one in the apparatus denies this but what can the System do?

As Shipman's murders unfolded, America was sinking into a prescribed opioid epidemic. This later led to 100 deaths per day, 50,000 per year, over half a million to date, with projections for half a million more in the next decade. Every year there are as many deaths from opioids as there were from AIDS at its worst, or from preventable medical errors. These deaths are a product of the system, not the lack of a system.

The opioid crisis began in 1984 with Purdue Pharma's MS Contin a slow-release morphine. This was targeted at the pain of terminal cancer. As the patent wound down, Purdue looked to a successor, Oxycontin, oxycodone in slow-release form. Another derivative of opium, oxycodone had been available since 1917.

Oxycontin launched in 1996 aimed at a market in pain beyond terminal cancer. There was an astute marketing of a linked set of ideas, namely that chronic pain is common and undertreated, that doctors suffer from opiophobia, and that people with real pain do not become addicted to opioids. The slow-release machinery, Purdue claimed, made Oxycontin unattractive to addicts. This was branding as sentiment rather than a reflection of the fundamentals. It echoed the marketing of non-addictive Heroin in 1896.

Within months of launch, the figures for addiction to Oxycontin and other opioids exploded. Deaths did too. Oxycodone is more likely to cause respiratory depression than morphine or Heroin. The FDA and the Drug Enforcement Agency (DEA) were onto the issue. Writing *Pain Killer* in 2003, Barry Meier, a *New York Times* journalist, thought the worst was over. But Oxycontin abuse continued, and other prescription drugs like fentanyl and homemade opioids rushed in to feed demand. Heroin use rose as it was cheaper and safer. Prescription drug abuse entered the lexicon.

In response, Purdue and other companies claimed the treatment of pain with opioids does not cause addiction. Anyone who became addicted had another disease in need of other specialist input. A series of professional bodies such as the American Pain Foundation, the American Pain Society and American Academy of Pain Medicine issued standards of care which, hinging on RCTs, endorsed Oxycontin and other opioids as effective for chronic pain. The International Association for the Study of Pain stated that "all patients with chronic pain are entitled to appropriate treatment including opioids." Bodies like this can be conjured out of thin air to suit a marketing purpose. The Institute of Medicine however had been around a lot longer, and it also bought the claim there were 100 million Americans in chronic pain deserving of effective treatment.

(America's continuing love affair with spinal fusions and other surgery may be one source of this pain. Nice of the ten most profitable medical device companies are American, 40% of the world market for devices is American, and over 70 million Americans have devices in their bodies, almost as much as the rest of the world combined).

The Federation of State Medical Boards (FSMB) stated doctors would not be prosecuted if they prescribed opioids for pain and doctors who undertreated pain should be punished. The FSMB published a pain management book (funded by Purdue and other companies). The Joint Commission on the Accreditation of Healthcare Organizations supported pain management educational programs that endorsed opioid use in materials stating: "some clinicians have inaccurate and exaggerated concerns about addiction, tolerance and risk of death…. This attitude prevails despite the fact there is no evidence that addiction is a significant issue when persons are given opioids for pain control." The materials were sponsored by Purdue. The only way for a doctor to get into trouble with opioids was to operate a pill mill, with cars from out of state backed up in the parking lot.

Trapped between clinical wisdom and the risk of being sued for non-adherence to a standard of care, doctors and patients engaged in a dance about pain management. Pain centered patient groups aggressively tackled physicians who advocated caution or pointed to evidence that treatment with an opioid beyond 4 weeks would leave the patient more sensitive to pain and seeking higher doses. In 2017 the Center for Disease

Control (CDC) was criticized for characterizing the opioid deaths as an epidemic. CDC responded that this was the worst drug epidemic in American history.

Lawsuits finally caught up with Purdue who in 2020 filed for bankruptcy. This and ongoing efforts to make the Sackler family pariahs will please many who lost loved ones, but it won't solve the hypnosis that leads to death and disability from all drugs.

The Act of Hypnosis

The opioids bring out a set of one-dimensional dynamics that feature in all drug wrecks. In the case of SSRIs and suicide, companies blamed suicide on the underlying depression or a latent bipolar disorder. In the case of statins, side effects are put down to a nocebo effect. Branded drugs can only benefit. Any problems must stem from another disease, never the drug. In Court, company lawyers apply to remove any reference to medical quotes such as Paracelsus's "the dose makes something a remedy or a poison."

This split into good and bad is incompatible with the maturity needed to bring good out of the use of a poison. As F. Scott Fitzgerald put it: "The test of a first-rate intelligence is the ability to hold two opposed ideas in mind at the same time and still retain the ability to function." Until recently, less qualified and less research savvy doctors than today's bright young things did this routinely. Veterinarians still do it, giving pets better care than their owners.

Concealing RCT data, ghostwriting articles to ensure messages about treatment benefits stand out and there is almost nothing about harms, and providing guidelines that mandate treatment and potentially put doctors at risk of losing their job if they don't comply, produces a perfect stage for hypnotizing doctors. Once induced, the way to deepen hypnosis is to get the subject to do something stupid—such as view addiction or suicidality as another disease rather than treatment induced. To maintain the trance, relating should be impersonal rather than personal, as when doctors use rating scales rather than chat freely. Finally, nothing should happen that requires the doctor to make a judgment call or use discretion.

Eighteen years after the launch of Heroin, prescription-only status for drugs was introduced in America in 1914 to control opioid use. Eighteen years after the launch of Oxycontin, in 2014 FDA made an opioid, naloxone, available without prescription to reverse the effects of opioid overdoses. The 1896 opioid epidemic was portrayed as an issue for minorities. The 1996 opioid epidemic was a whites' problem. A dream-like sequence befitting a trance.

Angus Deaton has portrayed the opioid deaths and deaths from suicide as Deaths of Despair driven by inequality. The *Shipwreck* argument is another form of grim.

SILENCING DISSENT

The scientific breakthroughs of the 1950s and 1960s converted many to a belief in modernity and progress. No one expected a medical world dominated by brands that accentuate the positive and eliminate the negative, any more than they expected death camps.

The creation of bacteriology was one of the glories of nineteenth century medicine. It set up alliances between business and medicine. The epidemiology of the 1950s which identified the harmful effects of tobacco, lead in paint and fuel, asbestos, vinyl chloride, benzene and other chemicals on respiratory and brain function or tumor growth, was one of the glories of twentieth century medicine. But it put medicine on a collision course with business.

Koch and Pasteur faced the typical resistance to new scientific ideas. Doll, Peto, Carson and others, however, faced corporations producing vinyl chloride, benzene and tobacco who challenged evidence linking their products to cancer or other disorders. These companies rapidly became adept at producing 'research' in a "doubt is our product" strategy that transformed scientific doubt from a means to detect truth into a means to conceal it.

Linking pollution and disease is difficult but easier than linking therapeutics and disease. People injured by chemicals are healthy before exposure. While chemicals and related products are good for the economy, no one expects them to be good for individuals. The conditions chemicals cause also cluster in ways that aid detection. Most importantly doctors don't make a living from prescribing benzene, tobacco, or lead.

When a drug causes a difficulty, defenders of the product can blame a disease and avail of a bias to see medical chemicals as curing rather than causing conditions. Drug-induced conditions are distributed across the developed world making links harder to spot. Critically, the doctors, who might spot any condition, make a living from these chemicals and prescribe them believing they are doing good. Exploring a drug wreck sets up a clash with industry, in which doctors and patients take industry's side.

Just as with the tobacco and chemical industries, anyone attempting to raise awareness of a hazard linked to a drug can face problems. Companies use gag orders, appeal to trade secrets, conceal risks their drugs pose behind a veil of attorney-client privilege, settle legal actions out of court to hide data and documents, stalk and harass critics, and co-opt universities with funding.

There is yet another factor. With industrial chemicals, the best studies typically point to hazards, with some company-sponsored "pseudo-studies" creating doubt. With medicines, the only studies are those companies run and these can only reveal benefits from chemicals that may be killing or disabling us.

September 20 1991

The phrase, the plural of anecdote is data, central to Google now, was coined by Raymond Wolfinger, a polling expert in 1969. Two years later the CEO of Nutrasweet claimed "the plural of anecdotes is not data" when his company's sweetener, aspartame, was linked to cancer. The related phrases "anecdotes are not science" and "harm has not been proven" were also coined at this time and used in media interviews by the Pedophile

Information Exchange defending sexual relations between adults and children. They are now the stock in trade of corporate risk management.

On September 20 1991, these phrases were weaponized. In February 1990, an *American Journal of Psychiatry* article outlined 6 cases in which people had become suicidal on Eli Lilly's SSRI antidepressant Prozac (fluoxetine). Prozac was then on its way to blockbuster status despite minimal RCT evidence for benefits. The suicidality appeared on treatment, stopped when treatment stopped, and reappeared on restarting. By all canons of causality, Prozac caused suicidality. FDA were forced into a hearing on Prozac. In preparation for this, Lilly submitted its RCT data in an article to the *BMJ*.

The editor of *BMJ*, Richard Smith, was an early fan of Evidence Based Medicine (EBM) as a way to control the pharmaceutical industry. Faced with this article, Smith saw Lilly seemingly embrace EBM. He missed the small print showing an increased risk of suicide on Prozac compared to placebo. *BMJ* ran Lilly's article on Prozac on September 20, the day of the FDA hearings. The article became a key exhibit in Lilly's media defense the plural of anecdote is not data. Who are you going to believe the anecdotes or the data? Lilly also deployed a mantra: "it's the disease not the drug."

FDA was sitting on RCTs showing older antidepressants were more effective than SSRIs, and that the soon to be released Zoloft (sertraline) and Paxil (paroxetine) also increased the risk of suicide. The combined evidence made the risk of suicide indisputable. FDA concealed this and cleared Prozac, saying the fuss was a public relations issue and warnings would deter people from seeking treatment. Up to 15% of the population in many countries now take SSRIs chronically, a large proportion of whom are physically dependent.

Medicine changed on September 20. After this, journals faced a choice between articles reporting RCTs or meta-analyses of RCTs, for which companies would pay a fortune for reprints, or case reports which up till then had been the mainstream of medical publishing, but which sold few reprints. Journal lawyers advised against publication of articles on treatment hazards when the traditional methods of establishing cause and effect no longer seemed to apply. Up till 2000, most doctors had a stream of drugs' bulletins assessing new drugs and detailing their hazards, but these became unprofitable and vanished. They were replaced by Guidelines, which list drug benefits but not hazards. As a result, it can now take 20 or 30 years for doctors to link treatments to significant and common hazards.

Twenty years later in 2011, under a new editor *BMJ* ran a celebrated campaign centered on the efforts of Peter Doshi and Tom Jefferson to access something closer to the data on the antiviral drug Tamiflu. On the back of articles claiming it was effective, governments had stockpiled billions of dollars' worth of Tamiflu to handle pandemic flu. Every time Doshi and Jefferson accessed the results of another study, Tamiflu's apparent efficacy slipped toward grin of a Cheshire cat status. Sales of Tamiflu, however, held up. Why? Because there were still no adverse event data and just as water will flow down the most minimal of gradients in the absence of bumps, so in the absence of harms even hints of efficacy sell drugs.

The various NGOs and purchasing bodies now seeking access to high-cost drugs have not understood this point. Refusing to buy because the price is too high puts them in a position of rationing treatments. Accessing the adverse event data would change the game.

The literature on drug wrecks dried up, just as they became a leading cause of death and drug prices escalated. Few doctors believe scientific journals and meetings are censored, although many concede it would be politically mature to accommodate to commercial sensitivities. Journals and meetings, however, self-censor. Adverse events appear only when one company is attacking the product of another and covers any liabilities.

Where doctors were once the customers of the medical media, these media now accept, as other media do, their advertisers are their customers. These advertisers produce both standard adverts and factsimiles. The medical media now embody the aim of propaganda, never achieved so well elsewhere, which is to become invisible.

Simply stating an RCT has not been done ends most discussions, notwithstanding that it would be unethical to run an RCT about a serious hazard. For instance, despite convincing epidemiological and biological evidence SSRIs increase miscarriage rates, cause cardiac and other birth defects, and lead to neurodevelopmental delay, all companies need to do to get doctors onside is to say no RCTs have shown these conditions.

Faced with reports of autistic spectrum disorder (ASD), SSRI companies set up teratology, pharmacology, epidemiology, pharmacovigilance, and psychology groups, each tasked to review the evidence from their area of expertise. While the overall picture may be compelling, the chances of any one box containing slam dunk evidence is less so. In addition, for "the sake of objectivity," the work is likely to be coordinated a person with no background in these issues, who if asked whether the workgroups considered studies showing developmental delay on SSRIs, can respond: "I have no expertise to decide whether we should do that or not, my brief was to get the groups to review any published articles that had the term ASD in them." This is not psychopathic; it's a technical issue.

Against this background, Lasagna's judgment calls on adverse events stand out. Companies, regulators, and academics now intone the mantra that lay judgment is prone to a *post-hoc ergo propter hoc* fallacy. He, in contrast, could say that young women with DVTs are as rare as snow in the Sahara and if we get faced with a rash of DVTs and the common factor is the women have been taking The Pill, then the pill is causing it.

Since 1991, doctors facing women with DVTs check the evidence base and finding nothing placebo controlled there defer to a bureaucrat in FDA. The regulator is there because they don't like engaging with people. He may have briefly practiced orthopedics and is now faced with a contraceptive. On consulting company reports from the selected RCTs sent to FDA, he has no incentive to spot a hazard hidden under a coding rubric in the way he might have if the data were in the public domain.

The consequence for us is that, when we need doctors to be able to see us, we have become invisible. We and our doctors are up against the 'science'. The scientific job is to decide the likeliest cause of this suicidal event, fracture, or cognitive failure. Clinical science is first and foremost judicial. If the conclusion is that treatment probably caused the event, but the academic literature gives no hint of this possibility, the next scientific task is to account for the mismatch. In the case of the SSRIs and suicide, mismatches stemmed from a lack of access to the data and ghostwritten articles. With access it became clear that the clinical events and the science lined up.

Bureaucrats and judgment calls don't go together. Medicine, law and daily life had stood out as areas where judgment remained critical. Without judgments, our legal systems wouldn't work. If we don't make judgment calls, we can't cross the road. Since 1991, spotting a medical chicken crossing a road has become an ever-rarer event.

Outsourcing PR

Creating awareness of medical conditions sells drugs. But it's difficult to sell a product that gets a bad reputation. The marketing mission at a meta-level is to manage the wider risk debate. This needs input from ex-regulators turned consultants, streetwise academics, and the best lawyers money can buy. The regulators advise on how to get a drug approved even if it doesn't work. Academics advise on trials that use a hazard a drug causes to hide the same hazard. Lawyers advise on what is needed to defend the product in legal settings. All are involved years before any public concern, briefed by a company right hand that knows what the legal or media issues will be, even though the left hand concedes nothing, even after the drug is removed from the market.

When marketing a new brand, companies gear up to produce an average of 2-3 articles per month in significant journals. In the case of drug groups like the bisphosphonates, statins, or dopamine agonists, where there may be 4 or more drugs in the group, this means up to 10 articles per month. If difficulties arise, therefore, companies will always have new studies that portray their brand in a good light. They are also more aware of the dates of legal cases, regulatory hearings, and the publication timelines of journals than academics. They can engineer statements from professional bodies to coincide with regulatory or legal events because these are usually drawn up by a small group of insiders and rarely go through peer review. When it comes to debate in the public domain about a hazard of treatment, it is always going to take a lucky slingshot to make a difference.

Besides the hidden consultants, there is a semi-visible set of newcomers. In medicine there is Sense about Science. Environmental and climate issues have Sound Science. These groups are linked to a disappearance that would have pleased Sherlock Holmes. When a controversy arises about a medicine now, companies don't bark. Just as ghostwriting, clinical trials and drug discovery have been outsourced, so too with public relations.

Sense about Science began in England in 2002, and has spread to Australia, Canada, and the US. It acts as a think-tank on risk issues, portraying the precautionary principle as the cowardice of a pampered society. It believes we need GM foods, and that RCTs get the right estimate of any hazards linked to medication. It manages risks to corporations.

Sense about Science outfits are closely tied to groups like the Science Media Centre (SMC), which also began in the UK and is now franchised to most English-speaking countries. These groups liaise with medical journals who send them preprints of articles. SMC then organize for independent experts to offer the lay media a view on what the article claims, and a guide on whose views to avoid, free from the constraints good public relations practice might impose on industry. Where mainstream media think nothing of tackling groups like the National Rifle Association, the Church of Scientology, and the Israeli Secret Service, they steer clear of these PR groups.

The luckiest break for these agencies came with the 1998 publication of a British paper on autism and gut disorders. There were prior concerns about MMR vaccines, the mumps component of which had been withdrawn in Britain because it was defective. In media coverage of the paper, a link was made by one of its authors, Andrew Wakefield, between autism and the MMR vaccine. This led to a drop in MMR vaccine uptake. A 2004 series of articles in the *BMJ* and other outlets accused Wakefield of fraud. This claim was not substantiated at trial, but it proved easy to mobilize people to turn on him, and anyone else who questioned vaccines. Ever since, governments and the media point to Wakefield's head sitting on a spike on the city walls in the name of stopping someone spreading concerns about a treatment or procedure.[51]

The hounding of Wakefield ran in parallel with concerns about bioterrorism after 9/11, which led to a Project Bioshield Act in 2004. Vaccines were going to be weapons of defense. They were also profitable. Between 2001 and 2014, the cost of vaccinating a single child in Britain rose 68-fold. In Britain, as of 2014, children got 14 shots under the age of 1. American children got 26, the highest rate in the world. Across 34 developed countries, the more shots an infant is given the higher the infant mortality.

A False Balance strategy, the mirror image of Doubt is Our Product, took shape. The media found themselves pressured to deny airtime to anyone concerned about treatment hazards. Where a scientific consensus existed, endorsed by regulators, it would be injurious to the public health, the argument went, to give scaremongers airtime. It would also risk jobs, as the pharmaceutical industry might pull out if the climate became unfavorable. The BBC formally adopted a policy of avoiding a False Balance in its science reporting in 2011.

In January 2013, Sense about Science set up AllTrials, a campaign to register all clinical trials. This looks like a model of transparency. Many pharma-critics signed up and even donated money. AllTrials began a month after GlaxoSmithKline (GSK) were fined $3 Billion by the US Department of Justice, for misrepresenting their clinical trial findings. Leading figures in AllTrials had close ties to GSK. Within weeks of its launch, GSK signed up. A few weeks later in March 2013, Andrew Witty, GSK's CEO, featured on the front cover of *BMJ* as the acceptable face of the pharmaceutical industry. Crucially AllTrials does not support access to trial data. It is not AllData. This is a win-win for pharma. It appears to commit industry to transparency while channeling the efforts of critics into a water-into-sand exercise unlikely to slow the prescription of a single drug.

---

51 This is not a defence of Wakefield. It's an effort to get the historical sequence right. But his misdemeanours, whichever way the story is cut, were minor compared to Nemeroff and others.

Where the brief for Sound Science is to take the risks out of environmental toxins, Sense about Science's mission is to make not taking them the greatest risk of inevitably risky chemicals. To ensure, doctors are afraid to speak about the hazards of treatment. To brand questioning of treatments as a War on Science. This McCarthyism has clinicians worldwide palpably scared.

We are now caught between business masquerading as science in the case of drugs and public policy masquerading as science with vaccines. On November 4 2016, days before the Clinton-Trump vote, Obama signed Executive Order 13747, advancing a Global Health Security Agenda, whose brief was to support vaccine production as a core feature of US defense strategy.

The War on Science

In March 2015, the cover of *National Geographic* featured a picture of the moon-landing with a title "The War on Science". A strapline said: climate change does not exist; evolution never happened; the moon landing was fake; vaccination can lead to autism; genetically modified food is evil. Even before the 2016 American election gave us Fake News, a progressive commentariat had lumped climate change deniers and anti-vaxxers together as a threat to rationality and science.

The early development of science hinged on an accommodation; God's truths were revealed in The Book (Biblos) and in the Book of Nature. Religion offered a framework for belief. Science operated through doubt. As this doubt spread to the Bible itself, the belief lost by viewing the Bible as just another text or map transferred to science.

The Second World War, Nazi death camps, and the Atomic Bomb produced a crisis for those who believed in progress, as did the history of science which pointed to a continual turnover of the 'truths' at the heart of science. Post-modernism arrived with Jean Baudrillard who traced it roots to Borges' 1946 parable *On Rigor in Science.*

Post-modernism contested science's claims to truth. Knowledge, it claimed, arises in a socio-political context and accepted truths always confer power on some to the disadvantage of others. The word truth derives from trust. Postmodernists asked if science, especially the human sciences, could flourish in a society that was not true or free. Lacking an anchor in philosophy, science could not be assumed to have a meaning, and certainly not a moral arc bending toward truth.

Cybernetics also shaped post-modernism, as caught by Marshall McLuhan's phrase, "the medium is the message". Information had begun to hyper-circulate and instant feedback rather than the content of messages increasingly dictated how we behaved. If the signifiers were as important as the signified, could there be any objectivity in either science or history?

This questioning triggered the Science Wars. Physicists and physiologists faced post-modernists, for whom scientific articles had become texts of uncertain truth value. The scientists called post-modernism a Cargo Cult. In World War II, US Air Force planes flying into Pacific islands disgorged all sorts of goods. Impressed by these flying cornucopias, after the military left, the islanders maintained the runways, control huts, and the American flag, believing the right appearances would lead to the right results. These were the Cargo Cults.

The scientists turned to the Latin word for truth, Veritas, from which we get verification. We may add to verification procedures but cannot reverse or undo them. It is this that means planes fly. Conjuring up airstrips and a flag can't get a post-modernist off the ground.

Medicine involves both trust and verification. Medical modernism began in Paris around 1800 with Pinel and Bichat. Although slow at first, there was extraordinary progress, culminating in advances that seemed far removed from a Cargo Cult.

Nevertheless Ivan Illich, Michel Foucault and others claimed a new technical medicine was arrogating to itself the right to pronounce on life, death, and disability. Medicalization was alienating us from our true selves rather than liberating us. An apparatus was replacing our natural moral instincts with a bureaucratic morality.

Battle lines were drawn over 'the medical gaze'. One side saw this gaze as good, the other as dehumanizing. The rhetoric pitted scientists, physicians and capitalism against post-modernists and socialism. The issues were vigorously contested up to 1990 when 'critique' fractured into post-ism—post-structuralism, post-modernism, post-humanism.

While there is now a growing appreciation of the originality of the historical Marx, from 1890 onwards, despite his 1847 challenge in *The Poverty of Philosophy* that the point is to change society, not interpret it, Marx's work spawned various forms of discourse analysis as empty as psychoanalysis. Now when it is possible to show that what passes for biomedicine offers the appearances of science rather than the real thing, with drugs obviously fetished, and health service planes stalling in flight, no one seems equipped to engineer change.

Instead with Foucault we got a babble about biopower and biopolitics. After his death, with the marketing of Prozac and talk of the Human Genome Project, social scientists embraced the New Human, and turned to RCTs.

Our Treatment Maps now recommend medicines that are less effective and more expensive than older drugs. Caring has been replaced by conformity to mission statements that say: "Because our name is on it, We Care." Any questioning of the changing climate in health is resisted by pro-vaccine and pro-drug climate change denialists who mobilize the media and politicians to quarantine people with conditions that have arisen from vaccines and drugs. Taken self-evidently because the takers were originally pro-vaccine and pro-drug.

The original post-modern critique of claims for the reality of diseases and efforts to force doctors to justify themselves should have grown in force as more drugs were given for non-diseases. Instead, pharmaceutical marketers now rewrite the text that is the human body from year to year with afflictions such as osteopenia, erectile dysfunction, and pediatric bipolar disorder with not a pipsqueak to disturb them.

Marketing Zyprexa for bipolar disorder in 2002, for instance, Lilly produced Donna:

> *a single mom, in her mid-30s appearing in your office in drab clothing and seeming somewhat ill at ease. Her chief complaint is*

> *'I feel so anxious and irritable lately.' Today she says she has been sleeping more than usual and has trouble concentrating at work and at home. However, several appointments earlier she was talkative, elated, and reported little need for sleep. You have treated her with various medications including antidepressants with little success... You will be able to assure Donna that Zyprexa is safe and that it will help relieve the symptoms she is struggling with.[52]*

Up to 1987, Donna was a poster case for treatment with Valium or Xanax. From 1988, the same symptoms made her a case of Prozac or Zoloft. Nothing in science warranted diagnosing her as bipolar in 2002.

Zyprexa greatly elevates cholesterol, so Donna may need a statin. It causes massive weight gain, so she may need Celebrex for arthritis, and Januvia for diabetes. Any doctor linking these conditions to Zyprexa will find other doctors unwilling to concede causality. He may be fired for refusing to prescribe the standard of care, Zyprexa. (NICE Guidelines put Zyprexa top of their list of antipsychotics in 2002 after Lilly threatened to pull out of Britain). Donna and her doctor are up against a post-truth skepticism embodied in "doubt is our product".

Zyprexa is like taking communion—there can only be benefits. There is no concession to the differences among patients. But differences among 'consumers' are recognized. One message is tailored for early adopting doctors, whose sense of personal heroism needs polishing. Another for those who want to keep to guidelines, and yet another for those who warm to the practicalities of a dissolve in the mouth wafer that forces patients to comply.

Donna will not find a champion inside or outside medicine. At best she will get a limp-wristed blaming of conflict of interest. But this leads nowhere. The implication is that government should run trials and fund academics. If there is no access to trial data, government control, as with

---

52 "Zyprexa, Primary Care Sales Force Resource Guide" (2002). Zyprexa MDL 1596, Plaintiffs' Exhibit 01926, 7.

vaccines and the control of tobacco in China, looks as bad as company control.

Through to 2000, Donna was at risk from a marketing that could conjure up airstrips and flags that fooled doctors. Her difficulties were compounded when social media companies weaponized ideas put forward by John Locke and Alexander Bain, and later Ivan Pavlov and B. F. Skinner. These produced human science techniques good enough to keep planes flying. Donna and her doctors can now be tracked and manipulated nearly as precisely as the particles in CERN's Hadron particle collider.

Big Panacea can be confident that even if outcomes on treatment get worse there will be no consumer (medical) concern, because the consumers cannot conceive of alternatives. There is almost no possibility of discrepant data emerging to trigger an unwelcome thought. The control of information in this market is total.

The climate within this totalitarianism was well caught in Friedrich Hayek's description of Eastern European science in 1944:

> *The general intellectual climate which this produces, the spirit of complex cynicism as regards truth which it engenders, the loss of the sense of even the meaning of truth, the disappearance of the spirit of independent inquiry and of the belief in the power of rational conviction, the way in which differences of opinion in every branch of knowledge become political issues to be decided by authority are all things which one must personally experience—no short description can convey their extent*[53]

There is a War on Science, most clearly seen in medicine. Postmodernists failed at a critical moment. They originally advocated pitching patients' lived experience against scientific truths. But they never engaged with a drug wreck. None of those now agonizing about the objectivity of history or qualitative research have looked at the history taking or qualitative interviewing critical to caring when someone presents with a treatment-induced condition. No post-modernist, historian, ethicist, or social

---

53 Hayek F, *The Road to Serfdom* (University of Chicago Press, 1992), 179.

scientist ever steps out of line and says that a drug has *caused* this person the condition they think it has caused.

THE APPROACHING STORM

Following Prussia's defeat by Napoleon, Johann Gottlieb Fichte challenged German academics to leave their ivory towers and engage with the world. They needed to make a real difference rather than use words rhetorically to pervert rather than advance truth. They should put forward theses that generating contrary observations (antitheses) might lead to a dynamic synthesis. They should educate their students in dialectical thinking. Philosophy didn't gain as he hoped but Germany overtook France in developing science.

Marx brought dialectical materialism into the university of life. The new factory techniques would antithetically change the experience of workers in a dialectic that would lead to a new synthesis of what we knew and could do to advance humanity. But the proletariat never graduated.

In the mid-1980s, as fee for service was being brushed aside by managed care, American rather than European physicians openly worried about an industrialization of medicine and their imminent proletarianization. Physicians, who had been sheltered from the gale-force winds of capitalism, could sense they were about to feel its full force.

Evidence Based Medicine (EBM) emerged in the early 1990s as a savior able it seemed to mobilize science as a bulwark against business. It championed a dialectical operationalism. Doctors would learn to think for themselves by combining clinical trial evidence (theses) with the contrary instances of adverse effects in clinical practice and patient values (antithesis) and would arrive at a new synthesis. Revolution was in the air, or perhaps just relief at the prospect of a shelter from the storm.

Not since the Trojans let a horse into Troy has a group under siege made such a mistake. It didn't have to be this way. Unlike the delivery of service packages, Care cannot be commoditized or proletarianized. Not at least, a Care that hinges on shared judgment calls between doctors and patients.

Instead of an entrepreneurial embrace of the risks involved in making judgments under uncertainty, doctors slipped into a risk avoidant bureaucratic apparatus that regards people as interchangeable. In this Kafkaesque environment, everyone has targets on their back, everyone is proletarianized and there is a striking increase in burnout among staff.

Every time we take an RCT informed pill we send a message that the risks health services seek to manage lie within us rather than in society. We make lepers of ourselves. The role of our doctors, like that of engineers, used to be to reduce the risks to us of the options we chose to take to an acceptable level. Now their role is to immunize corporate bodies from the risks we pose them. The increasingly Kafkaesque nature of our contacts with health services betrays the bureaucratic rather than entrepreneurial fundament to these services.

Meanwhile in 2011, the major pharmaceutical companies publicly pulled out of mental health. The profits were greater elsewhere and they had a duty to put their money where it would earn the best return. Auto-immune disorders and cancer, where high-cost niche-busting drugs could be brought on stream seemed the best bet. This didn't mean finding a cure for auto-immune disorders or cancer. It meant this was where the money lay. No psychiatry grandee argued for any contract between society and industry that warranted companies side-stepping their fiduciary duty to their shareholders. Medicine no longer has an establishment that pharma worries about.

By 2018, Solvadi and related antivirals looked like they might cure Hepatitis C. These are among the few drugs since Triple Therapy for AIDs that save lives as the first antibiotics once did. Poorer countries with high Hepatitis C rates pushed for access to Solvadi as they had for Triple Therapy. The price for a 12-week course dropped, as the price of Triple Therapy had, from $84,000 to $900. The share-price of Gilead who marketed Solvadi fell too. Goldman Sachs commented that curing patients is not a good business model.

Industry is no longer entrepreneurial. While pitching its activities to politicians as innovative, it prefers to collect rents than to innovate.

Hayek conceded that a private monopoly might be worse than a public monopoly, but he never thought this possible. Fifty years later, Milton Friedman prefacing a re-issue of *The Road to Serfdom* could not see the private monopolies all around him claiming:

> *The present discussion of a national program of health care provides a striking example. The intellectuals may have learnt the words but they do not yet have the tune… On both sides of the Atlantic, it is only a little overstated to say that we preach individualism and competitive capitalism, and practice socialism.*[54]

In health services now, there is nothing other than central planning. This is neither a socialism that seeks to secure a seat at the table for ordinary folk nor an enterprise seeking to produce better health.

For Veblen business posed a risk to science. When working properly, science opens up questions rather than provides answers. This is not a useful business or political strategy but claiming to be following the science is.

Since 1990, millions of sophisticated people have been hypnotized and have slept-walked off the common ground that used to be medicine. As this happened, the private monopolies of Google and Facebook emerged. Their mission statement could be the plural of anecdotes is data. When it comes to drug wrecks, there is no sign that it is.

The question now, as it was for Fichte, is how to wake the sleepwalkers up. The hypnotist on stage can undo the spell. Triggering a stampede in a crowded theater by crying fire can undo a spell. Sleepwalkers can also wake if they bump into an antithesis. But waking to find everyone else entranced is nightmarish.

---

54 Friedman M, *Preface to The Road to Serfdom* (1994).

CASTAWAYS

12: HITTING THE REEF

Nothing can describe the confusion of thought which I felt when I sank into the water; for tho' I swam very well, yet I could not deliver myself from the waves so as to draw breath.
   R Crusoe

A 1990 article reported Eli Lilly's SSRI antidepressant Prozac triggered intense suicidality in 6 adults (chapter 11). The symptoms cleared on stopping the drug and re-appeared on re-exposure. By all laws of cause and effect, Prozac caused suicide. Convincing reports later emerged of adolescents given Prozac and related drugs who had committed suicide.

Few clinicians in America or Europe in 1990 thought children or adolescents got depressed. Unhappy and miserable yes but not melancholic. Support from an understanding adult was viewed as the best remedy.

Neal Ryan from Pittsburgh, Marty Keller at Brown, and others drew up a protocol for an RCT in children comparing paroxetine (Paxil) with imipramine, and placebo. SmithKline Beecham, whose Paxil had just been approved for use in adults supported Study 329.[55]

Despite many open-label articles by clinicians reporting benefits to minors from SSRIs, none of the 15 RCTs of older antidepressants had shown a benefit. The first pediatric RCT of Prozac was also negative.

---

55 Documents and media linked to Study 329 are on Study320.org and linked to *Children of the Cure* (Samizdat Health Writer's Co-operative, Inc., 2020).

The challenge to the 329 group was to see if using a specific Childhood Depression Rating Scale, in a longer than usual trial, they could show a benefit. Paxil was pitted against up to double the adult dose of imipramine, and placebo, in an 8-week trial of 275 12-18-year-olds, with a 26-week continuation phase.

The first child entered the study in April 1994. Recruitment was slow. More centers were added. A Study 377 also began with centers in Europe, Canada, South Africa, United Arab Emirates, Argentina and Mexico. The last child entered Study 329 in 1997.

The results were published in July 2001 in the *Journal of the American Academy of Child and Adolescent Psychiatry* (JAACAP), the highest impact factor journal in the field. The article, with Martin Keller as first author and a distinguished authorship line lauded the benefits and safety of Paxil.

SmithKline Beecham and Glaxo Wellcome became GlaxoSmithKline (GSK) in January 2001. In September 2001, Panorama, BBC TV's flagship investigative program, began researching GSK, a British company, then the world's biggest drug company, whose paroxetine (traded as Seroxat in the UK) was one of the best-selling drugs in the world. Three months earlier, in June, Paxil and GSK had been on the wrong end of a verdict in Cheyenne, Wyoming. Don Schell a 58 year old oilman, after 48 hours on Paxil, put three bullets through the head of Rita, his wife, Deborah, his daughter, and Alyssa, his grand-daughter, before killing himself. This was a first verdict against a drug company for a behavioral effect of a drug.

The proposal for the *Panorama* program came from Ed Harriman, an American working in London. He claimed the investigation would reveal that GSK and other companies were recruiting children from minority and deprived backgrounds to studies like 329.

The 'lips' on the program was Shelley Jofre. On the plane to an American Psychiatric Association meeting in Philadelphia in May 2002, Harriman gave Jofre Study 329 to read. Her brief was to interview authors at the meeting and nail down where the children had come from. Reading the paper, her eye was caught by references to children becoming emotionally labile on paroxetine. Questions about whether the children were from deprived backgrounds got nowhere with interviewees. In a final interview, short of questions, she asked Neal Ryan about emotional lability. Ryan looked uncomfortable and cut the interview short. Panorama changed tack.

GSK were in the process of availing of a 1997 amendment to the FDA's Prescription Drug User Fee Act. This offered six months patent extension to companies who provided safety data on their drug in children even if the drug hadn't worked. With Paxil heading towards sales of $2 billion per annum, a six-month patent extension was worth a lot. In August 2002, GSK submitted their Paxil pediatric depression trials to FDA, including studies 329 and 377. FDA had a seven-week deadline to respond.

On October 7 2002, the front cover of *Newsweek* featured an unhappy teenage girl and a headline "3 million kids suffer from it. What can you do? Teen depression". The message was depression would cost children their careers, relationships, lives and would lead to drug abuse and worse. The answer was Prozac had just been approved for teenage depression and Paxil and Zoloft (sertraline) were about to be.

On October 10, World Mental Health Day, and the fortieth anniversary of the 1962 FDA Amendments, FDA sent a letter to GlaxoSmithKline stating: "we have completed the review of this application [for approval to claim a benefit in depressed children] and it is approvable."

Panorama's *The Secrets of Seroxat* aired on October 13. The program covered suicidality from and addiction to paroxetine as well as the testing of the drug in children. GSK flat out denied there were any risks. BBC were flooded with thousands of calls and emails, linking paroxetine to suicidality and addiction. *Panorama* who had never in fifty years repeated a topic did three more programs on GSK and paroxetine.

The calls and emails laid the basis for *Emails from the Edge* on May 11 2003. This program led Britain's leading patient mental health advocacy group to protest outside the HQ of Britain's drug regulator, the Medicines and Healthcare Regulatory Agency (MHRA), calling for a ban on the drug.

Under pressure, GSK prepared a "Science with a Conscience" brochure and advertisements directed at their own staff, whose themes were:

- Were the UK doctors who wrote 4,580,000 prescriptions for Seroxat last year right?

- At GSK we believe that the best people for patients to consult about their treatment are their own doctors.

- The safety [of drugs] is constantly monitored by the MHRA—a rather more expert body than the producers of Panorama.

- If you are depressed who should you consult? A TV presenter or a doctor?

- We have total faith in Seroxat. So can you.

- Depression affects 5 million people in the UK. Seroxat is a highly effective answer.

- Judge Seroxat on clinical trials not trial by media.

In its October 10 approvable letter, FDA had asked GSK for details on all behavioral adverse events and the company rationale for coding events as emotional lability. On May 22, 2003, at odds with its 'Science with a Conscience' brochure, GSK's response to FDA showed a doubling of the suicidal act rate in children on Paxil in Study 329 and other pediatric trials. Where their brochure stated there was no evidence linking paroxetine to violence, their response to FDA showed a doubling of violent acts on paroxetine compared to placebo. Where the brochure denied risks of addiction, other company data showed healthy volunteers displaying symptoms consistent with dependence after brief exposures to Paxil.

On June 2, after receiving GSK's response, FDA called for data across 15 pediatric antidepressant trials from 7 companies seeking approvals and patent extensions. It also issued a caution about prescribing of antidepressants to children. But in October, the agency began downplaying the risks. It called a Psychopharmacological Drugs Advisory Committee (PDAC) meeting for February 2, 2004, at which all pediatric trial data would be made available.

On January 27, an American College of Neuropsychopharmacology working group, including a number of the 329 authors, issued a paper denying a link between antidepressants and suicide. This got national coverage, which was part of the deal offered by GYMR (Get Your Message Right), the PR agency, who had written the paper.

On February 1, the *San Francisco Chronicle* claimed FDA's pediatric reviewer, Andy Mosholder, had been barred from presenting findings of a statistically significant doubling of the risk of suicidal acts on antidepressants at the PDAC meeting the next day.

In the middle of the February 2 hearing, Panorama released a 6-page GSK document dated October 1998. The summary stated:

As you well know the results of the studies were disappointing in that we did not reach statistical significance on the primary end points and thus the data do not support a label claim for the treatment of adolescent depression. The possibility of obtaining a safety statement from this data was considered but rejected. The best which could have been achieved was a statement that although safety data was reassuring, efficacy had not been demonstrated. Consultation of the marketing teams via Regulatory confirmed that this would be unacceptable commercially..."

Addressing the results of Studies 329 and 377, the document stated:

- *There were no differences in the safety profile of Seroxat/Paxil in adolescents when compared to that already established in the adult population.*

- *The efficacy data from the above clinical trials are insufficiently robust to support a regulatory submission and label change for this patient population.*

- *Based on the current data, and following consultation with SB country regulatory and marketing groups, no regulatory submission will be made for either efficacy or safety statements relating to adolescent depression... [because]:*

- *regulatory agencies would not approve a statement indicating that there are no safety issues in adolescents, as this could be seen as promoting off-label use.*

- *It would be commercially unacceptable to include a statement that efficacy had not been demonstrated, as this would undermine the profile of paroxetine.*

Target: *To effectively manage the dissemination of these data in order to minimise any potentially negative commercial impact.*

Proposals: *Positive data from Study 329 will be published in abstract form … and a full manuscript of the 329 data will be progressed.*

The positive data became the 2001 Keller et al JAACAP article.

GSK claimed the 6-page document did not reflect the company position, even though in their approvable to GSK in October 2002 FDA had noted that:

> *We agree that the results of Study 329 failed to demonstrate the efficacy of paroxetine in pediatric patients with MDD [Major Depressive Disorder]. Given the fact that negative trials are frequently seen even for antidepressant drugs that we know are effective, we agree that it would not be useful to describe these negative trials in the labelling.*

At the PDAC meeting, FDA presented its assessment of the data from the 15 trials. It logged two Prozac trials as positive—the basis for its approval of Prozac for children. The combined data from all trials pointed to a doubling of the risk of a suicidal event. Taking a time out, FDA asked a Columbia University group to review all events in the trials to make sure they really were suicidal events. A second meeting was set for September 14 to review the Columbia findings.

In March, Panorama's GSK document came to the attention of Rose Firestein working for New York State's Attorney General, Elliott Spitzer.

In June, Spitzer's office initiated a fraud action against GSK, claiming the company made money from Paxil for children on the back of an article claiming it worked, even though it knew the results of Study 329 showed Paxil didn't work. The lawsuit was resolved in August 2004 with GSK agreeing to post details of all its clinical trials on their website.

At the September 14 meeting, although the Columbia report pointed to findings very similar to the February findings, a string of academics lined up to claim that a warning would put a chill on clinical care. Nevertheless, the meeting voted in favor of a Black Box Warning for suicide. Russell Katz, the Director of the FDA division responsible for psychotropic drugs, stated that FDA accepted that antidepressants cause suicidal behavior in minors. Two years later in December 2006 the warning was extended to 25-year-olds.

On September 20, 1991, faced with equivalent RCT data on suicidality in adults, FDA had stated there was no scientifically established risk of suicide and professed concern that a warning might put a chill on saving lives by deterring people from seeking treatment.

The 2004 data were almost identical to the 1991 data, with two differences. The drugs were going off patent. And there was a lack of even minimal benefit in minors against which risks could be discounted.

In the event psychotropic prescriptions to minors increased, perhaps aided by warnings. Company marketing of on-patent antipsychotics and anticonvulsants for bipolar disorder spun a line that suicidality on antidepressants pointed to an activation of bipolar disorder by antidepressants. The undiagnosed illness not the drug produced the difficulty. Give Zyprexa (olanzapine) or Depakote (semi-sodium valproate) instead.

Over a decade later, few physicians believe SSRIs cause suicide or even dependence. Many assume FDA bowed to pressure from some lobby like the Church of Scientology.

Ghosts

Study 329 was in fact authored by Sally Laden of Scientific Therapeutics International (STI). The final text was polished to a point where the GSK liaison writing to Laden seems to have felt uncomfortable:

> *It seems incongruous that we state that paroxetine [Paxil] is safe yet report so many SAEs [serious adverse events]. I know the investigators have not raised an issue… I will again review all the SAEs to make myself feel comfortable about what we report in print.*

Complete with covering letter from Martin Keller, also written by Laden, Study 329 went to *JAMA*, who rejected it. It then went to Mina Dulcan, the editor of *JAACAP*, who accepted.

The figures for suicidal events in the article were completely wrong but not even Laden had access to the raw data. GSK alerted Cohn and Wolfe, handling the PR for the article, that the study was a dud. Nevertheless, the message crafted for doctors was:

> *This "cutting-edge" landmark study is the first to compare efficacy of an SSRI and a TCA [tricyclic antidepressant] with placebo in the treatment of major depression in adolescents. Paxil demonstrates REMARKABLE Efficacy and Safety in the treatment of adolescent depression.*

In the wake of the FDA hearings, it became clear that as of 2004 the entire literature on antidepressant trials in children was ghost or company written.

A study the year before had provided clear evidence that between 50 and 100% of the antidepressant adult literature was also like Study 329 ghostwritten[56]. A later study by Erick Turner, an ex-FDA staffer, showed that nearly half of adult antidepressant trials done at the time of licensing remained unpublished. One third of the published trials had been viewed as negative by FDA but appeared as positive in medical journals.

---

56 Healy D, Cattell D. "The interface between authorship, industry and science in the domain of therapeutics." *British Journal of Psychiatry* 182, (2003), 22-27

Study 329 is company modus operandi. It applies to the literature for all on-patent drugs, whether cancer chemotherapies, antibiotics, or drugs for cholesterol, osteoporosis, or diabetes. It is difficult to establish just what proportion (90% or more) is ghost or company written, but in 100% of cases access to trial data is blocked

An Event

New York's fraud action against GSK in 2004 produced an agreement that GSK would post details of its trials on its website. This led to the publication of a set of Clinical Study Reports (CSRs) for the pediatric Paxil trials, including a 782-page CSR for Study 329.

Summary reports of trials for other GSK drugs, including trials of rosiglitazone (Avandia), for diabetes, were also made available. These were only 3-7 pages long. The reports, however, contained enough for Steven Nissen of the Cleveland Clinic to show an increased mortality rate on Avandia, leading to its withdrawal in Europe and restriction in the US.

The US Department of Justice took an action against GSK for promoting Paxil and Wellbutrin for unapproved uses and failing to report Avandia safety data. GSK resolved this case in 2012, paying $3 billion, then the largest such payment in corporate history. Their CEO, Andrew Witty, defended the company saying the 100,000 people who worked for GSK were as ethical as anyone else. A few rotten apples were the issue.

In January 2013, an AllTrials initiative, coordinated by Sense about Science, launched. AllTrials ostensibly would force companies to make their clinical trials available so that doctors could make properly evidence-based decisions. AllTrials favored a responsible method of accessing a limited set of company documents that would not compromise corporate privacy rights or patient confidentiality. This was AllTrials, not AllData.

Andrew Witty committed GSK to AllTrials. Transparency campaigners lauded the company. Three months after the *BMJ* noted GSK's $3 Billion settlement, it featured Witty on its March 9, 2013 front cover as the acceptable face of Big Pharma, with an image of an Obama-like candidate of hope figure.

Meanwhile, in July 2012, Peter Doshi, a key mover in transparency circles for his Tamiflu work (Chapter 11), noted that the CSRs for Paxil posted on GSK's website listed appendices A to H but these were unavailable. He wrote to New York State's Attorney General's Office about this. GSK agreed to add appendices A-G, but not appendix H. In the case of Study 329, appendices A-G contain the protocol and summary data tables. They amount to 5,494 pages. Appendix H contains Case Report Forms (CRFs), closer to the data.

In June 2013, Doshi and colleagues proposed a Restoring Invisible and Abandoned Trials initiative. Where there was sufficient data in the public domain, the idea was to author trials never published, or re-author published studies where there were grounds to think the original publication was misleading.

Study 329 was an obvious candidate for restoration. Invited to restore it, GSK replied that the published version was perfectly good. None of its authors had indicated a wish to change anything and JAACAP saw no reason to retract it.

Work began on the restoration in July 2013 using material on GSK's website, minus Appendix H. In December, the restorers applied to GSK for access to Appendix H for audit. Perhaps fooled by the word audit, GSK offered access through a portal with a triple identification access system to a remote desktop in GSK. There was no ability to download or print anything. The system routinely chucked the restoration team off in mid-task, which made interrogating the 77,000 pages of Appendix H difficult.

Despite the difficulties, on September 1, 2014 the team submitted a Restored Study 329 to the *BMJ*. *BMJ*'s website states that it takes an average of 8 weeks from study submission to publication. The paper had six reviewers, instead of the customary two. It went through seven reviews rather than the usual one. A year later it had not been published. *BMJ*'s editors were in agony. They queried a myriad of minor details, paying little heed to the responses. They repeatedly accepted and unaccepted the paper.

BMJ finally came clean. They were stuck on the conflicts of interest of the restoration team, two of whom had been experts for plaintiffs in SSRI lawsuits. *BMJ*'s lawyers said this fatally compromised the journals position should GSK take an action against it. But it turned out the partner of the *BMJ* editor handling the paper was also partner in Ropes and Gray, a Boston law firm, who handled GSK's defense against the US Department of Justice and also legal difficulties GSK were then having in China.

In the resulting duel, *BMJ* cracked. "Restoring Study 329" was published on September 15, 2015. Regardless of how the data were cut, paroxetine could not be shown to work.[57]

The Keller-Laden paper had reported 6 cases of emotional lability in 2001. In response to FDA's 2002 letter asking for all cases of suicidality, GSK reported 10 cases. FDA found one more. The restoration showed 14 cases, and others have since come to light. Appendix H was critical to revealing the location of these drug wrecks.

The never published 26-week 329 continuation phase was published in 2016 and revealed even more suicidal acts. These data generated in 1997 showed that the withdrawal arms of both acute and continuation phase were highly dangerous. SmithKline in 1997 was publicly denying any withdrawal or dependence issues on Paxil.

The restored study offers a compendium of ways in which companies hide adverse events. There was a use of obscure codes like emotional lability to hide suicidal events. Common and less severe symptoms like headache or dizziness were grouped with agitation or suicidality to hide the difference between Paxil and placebo. Some suicidal events simply never made it from Appendix H to the clinical study report (CSR). Both Paxil and placebo subjects were allowed other medication, such as antihistamines, some of which are serotonin reuptake inhibitors, which hid the difference between treatment and placebo.

The maneuvers were egregious but there is little here that health service managers don't do every day of the week. The difference lies in the claims that Study 329 is science and the impossibility of accessing the data.

---

57 See: Study320.org and *Children of the Cure* for details.

The Restoring Study 329 message is that scientific articles are not Biblical texts. Trials generate outputs not truths. Companies hide outputs, figures and data—the identity that is of the participants. All interpretations of the outputs are provisional although some may command greater assent. Studies should open up questions rather than close them down. Journal texts are prescriptive rather than descriptive. They hand down commandments. This has been shown to work; Your job [clinicians] is to prescribe and your job [patients] is to take.

Study 329 is about authorship and scientific authority. It is the only study with divergent analyses in print simultaneously. One, the subject of a fraud action and a $3 billion fine; the other, the only company study in a major journal complete with outputs others can analyze and interpret. The Keller paper and other papers from this period remain built into guidelines and articles on childhood depression that still recommend the use of SSRIs.

AllTrials, Sense about Science, and GSK dismissed the Restored Study as irrelevant. Iain Chalmers, the founder of the Cochrane Collaboration, claimed GSK had shown themselves to be enlightened. But while trumpeting transparency, GSK (and other companies) continued to block access in usable form to the outputs and data from their trials, insisting patient confidentiality forces them to block access.

There is a statistically significant increase in the rate of suicidality on paroxetine in Study 329. In normal clinical practice it is appropriate to tell a patient about links between a hazard and treatment, so they can avoid this and related drugs in future. Knowing the cause of a suicidal event is important for the self-image of any of us, especially a teenager. GSK say the patient's doctor must decide what to tell their patient. But the Study 329 doctors are wrapped into a fraudulent interpretation of data they never had. Unless GSK reach out to patients injured in this trial, claims that their refusal of access to the data is based on a concern for patients ring hollow.

Shelley Jofre made clear how easy it is to spot warning signs in a study that fooled many. It takes a lack of deference to the reputation of a journal and the distinction of names on an authorship line, an unwillingness to be fobbed off with statistical jargon, and an ability to insist on sensible answers to questions.

These are the qualifications needed for dealing with a politician. The presentation of RCTs in medicine has now more in common with politics than science. Neither consumers (doctors) nor the media have caught up with this.

RCTs arose from a realization we are biased toward hope. If a cancer treatment has only a 3% chance of success many of us will grab it. This hope creates a spin that may be difficult to overcome. RCTs were once about countering this spin with data, countering a pleasure principle with a reality principle. Not now. Sally Laden, the doyenne of ghostwriters, caught it when, faced with a SmithKline decision to abandon a manuscript on Paxil withdrawal effects, she wrote: "there are some data that no amount of spin will fix."[58]

Study 329 remains unretracted. The editor of the *New York Times* would have been fired for publishing it, or at least not retracting it when the background story came to light. Mina Dulcan, the *JAACAP* editor was unfazed by the Fraud case or the $3 billion fine. We might all be safer if RCTs were published in the *New York Times* rather than in medical journals.

Study 329 points to a totalitarian control of the medical literature and a failure of authenticity beyond anything the Old Left, New Left, Third Way, or Religious Believers could ever have imagined. Anyone taking any medication brought on the market since 1990 is part of an alienated class whether they know it or not, at risk from manufactured risks. The authors featuring on these articles are the epitome of celebrity culture, famous only for being famous.

The Bigger Picture

This is not an ivory tower matter. Even doctors who accept the risks of SSRIs are under pressure from guidelines and insurers to prescribe

---

58 Email from Sally Laden to Daniel Burnham. Subject: Re Par 222 manuscript. (December 14, 2000).

antidepressants from the first day of conception to the last day of life. Doctors wary of bisphosphonates, statins, or adding a third antihypertensive, when blood pressure has not come down to a target level, are under the same pressure from an apparently scientific literature.

As of 2020, there have been 30 RCTs on antidepressants involving over 10,000 children. All negative. Even the two Prozac studies listed by FDA as positive and the basis for an approval of Prozac for children were negative. In one NIH study, there were 34 suicidal events on Prozac compared to 3 on placebo, but no mention of a suicide risk in any of the 7 published articles from this study. The material from this study has since been destroyed.

Studies continue, recruiting thousands of children in settings from the Russian Federation and Mexico to American foster-homes or correctional facilities. These make Study 329 look ethical. Articles claiming the drugs work continue to be published. One such article appeared in Frontiers in Psychiatry in 2020. Meta-analyzing ghostwritten articles without any access to the underlying 'data', it extracted a positive result from these negative trials and on this basis claimed antidepressants worked for children.[59]

In 2001 when the Keller paper was published, over 70 articles claimed benefits to minors of antidepressants in largely individual cases. The reason for RCTs is to curb the enthusiasms and selection biases that can affect clinicians' assessments of new treatments. Despite 30 negative RCTs, by 2018 antidepressants had become one of the most used drugs by Western adolescent girls.

In 2016 Britain's Health Secretary billed the state of children's mental health services as the greatest failing of Britain's NHS. Children were attempting suicide while waiting for appointments, despite large amounts of money being pumped into the services. The money was going into screening, auditors, and managers rather than coalface staff. The suicide attempts came from children put on antidepressants by family doctors

---

59 K Boaden et al. "Antidepressants in Children and Adolescents: Meta-Review of Efficacy, Tolerability and Suicidality in Acute Treatment." *Frontiers in Psychiatry*, doi: 10.3389/fpsyt.2020.00717

while they waited for appointments. These drugs disinhibit, create risk taking behavior, cause suicidality and aggression, and change personalities. When finally seen, children risk being incorrectly diagnosed, inappropriately treated, and further damaged.

This is identical to the osteoporosis scenario featured in these pages except that aging cannot be blamed. The mantra that health costs keep escalating because of our aging populations comes unstuck here. Both children and the elderly are caught by the same dynamic. Fraudulent studies lead to guidelines that mandate treatments more likely to harm than help. This leads to more screeners, auditors and managers, whose employment hides the growing spend on drugs that increase rather than reduce risks to us.

The Panorama programs happened when a narrative about whistleblowers the media are comfortable with could be spun. It is now clear that we have a rotten barrel rather than just rotten apples. There is no access to any data, the entire literature is ghostwritten and, rather than let the public know they should never have licensed Prozac for children, regulators and politicians refuse to take questions.

The media cannot tackle rotten barrels. They like to blame doctors who do not keep to the guidelines or who prescribe off-label. They get a warm glow from suggesting putting more money into talking therapy rather than drugs. They cannot cope with the idea their answers will only fuel the use of psychotropic drugs.

The media are also shackled when it comes to rotten barrels in that the third estate are no longer companies with a vocation to engage citizens. They are largely outsourced media-service operations that deliver products to consumers, keeping to false-balance guidelines. Study 329 offers a window on something that needs an extra-ordinary response.

Murder or Accident

Two weeks short of fifty years from the day Marilyn Monroe committed suicide on sleeping pills, James Holmes walked into a movie theater in Aurora, Colorado, showing Dark Knight Rises. He opened fire, killing twelve and injuring seventy.

A few months earlier, as a quiet introvert, anxious at speaking in public, at the suggestion of his first ever girlfriend, he walked into a university clinic and was put on the SSRI sertraline. Despite complaining of side effects in successive visits, his doctor hiked his sertraline. As the dose increased, his personality changed. His shyness vanished. He visited dating sites, approached attractive women, and bought a motorbike. Ideas of violence emerged, took root, and grew in force. He bought guns and went to a shooting range to practice. He made plans. His efforts to warn acquaintances and his doctor of the risk he posed went unheeded. In a diary he charted the evolution of what he called dysphoric mania.

He previously had a related but mild reaction to a serotonin reuptake inhibiting antihistamine. After the shootings, both his parents had disturbing and violent reactions to SSRIs at a time when they had no inkling their son had been on an SSRI. When re-exposed to an SSRI several months later in jail, Holmes became suicidal.

Holmes had a compelling drug defense, but despite believing his medication played a role in the shooting and a strong expert report in support of this, his public defender lawyers didn't mention sertraline, perhaps as part of a deal with the prosecution. They ran an insanity defense and tried to persuade a jury he had schizophrenia. The record didn't bear this out and he barely escaped execution, ending up with the third longest jail sentence in US history, locked away somewhere with a changed identity.

England's Lord Chief Justice, Matthew Hale, outlined Holmes' defense, in 1736 in a book even more central to American than British criminal law:

> *if a person by the unskilfulness of his physician or the contrivance of his enemies, eat or drinketh such a thing as causeth such a temporary or permanent frenzy, as aconitum or nux vomica, this puts him into the same condition, in reference to crimes as any other frenzy, and equally excuseth him.*[60]

---

60 Hale M (1736/2003) *Historia Placitorum Coronae. Vol 1 Lawbook Exchange.* Clark, (New Jersey), 30.

But today, despite small-print concessions by companies their drugs can cause homicide, our legal systems have no idea how to handle an event like this. Few forensic psychiatrists can distinguish insanity from a drug-induced delirium.

The data that drugs like sertraline can cause homicide are compelling. All drugs in the SSRI group cause akathisia (mental turmoil—dysphoric mania) in a significant proportion of those who take them, along with disinhibition and delirium. These mechanisms, singly or in combination, lead to inner-directed violence, suicidality, or outer-directed homicidality.

As early as 1982, Pfizer accepted sertraline had made healthy volunteers aggressive. In later clinical trials, it caused more aggression than placebo. The 2004 paroxetine and sertraline data showed increased rates of aggression in minors. At the time of the Aurora events, the SSRIs came with Black Box warnings about the risks in those 25 and younger. Holmes was 24.

There is a compelling case that sertraline can cause homicide and in Holmes' case it did. No reader can judge the validity of this claim. Every reader can however reflect on the issues for a defense team, who believed the drug had played a key role. They had a supportive report. They faced prosecution experts with no psychopharmacology expertise. Yet they did not feel able to raise the issue, even in mitigation, for a client who faced execution.

A sertraline defense would have brought ghostwriting and the lack of access to trial data into play, and evidence that Pfizer and other companies had known about treatment induced homicidality for thirty years.

When a jury in Cheyenne in 2001 convicted GSK in a homicide case, they didn't have to let anyone who pulled a trigger walk out of court free. In a 2001 case in Australia, a judge took it upon himself to bypass a jury completely and declare that but for the sertraline David Hawkins had been put on he would not have killed his wife. Hawkins walked free. But had Holmes' lawyers succeeded in acquitting their client, both they and he might have had real worries he would have been torn apart had he walked out of court.

Holmes was in a similar situation to the Guildford Four. In October 1974, in the middle of an IRA bombing campaign in England, two bombs went off in pubs in Guildford. Four innocent Irish people were picked up and jailed. English lawyers working to free them were up against the system. As England's Chief Justice, Tom Denning, put it:

> *If their story is right, it is such an appalling vista it cannot be. Wrongfully convicted prisoners should stay in jail rather than be freed and risk a loss of public confidence in the law.*[61]

Treatment induced homicides, and terror cases like the Guildford Four, might seem to belong to worlds far removed from ours. Everyone who is drug wrecked, however, is up against the same dynamic. There are over 100 drugs from antibiotics to skin drugs and statins that companies accept can cause enough agitation to lead to violence or suicide. But in the event of a death or disability on treatment, health services have no boxes for the things that regularly go wrong when good staff keep to guidelines. The managers who supervise root-cause analyses after a death or injury will not snarl at us the way a prosecutor might or incarcerate us the way a judge might. They are, though, just as capable of locking us into a cage of bewilderment and resentment, with as little chance of clearing a loved one's name.

One hundred and fifty years ago faced with a predictable number of deaths from anesthesia each year, American surgeons faced questions about the ethics of doing evil in order to do good. If the patient died from the anesthetic, were they murderers? We collectively decided they aren't murderers, even though roughly one per thousand anesthetic events today still lead to death. Patients are warned of this risk beforehand.

In the case of the miners in Lens in 1970 (chapter 9), if there were decent efforts to make the mine as safe as possible, most people were prepared to regard the deaths from a disaster in a mine as unfortunate.

What do we call the deaths of minors or others triggered by an SSRI taken on the back of studies like 329? Is the consent these minors or their

---

61 See Healy's comments: bmj.com/content/358/bmj.j4196

families give to taking the medication valid? Unlike the miners in Lens, these minors are not paid to take risks, and are not covered by insurance. Unlike anesthesia, the odds of being harmed are greater than the chance of benefit. Key to these deaths is information put in place to facilitate the sales of tablets rather than the safety of those who take them.

We want to see monsters in the dock rather than people who are just doing a job. That otherwise good people in GSK and Pfizer, bureaucrats in FDA, and on the editorial boards of medical journals, can be linked to such an outcome is the essence of what Hannah Arendt termed the banality of evil.

Like the mining disaster in Lens, the restoration of Study 329 is an Event. The details of how many articles are ghostwritten, or the rate at which patients are hospitalized for treatment induced conditions are now known. Events make history. They create a before and after, but not necessarily right here and now.

All politicians, regulators, guideline writing bodies, medical associations and senior figures in the legal establishment know about the ghostwriting of the medical literature, and lack of access to trial data. Their response is "yes we know but what can we do about it?" Or, "it's not our job to police the medical literature."[62]

James Holmes' Drug Wreck is billed as murder. Wrecks like these challenge the validity of the Liberal State central to which is its reservation of the right to violence to itself. We give up our right to retaliate in favor of due process. Due process in this case though seduces us into taking a drug that can cause us to kill without warning this might happen. If we try to defend ourselves, due process pits us against a ghostwritten literature without access to the data that might prove our innocence. To find us not guilty, jurors would have to become aware of an abyss and then traverse it.

---

62 For copies of letters to and from all these bodies following the death of Stephan O'Neill, see: davidhealy.org/the-perfect-killing-machine/ with posts before and after.

13: ONCE IS NOT NEVER

This generation thinks that nothing faithful, vulnerable, fragile can be durable or have any true power. Death waits for these things as a cement floor waits for a dropping light bulb. The brittle shell of glass loses its tiny vacuum. This is how we teach metaphysics on each other.
Saul Bellow, Herzog, 1964.

FDA licensed Chloromycetin in 1949. By 1952 the latest wonder antibiotic had made Parke-Davis the world's most profitable pharmaceutical company. That year in Los Angeles Dr. Albe Watkins turned to Chloromycetin when his son James developed a urinary infection. Shortly afterwards, James began to bruise. He had aplastic anemia, a disorder that turns blood into water and kills gruesomely. While his son was dying, Watkins learnt that Parke-Davis knew of other cases in Los Angeles. After James died, he drove his family across country to FDA. Tracking down doctors in towns they stayed in, he enquired about aplastic anemia and found 12 deaths and more later. FDA had been notified of 75 others.

Parke-Davis began hunting through individual histories and circumstances for factors on which they could pin the aplastic anemia. They created an "Anything But the Company Drug" (ABCD) playbook that all companies now use.

FDA convened a panel to investigate, which agreed Chloromycetin could cause aplastic anemia. Parke-Davis spun its emergence on the far side of FDA's review into an FDA endorsement of their drug. Sales boomed.

Leo Meyler published *Side Effects of Drugs* that same year. Along with Watkins' efforts, this convinced FDA they needed an adverse event reporting system. The agency tried but failed to get doctors and hospitals on board. In 1968, FDA asked companies to submit Periodic Safety Update Reports on their drugs covering all serious adverse events reported. This offers companies an opportunity to hone their ABCD skills. FDA gets details of all other factors the company believe make it impossible to link their drug to whatever effect.

FDA created MedWatch, an Adverse Event Reporting System aimed at doctors in 1993. It was revamped in 2004, and in 2010 the public were encouraged to report. Most reports in the US, however, still come from companies. In other countries they are more likely to come from doctors. But no country does anything with enthusiasm. FDA state that little more than 1% of serious adverse events are reported to them. All regulators categorize these reports as anecdotes or hearsay and caution against inferring causality.

Neither Daniel Carpenter's 800-page history of FDA, *Reputation and Power*, nor Philip Hilts 460-page volume, *Protecting America's Health*, mention MedWatch. To have histories of an agency largely shaped by its Wrecks, thalidomide, sulfanilamide, Chloromycetin, Panalba, Vioxx, feature nothing about safety systems is like encountering the Marie Celeste—an American ship discovered adrift in the Atlantic in 1872 with no-one onboard.

The silence is even stranger given that Drug wrecks are now a modal form of death and disability. A dwindling band of clinical pharmacologists have published papers claiming treatment is the third most likely cause of deaths in hospitals, even when all cancer deaths are put down to the cancer rather than the drugs used to treat it. Cancer drugs are among the most toxic in medicine but are never listed as the cause of death. Cause of death is less likely to be investigated outside hospital where, given that people are not acutely ill, drugs are even more likely to be a lethal factor and source of disability. None of these estimates include the 50,000 deaths per annum linked to opioids in the US—more than happen on the roads, or at the height of the AIDS crisis.

The silence is linked to a lack of rescue options. Outside the United States, it is close to impossible to take an action against a pharmaceutical company or a doctor for a Drug Wreck. Within the US, actions rarely succeed. The hit to companies is so minor it can be factored in as a cost of doing business.

Something leads doctors not to report drug wrecks. It leads nurses and pharmacists not to report. Psychotherapists bitterly hostile to the medical model don't report. Now that the public can report, we don't. Our families won't support us in taking these issues to doctors. Most of us sense that even pleasant doctors are likely to get nasty if we raise things. If not nasty, we will be viewed as driving the wrong way on the motorway. We share an experience with Holocaust survivors that Primo Levi noted, if we start talking, we are just not heard or seen. From time immemorial, misfortune has been shunned.

Mapping the Island

In 1952 clinicians and regulators had no idea who was taking Chloro-mycetin. This remains the case today for all drugs. In contrast, by 1970 drug companies knew just who prescribed their drugs. In the 1950s, the McAdams Agency, with Arthur Sackler at the helm, was emerging as the leading advertising agency for pharmaceuticals. Its closest competitor was the Frohlich advertising company. In 1954, Bill Frohlich and David Dubow set up Intercontinental Marketing Services (IMS), a market research company offering to enable companies to make informed strategic decisions about the marketplace.

In the early 1950s, some companies collected pharmacy sales data. When medicines were made prescription-only in 1951, IMS were the first company to collect prescription data. The operation grew. Frohlich hived it off as a separate business.

With IMS data a company salesperson who visited a doctor knew exactly what she was prescribing and could arrive at her office with a tailored marketing pitch. When Purdue marketed Oxycontin in 1996, IMS data showed which doctors were receptive to their message about pain and which weren't. At the same time, pain specialists and patient groups complained about mandatory opioid tracking schemes that would let the Drug Enforcement Agency (DEA) establish what was going on.

Oxycontin attracted attention to Purdue. A hidden story emerged. IMS was Arthur Sackler's brainchild and David Dubow had transferred from McAdams to Frohlich to run IMS. With Frohlich's death in 1971, IMS was solely owned by Raymond and Mortimer Sackler. It made the Sacklers wealthier than Purdue did.

Skin in the Game

Parke-Davis began in Detroit Michigan in 1866 as a small pharmacy business. While the names of Hervey Parke, an early investor, and George Davis, an early employee, stuck, it was never a family business. Shrewd management kept it in business long enough to take advantage of the post-War pharmaceutical revolution. It was much bigger than Pfizer when the opportunities to become a modern pharmaceutical corporation emerged in mid-century.

After a dip in sales linked to aplastic anemia, Chloromycetin prescribing picked up again. Lasagna noted in 1968 that this drug, by then supposed to be targeted at severe infections only, was given by doctors for common colds and put by veterinarians in feed for livestock. But decades defending Chloromycetin rather than finding new products left Parke-Davis vulnerable to a take-over by Warner Lambert in 1976, who were swallowed by Pfizer.

In contrast to Parke-Davis, Maurer and Wirtz, which began in 1845 as a chemical company in Germany, remained a family business. In 1945, Hermann Wirtz, who inherited a place on the family board, was its driving force. The Wirtz family were among the most notable Catholic families in Aachen. They were also National Socialist party supporters.

In 1946 Wirtz hived off Chemie-Grünenthal as a pharmaceutical company. Somehow, he became the first German supplier of penicillin.

The company grew rapidly. Heinrich Mückter, who had spent the war testing typhus vaccines in Polish concentration camps, was recruited as chief pharmacist.

Otto Ambros, who had developed sarin, soman and other nerve gases as a chemist in IG Farben, and was imprisoned at Nuremberg, joined the Grünenthal board in 1952 after his release. By then the post-war West German economic miracle was taking shape, and there was a dense amnesia about the Nazi period. Ambros became a consultant to Konrad Adenauer, the German Chancellor, and the US Army Chemical Corps.

Ambros briefed Mückter on a series of compounds developed by a team under Ernest Fourneau in the *Institut Pasteur* in Paris. Allied to the Rhône-Poulenc pharmaceutical company, in 1936 Fourneau had robbed Bayer of the sulfa drugs (chapter 5). This collaboration also developed the first antihistamines, Antergan, Neo-Antergan, Multergan and Phenergan. Fourneau was jailed after the War for collaboration with the Nazis. Ambros suggested acquiring K 17 from Rhône-Poulenc. Mückter wrote up a way to mass produce this. In May 1954, this gave Grünenthal a process patent on the compound. On October 1, 1957, K 17 was marketed as Contergan, a sleeping pill.

Grünenthal billed Contergan as absolutely safe. It is now clear it has an SSRI-like profile with agitation in some, sexual dysfunction, and peripheral neuropathy in others. By early 1958, the company was stonewalling enquiries about peripheral neuropathy. Instead, they ramped up their marketing effort and made the drug up in syrups and suppositories also. Kinesaft was promoted as a sleeping juice to give children before parents went to the cinema (Kine).

The first baby with deformities was born at Christmas 1956 to a Grünenthal employee. Others followed. Peak Contergan sales in November 1960, coincided with a letter from a pharmacist asking about birth defects. The company claimed it was safe in pregnancy.

In June 1961, William McBride, an obstetrician in Sydney, reported 3 cases of birth defects linked to Distaval (thalidomide) to the Australian company marketing the drug. He sent an article to the *Lancet*, which was rejected. In June, Widukind Lenz, a pediatrician in Hamburg, also made a link to babies with birth defects. He found hundreds of cases in the Hamburg area. On November 15, Lenz phoned Mückter stating thalidomide had caused hundreds of babies to be born with birth defects. He demanded the company withdraw it. Mückter refused. Grünenthal threatened to sue Lenz. They capitulated when the newspaper, *Welt am Sontag*, reported Lenz's views on November 26. The drug was withdrawn in Germany but not in Britain, Canada, Spain and elsewhere.

In late 1961, Frances Kelsey, a Canadian, began in the FDA when her husband moved to Washington. She was faced with Richardson Merrell's application to market thalidomide. Concerned about reports of peripheral neuropathy, she delayed its approval. Kefauver's Bill was close to dead in Congress. Emmanuel Celler, chair of a House Anti-Trust subcommittee where Kefauver's bill was in review, called Dr Helen Taussig, a recently retired professor of pediatrics, who had been to Germany and seen thalidomide babies. She testified on May 24, 1962. The US media paid no heed. On July 15, the story was repackaged by Morton Mintz in terms of the heroism of Francis Kelsey. The US paid heed. Kefauver's bill rose from the grave and was signed into law on October 10, 1962, delaying the US approval of thalidomide by 3 decades.

Several German states took action against Grünenthal. A legal trial, expected to be a second Nuremberg Trial, began in Aachen Casino in May 1968. Hermann Wirtz was too ill to come to court but not too ill to attend a secret meeting with the Government. In early 1968, the Social Democrats replaced the Christian Democrats in government on the back of growing awareness of the Holocaust and the role of National Socialists in government. Grünenthal's lead lawyer, Joseph Neuberger, a Jew, took over as Minister for the Interior. Neuberger promoted a deal that assigned minor guilt to the defendants. It awarded thalidomide victims a pittance, half of which came from the company and half from the government, in exchange for signing away all rights to take further action against the company.

Grünenthal produced thalidomide through to 2003. It took out 24 patents on it and related molecules between 1965 and 2001, filing some during the Court case. It put thalidomide into trials of vulnerable patients with learning disabilities, and Alzheimer's dementia. In 1961 it marketed the pain-killer Tramadol, Ultram, viewed as contributing to the opioid epidemic. From 2000, it marketed Purdue's Oxycontin in Europe and South America.

Jacob Sheskin, working in Jerusalem with leprosy patients, in 1965 claimed thalidomide eased the pain of the red and painful nodules that sometimes develop in leprosy called Erythema Nodosum Leprosum (ENL). Sheskin ran a trial of thalidomide in Venezuela and WHO ran a further trial in 1971; Grünenthal supplied the drugs. Both trials reported a benefit. Dapsone was the standard treatment for leprosy in 1965 in a dose of 20mg. Sheskin was giving this in doses up to 700mg. At these doses ENL is more common.

Grünenthal took out a patent on thalidomide for leprosy. Articles appeared co-authored by Sheskin and Grünenthal. One of Sheskin's colleagues was slated as an expert witness for Grünenthal in the 1968 trial. The media ran with a story about a cure for leprosy that led to a flourishing market for thalidomide in Latin America in the 1970s.

Through the 1970s, a string of breathless reports of benefits in skin conditions such as actinic prurigo, discoid lupus erythematosus and Behcet's syndrome, a condition with more articles written about it than patients who have it, maintained interest in thalidomide. Anti-inflammatory effects led to talk of benefits in auto-immune conditions and perhaps cancer. Its effect on skin conditions that sometimes didn't respond to other treatments brought it to the attention of patients with AIDS, when the epidemic struck in the 1980s. Buyers' Clubs formed and imported thalidomide from Brazil through Mexico.

Another path also took thalidomide to AIDS. The major German pharmaceutical companies, Hoechst and Bayer, merged to form IG Farben in 1925. After the War, Hoechst and Bayer were reborn. Hoechst took over the American Celanese Corporation, a chemical company, in 1985 and split off a pharmaceutical division, Celgene.

The story Celgene promote is that David Stirling of Celgene, looking for new drug leads, visited Gilla Kaplan, an Israeli, then working in New Jersey close to Celgene's headquarters. One of the consequences of the immune-deficiency AIDS caused was a re-emergence of tuberculosis. Thalidomide like everything in the 1940s had been tried in tuberculosis and its 1954 patent claimed it could help. Reviewing options for AIDS treatment, Kaplan suggested thalidomide. AIDS patients by then were already importing thalidomide from Brazil and claiming that it could turn around the wasting syndrome linked to the illness.

Kaplan worked on anti-Tumor Necrosis Factor (TNF) drugs as treatments for auto-immune conditions. She claimed thalidomide had anti-TNF effects, which might underpin anti-inflammatory and perhaps other effects. She reported increased T-cell counts, the same effects as with AZT. In the febrile atmosphere of the AIDS epidemic, thalidomide was talked about as the miracle drug that would cure AIDS. Kaplan joined the Celgene Board.

Celgene took out a product patent on thalidomide in 1992. In the wake of Lasagna's work to speed up access to the market for AIDS drugs, and the Orphan Drugs Act, Celgene opened negotiations with FDA. In 1996, FDA invited a submission for thalidomide for use in ENL, of which there were a vanishingly few patients in the US. A license was granted in June 1998. The drug was marketed with a System for Thalidomide Education and Prescribing Safety (STEPS) in place. This would now be called a Risk Evaluation and Mitigation Strategy (REMS), comprising a set of stern warnings, monitoring and consent forms for doctors, patients and pharmacists. Celgene patented the REMS package.

By the time thalidomide was approved, the AIDS wave had swept past. The illegal supply may have helped wasting by curing mouth ulcers and letting people eat. But no one ever asked whether an anti-TNF action, producing a state of immune deficiency, was a good idea in immune deficient patients. The drug causes neuropathy, thrombosis, heart attacks and strokes. Its informal use in AIDS was likely greatest just at the time when AIDS deaths were most common.

After supporting its use in Latin America for three decades without a REMS package, in 2003 WHO dropped thalidomide as a treatment option for leprosy. A 1993 BBC program claimed there were more thalidomide babies in Brazil than anywhere else in the world. They were born to women who received it through informal networks as a sedative and tranquilizer.

Perhaps to justify continuing production, in the 1970s and 1980s Grünenthal claimed to be researching possible uses for thalidomide in cancer. Another story has it an AIDS patient drew Celgene's attention to multiple myeloma, a cancer of white blood cells, after giving it to his father and seeing benefits. Within a year of its launch, Celgene was running trials for Thalomid in multiple myeloma, where it has minor benefits. They were later fined for promoting it aggressively for cancers in general.[63]

The REMS package did more than justify high costs. In 2009 Dr Reddy, a generic company challenged Celgene's patent on the drug. Celgene's successful defense was based not only on its product patent on thalidomide but also on a patent taken out on STEPS (REMS).

A tweak to the thalidomide molecule produced lenalidomide (Revlimid), which in some animal models is an even more potent teratogen. It also causes peripheral neuropathy, sexual dysfunction, and agitation. FDA granted lenalidomide orphan drug status for the treatment of multiple myeloma in 2001. Complete with a REMS program, it was licensed in 2005 and came on the market at a cost of $165,000 per year. By 2016 Revlimid was worth $7 billion per year to Celgene. Its price tripled between 2005 and 2020 for no reason other than to enhance the profitability of the company and its executives.

Another tweak to thalidomide produced apremilast (Otezla), which Celgene introduced for psoriasis in 2014. This was launched with images of women in swimsuits or wearing low cut dresses, who might have a touch

---

63 In 2018, Celgene settled a whistleblower lawsuit for $280 million linked to behaviour around 2000. See: youtube.com/watch?v=qYvW4pm0_fI

of psoriasis at the back of a neck. It costs a fortune. It causes suicidality. Its approval trials were run through a clinical trials' mill with the names of significant dermatologists attached to ghostwritten articles. Reports of suicidality were dismissed as down to the depression psoriasis causes. It also causes birth defects.

Forbes rated Celgene as the world's second most profitable pharmaceutical company in 2013. It had few drugs other than Thalomid, Revlimid and Otezla, but these had brand recognition to die for, making it a prime target for takeover by Bristol Myers Squibb in 2018.

Otezla is billed as a phosphodiesterase inhibitor. Whether this action has anything to do with its benefits in skin conditions is less clear. This mechanism of action was rolled out as the next big thing for treating depression in the 1980s, before the SSRIs came onstream. Several phosphodiesterase inhibitors came and went before Otezla reused this card.

Another phosphodiesterase inhibitor, Siliq (brodalumab), was also approved for psoriasis. The Siliq trials threw up so many suicidal acts that Astra Zeneca, its sponsor, withdrew. Valeant, a company few had heard of, picked it up. FDA approved Siliq, with a REMS package. Doctors, patients, and pharmacists all had to sign for each prescription, stating they had been told about the risk of suicidality on Siliq, just as they would if prescribing Thalomid or Roaccutane to women of child-bearing years

Why the REMS package? The SSRIs and opioids have a benefit in that doctors can blame any difficulties on a patient's disease rather than the drug. As a treatment for skin disorders, Siliq is more exposed. Valeant's adoption of Siliq may have just been aimed at making the money from the share-price jump that would come with approval. Or industry may be interested to see if the frisson REMS packages generate can add 'value'.

Skin was where the game was in 2015. Lilly's Taltz, Novartis' Cosentyx, and Centocor's Stelara, billed as interleukin antagonists, were rolled out for psoriasis, aimed largely at women. Patient panels were convened to bring the horrors of genital psoriasis in from the cold. All came with a potential to cause birth defects and suicide. There were no panels to manage these horrors.

The Manner of Our Dying[64]

Until recently a good death came with a warning. We could feel its approach and had time to set our affairs in order, take leave of family and friends, and reconcile ourselves with our creator. By 1900 a growing number of us had reasonable prospects of living beyond three score and ten years and an abrupt death was more likely to be viewed as good.

The change was caught in 1886 by Leo Tolstoy in *The Death of Ivan Illich*. Illich, a 45-year-old living a very ordinary life but feeling 'wrong' consulted his doctor. The then new quest for a specific diagnosis and treatment offered him hope. The doctor was unclear what was wrong. In the dark about his diagnosis and treatment, Illich felt trapped. Every hint of decay became a further horror. His doctor's management was a tissue of lies, cutting him off from family and friends and compromising his dying.

In 2002 Raymond Ilich, a 48-year-old man, who worked for Boeing as a computer specialist, was comfortably placed and living a very ordinary life with his wife Lois. He had no history of illness, was on no medication, and seemed unlikely to die.

Following 9/11 there was talk in Boeing about restructuring. On July 30, a day before his summer holiday ended, he told Lois there was a new divisional head and he was nervous he might lose his job. He was better placed than most to avoid this and colleagues helped him prep to meet the new manager. On Monday August 5, Lois suggested he have one of her Celexa, an SSRI, to help him settle. He took it. He became more agitated. Lois took him to their doctor who issued a prescription for more Celexa. Ray voiced thoughts of suicide.

The interview with the divisional head on August 9 went well, but afterwards Ray had a panic attack. He and Lois returned to the doctor, where he confessed to suicidal thinking. The doctor added further medication to calm him down. Lois removed the kitchen knives from the house, leaving only two steak knives. Over the weekend Ray's agitation grew; he felt like "crawling out of his skin." On Monday Lois teed up a psychiatric appointment for the next day. Ray was up before her. Going downstairs,

---

64 A phrase that stems from Dee Mangin.

she saw him race into the garden and fall on a knife. The police later found the other knife broken in attempts to stab himself.

Lois Ilich took a lawsuit against Forest, the company marketing Celexa in the United States. A pre-trial hearing was held for the judge to determine whether reliable scientific evidence could be brought to bear on the case. Forest's lawyers claimed no-one could come to a reliable judgment about what had led to Raymond Ilich's death. Depression kills, paranoid agitation kills, the other medication Ilich was put on can kill. So, the lawyers argued, there was no reliable scientific evidence to permit the case to go ahead.

The extension of this argument is that there is no valid way to diagnose the cause of death in any case. The existence of changes on scans or blood tests may simply be evidence of what we can live with. If it's not possible to diagnose the cause of Ray Ilich's death on the balance of probabilities, it's not possible to come to a verdict in any legal case or clinical case. But the pattern of Ray's death mapped much better onto the pattern of Celexa induced suicide than onto depression, paranoia, or his other medication. Diagnoses and verdicts are judgment calls. The judge threw out the company argument and Forest settled.

In fact, in the small print of drug labels that now run to 40 pages, under headings such as other reports, companies report events like depression and suicidality in over 300 drugs and psychosis or violence on up to 100 drugs. They assume medical and lay readers will infer these reports come from people who hate drugs and perhaps believe we never made it to the moon and will regard the company as wonderfully transparent for mentioning these reports. In fact, companies only include events in these sections when they have run through their ABCD playbook and are left with no option but to conclude their drug likely played a part. The label for sertraline (Zoloft), James Holmes' drug, included violence and psychosis at the time of the Aurora shootings.

Would any of us choose such a horrific death? There are over 300 drugs for which, based on cases like Raymond Ilich's, companies have decided there is convincing evidence treatment can trigger suicide. This includes many antibiotics, all antipsychotics, antidepressants and anticonvulsants, several analgesics, antihypertensives, contraceptives and statins. But when we take these, we are never told we might be choosing our death. A 2018 Chicago study found that even if we have no psychiatric history, our risk of depression and suicide goes up with each of these drugs, doubles if we are on two and triples if we are on three or more.[65]

It is not just death by suicide we don't get a choice about. While the statins have modest effects in reducing deaths from cardiovascular events in high-risk groups, they increase the risk of cancer leaving the number of deaths overall unchanged. We are not informed of this. Some might prefer an abrupt and pain-free death to a lingering and painful one.

Anonymous

In 1962 we put a premium on flights that get places 15 minutes faster rather than on flights that get there 100% of the time. We created a market in effectiveness rather than safety. Regulators put adverse event reporting systems (AERS) in place for doctors, just as pilots have air safety reporting systems (ASRS). But where pilots refuse to fly if their near misses are ignored, doctors report on no more than 1% of serious events that happen on treatment and accept that no-one heeds their reports. If we go down *en route* to New York, our pilot also goes down. If our femur fractures on a bisphosphonate, or we develop cognitive dysfunction on a statin, in contrast, our doctor flies on unaffected.

Key to the neglect of AERS reports is that reports to regulators from doctors or patients are anonymized. This transforms them into hearsay. The hearsay rule dates to the execution of Walter Raleigh in 1618 whose conviction was based on accounts of what he had said and done offered by people who would not come to court to be cross-examined. No lawyer arguing a case can get a court to take reports of prior injuries or deaths on a drug into account if no-one can be brought to court to be questioned in front of a jury.

---

65 See: samizdathealth.org/shipwreck/

In 1959, Frank Ayd, an American psychiatrist, discovered a second tricyclic antidepressant, amitriptyline. It was effective for melancholia, a condition where sufferers lose interest in everything including sex. The only treatment for melancholia then was electroshock, which Ayd had given his father on a kitchen table. Ayd had no wish to compromise his drug, but in 1960 he reported amitriptyline could cause a sexual dysfunction distinguishable from the effect of melancholia on libido.

George Beaumont joined Geigy in 1970. He was given a brief to find clomipramine a niche. Now regarded as the most potent antidepressant, it was then another molecule in a crowded field. Beaumont placed articles in newspapers featuring a minor celebrity, thrilled her boyfriend's premature ejaculation could be managed by 10 mg of clomipramine, a fraction of the 150 mg antidepressant dose, taken 30 minutes before intercourse.

Beaumont also established clomipramine as the premier drug treatment for Obsessive-Compulsive Disorder (OCD). It began to encroach on behavior therapy for OCD. Isaac Marks, the leading proponent of behavior therapy fought back. In lectures, he often mentioned the persistent orgasms a patient of his, a nun, experienced after withdrawal from clomipramine, a first description of Persistent Genital Arousal Disorder (PGAD).

Sandra Leiblum put PGAD on the map in 2001. Although a therapist, she was convinced the persistent genital arousal 4 of her patients reported was organic rather than psychological. PGAD is now linked to hormonal changes around the menopause and discontinuation from serotonin reuptake inhibitors, which includes many antibiotics, antihistamines, analgesics, anxiolytics and antidepressants. Women with PGAD have turned to perineal nerve ablation, clitoridectomy, and other drastic remedies for relief, but nothing helps.

The SSRI antidepressants stem from clomipramine. Launched around 1990, these are ineffective for melancholia. Melancholia however is a rare disorder compared to the nervous conditions for which doctors were then giving benzodiazepines. The marketing need was to transform cases of Valium, not amitriptyline, into cases of Prozac, and Zoloft.

Doctors heard they could be sued for prescribing dependence causing benzodiazepines. Rather than treat the superficial anxiety, they should treat the underlying depression, with non-dependence producing antidepressants. Prior to marketing, healthy volunteers in trials, however, had become dependent on SSRIs. Within 3 years of SSRIs being on the market, there were more reports in Britain about dependence on paroxetine than there had been in 20 years from all benzodiazepines combined.

The labels for SSRIs stated that less than 5% of patients in clinical trials reported sexual dysfunction. But in some healthy volunteer trials, over 50% of volunteers had marked sexual dysfunction that for some lasted after treatment stopped.

Over 50% can become less than 5%, and dependence disappear, simply because in RCTs investigators have to tick innumerable boxes, devoted to the question of whether the drug works, with minimal space and time to record adverse events. The healthy volunteer trials alerted companies to the need to manage investigators and so the only sanctioned questions about sex assumed changes stemmed from the condition rather than the treatment.

The 5% figure from clinical trials trumped later survey evidence that rates were over 50%. It trumped a marketing of the SSRI dapoxetine for premature ejaculation, which depended on the drug impacting on the sexual functioning of close to 100% of men. Patients on SSRIs were told any sexual difficulties would remit once treatment stopped. They could even take a break from treatment for a romantic weekend.

The first report to British regulators of PGAD dates to 1987. The first report of what is now called Post-SSRI Sexual Dysfunction (PSSD) was filed in 1991. The regulators told no-one, even though they at least notionally saw the pre-marketing healthy volunteer trials. PSSD came on my radar in 2000 when a patient said that 3 months after stopping treatment, she could rub a hard-bristled brush up and down her genitals and feel nothing.

The first publications on PSSD were in 2006. These made clear that some sufferers had the condition for a decade or more. Hundreds of women and men in internet forums have since exchanged information about the effects of drugs acting on serotonin or dopamine systems, phosphodiesterase inhibitors, herbs, metals, and operative procedures all of which had some rationale, many of which were dangerous, and none of which work. Some sufferers have committed suicide and assisted dying centers report people self-referring.

The core features of the condition are genital numbing, loss or muting of orgasm and loss of libido. Many are equally concerned by features like emotional numbing or derealization. Both sexes, all ages and every ethnic group can be affected. The condition may begin after only a few doses and leave someone affected for life. Or a relatively mild dysfunction can worsen dramatically when the person stops treatment.

An almost identical condition, post finasteride syndrome (PFS), was reported in 2011. Finasteride has been marketed since 1997 to young men with thinning hair. A post-retinoid syndrome (PRSD) following isotretinoin (Accutane) prescribed for acne appeared in 2014. PRSD has also been happening for decades previously. In Chicago in 2006, Hans Peterson killed Dr David Cornbleet for giving him isotretinoin and sexual dysfunction.

Having reported on 300 cases of enduring sexual dysfunction following antidepressants, finasteride or isotretinoin, I rounded up everyone who had published on PSSD or PGAD to petition the European Medicines Agency (EMA) and FDA to recognize enduring dysfunction on drug labels. The hope was that recognition might lead to research and treatment.

Another reason was because, in addition to direct treatment harms, many are harmed by doctors' responses. They are ridiculed for thinking a drug could cause difficulties after it has left the body. They are referred for therapy of childhood issues or offered antidepressants. They are also told that if they consult Google they will be ill forever.

All the while, regulators have been sitting on thousands of reports from doctors. These reports are anonymized, transforming them into hearsay. Unless a patient and doctor can be cross-examined it is not possible to establish causality. Aware of this, we sent EMA named patient reports and contact emails and letters from doctors to confirm the patient's identity, their treatment with an SSRI and lack of a competing explanation. Despite explicitly offering EMA the possibility to cross-examine patients or their doctors to establish causality, when the package arrived, EMA re-anonymized the reports before sending them to an assessor.

In contrast, companies are obliged to cross examine us if we report. They seek access our medical records to find ways to explain the issue away. When their drug is the only way to explain the condition, they include it on their label under "other reports," which for doctors translates as this wonderfully transparent company even lets us know about reports from Flat-Earthers. For PSSD, the patient's nervous disorder gives companies an escape.

EMA, however, agreed to ask companies to note the risk that sexual dysfunction can persist after treatment stops. Why? Perhaps because with SSRIs off-patent, flagging up hazards opens a door for companies to market new more expensive drugs for nervous conditions.

In the 1960s, it rarely took more than a few years between first reports of conditions to wider acceptance, but now common and obvious difficulties can take 3 decades to be accepted. The willingness of doctors and patients to put their names to reports and be cross-examined is key to reversing this increasing delay. Cross-examination, not clinical trials, is how to establish drug X causes effect Y. A judge who dismissed as hearsay reports signed by doctors and patients willing to be cross-examined in court would cause a legal crisis.

Doctors for the most part are too scared to engage. We need maps of where to find the one doctor in ten willing to stand behind a report. If any vestige of a market remains, the example of some may bring others around to an engagement that could restore healthcare and retrieve Friday from the health services pot in which she is about to stew.

It is also time to revisit a ruling that allows RCTs escape the hearsay rule. When first judged not subject to the hearsay rule, investigators who knew all the patients in a study could be summoned to court. There are no such investigators now; the patients may not even exist.

Meanwhile in 2019, a *BMJ* article "Declining Sex in Britain" fingered depression as a cause of this decline. Neither the article nor media coverage mentioned that antidepressants are more likely to wipe out our interest in or ability to make love than the nervous conditions for which they are given. Over 10% of sexually active people in the West take antidepressants chronically. Nearly 20% of the population, therefore, may not be able to make love the way they want. In deprived areas, the figure may be nearer 50%. Some likely comfort themselves with the thought that once they stop treatment, they will get back to normal, when in fact they may be a lot worse off. While sex normally sells, there is no media interest in these issues.

14: WHAT'S DONE CANNOT BE UNDONE

He who orders, does not buy.
And he who buys, does not order.

Whether from the political Right or Left, everyone cites this observation by Kefauver at the opening of his pharmaceutical industry hearings. Prescription-only status is a conundrum, he said, for anyone interested in monopolies and fixed prices as, no matter how high, prices are irrelevant to a consumer who doesn't pay for the product.

Fairy Godmothers

The sulfanilamide disaster in 1937 raised the question of how to impart information about drugs that can cure if used properly but can also kill.

US Courts stepped into the mix in 1948, in Marcus v Specific Pharmaceuticals, a lawsuit brought by the parents of a 13-month-old child who died after being given a larger-than-recommended dose of a prescription suppository:

> *[I]t is difficult to see on what basis this defendant can be liable to plaintiff. It made no representation to plaintiff… To physicians it did make representations… There is no reason to believe that a physician would care to disregard his own knowledge of the effects of drugs and hence of the quantity to be administered, and substitute for his own*

> *judgment that of a drug manufacturer. Nor is there any reason to expect that if a doctor did choose to rely on the information given by the manufacturer, he would prescribe without knowing what that information was. In the absence of any such grounds for belief there would be no negligence.* [66]

Three years later, the Humphrey Durham Amendments gave FDA power to decide which drugs would be prescription only. Doctors, viewed as skeptical about health fads, would be made our protectors in certain situations.

Our protectors were given the name Learned Intermediary in a 1966 legal case. A Learned Intermediary has nothing to do with medicine. He is a legal fiction:

> *We are dealing with a prescription drug rather than a normal consumer item. In such a case the purchaser's doctor is a learned intermediary between the purchaser and the manufacturer. If the doctor is properly warned of the possibility of a side effect in some patients and is advised of the symptoms normally accompanying the side effect there is an excellent chance that injury to the patient can be avoided.* [67]

This might appear to be about our good but it's about company convenience. It means the warnings about a medication's hazards need only go to physicians. This is billed as maintaining the sanctity of the physician patient relationship. It suits drug companies to claim they communicate with physicians only rather than with us.

> *Where a product is marketed solely to professionals experienced in using the product, the manufacturer may rely on the knowledge that a reasonable professional would apply to using the product.* [68]

---

66 Marcus v. Specific Pharm., Inc., 77 N.Y.S.2d 508, (N.Y. App. Div. 1948)

67 Sterling Drug Inc. v. Cornish, 370 F.2d 82, 84 (8th Cir. 1966)

68 Sterling Drug Inc. v. Cornish, 370 F.2d 82, 84 (8th Cir. 1966)

As a result, if there is something that can be portrayed as a warning, any injury from a drug is down to physician rather than company negligence. A company is immune if you are injured and your doctor, invoking the benefits a drug can bring, says they would have used it anyway. Aware of this, companies craft messages that palm off legal liability and ensure doctors see efforts to explore a drugs' hazards as an attack on them and patients hear talk of harms as an effort to deny them benefits.

When doctors primarily managed medical emergencies, there was something to be said for a Fairy Godmother to whom we can hand over responsibility. Since 1980 risk prevention, chronic disease management, has been the order of the day. In these situations, Fairy Godmothers become a hazard.

Taking a medicine is rarely healthier than working down a mine or in a chemical plant. When things go wrong on treatment, as they must if we take a poison for any length of time, the relationship we have with our doctor increasingly reflects the dynamics of our relationships with company doctors. From the mirror workers of Furth in 1860 to the miners of North Wales in 1920, employees who became ill at work have denied what is happening and concealed their difficulties (chapter 3). There are trade-offs to be made that can lead us to sing from the same song-sheet as employers, nudged that way by company doctors. As all doctors have effectively become company doctors, these industrial dynamics have worked their way into routine clinical care.

Taken Hostage

While doctors were still a revolutionary class, their involvement in assessing occupational injuries gave them a place in the emergence of socialism and liberalism. This changed around 1882, when Bismarck introduced Health Insurance, and co-opted medicine. That year, in *An Enemy of the People*, Henrik Ibsen, faced Dr. Thomas Stockmann with the dilemma we now pose doctors when we are drug wrecked. Stockmann had evidence the water supply to his town's new spa was contaminated and wanted this remedied before the season's tourists arrived. The newspapers, socialists, and townspeople were with him until the implications of missing out on the tourist kroner sank in. Then, they turned against him, and, unlike the Hollywood hero of *Jaws*, he had to leave town.

In August 1973, Jan Olsson, attempting to rob the Kreditbanken in the middle of Stockholm, holed up with four hostages, triggering a 5-day siege. After the siege ended, the hostages, as if hypnotized, spoke well of their captor. "Stockholm syndrome" was born. This is caused by isolation, a fear our life is at risk, and kindness on the part of a hostage taker. This is exactly what happens when we get ill, and doubly so if we face a drug wreck. Both disease and drug wrecks isolate us, put our lives at risk, and doctors control our escape.

Younger doctors, who have been trained to 'communicate', cannot imagine being a hostage taker. They have been trained to break the bad news of cancer to us. They have not be trained to hear about things they might have done to jeopardize us. They cannot imagine that keeping to the guidelines could deliver anything but the best possible outcome. The thought wouldn't occur to them that we might be able to teach them things.

Just as Olsson was, these young doctors are ringed by snipers. Speaking up about a new hazard, as Lasagna did about DVTs on contraceptives, once the material of medical advance, is now a recipe for professional suicide. Invitations to apply for jobs dry up. Where the hazards of treatment filled medical meetings in the 1960s, talk of them is now as rare as snow in the Sahara. Journals don't accept publications outlining new hazards. Worst of all, doctors who acknowledge a hazard can end up being seen by the patient or their family as a persecutor—Stockmann syndrome.

Rather than believe SSRIs cause osteoporosis, strokes, birth defects, and permanent sexual dysfunction, doctors now readily accept depression causes all of these, until recently such a claim would have seemed ludicrous. Families bereaved by suicide or violence, unaware of the role treatment may have played, become advocates for the early detection and treatment of schizophrenia,[69] depression, or the latest mental illness. They form pressure groups without any coaxing from Pharma, increasing the chances others will suffer the very outcomes that have wrecked their lives.

In the 1952 when Albe Watkins reported aplastic anemia on Chloromycetin he was taken seriously by FDA. When Lasagna reported DVTs on contraceptives in the mid-1960s, he was taken seriously. Nobody argued with women and their hairdressers when they reported hair change on contraceptives. As late as 1980, when investigated, over 80% of the 'anecdotes' reporting a new event on treatment turned out to be correct.[70] Almost all drug wrecks we know about came from direct observation.

Responding in 1983 to criticisms that spontaneous reporting is "the least sophisticated and scientifically rigorous method of detecting new adverse drug reactions," Lasagna said that "this may be true in Webster's dictionary sense of sophisticated meaning adulterated. But I submit spontaneous reporting is more worldly wise, knowing, subtle, and intellectually appealing than expensive [trials]."

RCTs don't discover drug wrecks. This isn't because close to 30% of the trials remain unreported, or almost all are ghostwritten and, in the process, adverse events disappear, or that the data from trials remains inaccessible. Even trials done by angels are not the way to discover most drug effects. The observations of hairdressers are more reliable.

But a doctor reporting a drug wreck now can get no traction. The report is designated an anecdote, uncertain and unreliable information. The mantra that only trials tell us what happens on treatment, allied to an assumption that bureaucrats get to see all the data, means doctors now defer to bureaucrats rather than go by the evidence of their own eyes. Unless a company opts to remove a drug from the market, regulators will

---

69 Such as J. Holmes' family persuaded that he had schizophrenia and that what happened to him offered a compelling case for screening programs and early intervention.

70 Venning G "Validity of anecdotal reports of suspected adverse drug reactions: the problem of false alarms." *BMJ* (1982), 284, 249-253

parrot a line that risk benefit ratios remain favorable. Doctors develop a low-grade psychosis.

Up the mid-1980s, there was a chance some doctors might apply the basic principles of cause and effect to drug wrecks—if it appears on treatment, clears when treatment stops and reappears on rechallenge, treatment is likely the cause. Now, we have decades of doctors educated to override both the evidence of their own eyes and the basic rules of causality assessment. As a result, major difficulties that came to light quickly in the 1960s, such as tardive dyskinesia on antipsychotics, now take 20 years or more to be accepted as caused by treatment. Many doctors will even view Black Box Warnings as evidence FDA has bowed to some consumer group rather than responded to real evidence of a hazard.

As this change happened, the value of our doctors for companies has grown. Direct to Consumer Adverts have shown it is possible to funnel complex information about medicines that can both save and kill to the public. Companies, however, still want a Fall Guy for distributing poisons to us when we are at our most vulnerable. Someone whom they can coach in the arts of persuasion to play on our anxieties so we take medications we might not take if left to ourselves. Someone with little of the resistance fighter about him.

Today's doctors have no training in marketing. Told Evidence Based Medicine takes care of marketing, few guess RCTs are the major marketing tool of companies. Few see RCTs are the Gold Standard way to hide drug wrecks. None appreciate RCTs opened up a way to engineer a medicine's informational component—control this and every risk from patients, doctors or politicians, manages itself. Few are aware the profession once viewed itself as a revolutionary class but now the minds of doctors are more colonized that those of women ever were by men, or a younger generation by an older one.

We have constructed systems and engineered adherence to processes that can produce mad, even evil, outcomes. No-one shaping the idea of a learned intermediary ever thought that the intermediary's learning might be entirely constructed for him.

Study 329 shows the cold limit to the Learned Intermediary calculus. In this study paroxetine unequivocally made children suicidal. Good care would have explained this to them and their relatives to repair their self-image and alert them to avoid similar drugs. No company has ever demonstrated care of this kind for any subjects in trials. They plead an unwillingness to be the Ugly Sister intruding on a Fairy-Godmother Cinderella relationship they have grossly distorted.

Talk to your Doctor[71]

This phrase has closed a million direct to consumer adverts (DTCA). It was born in 1997. Several blockbuster drugs, such as Zantac, Glaxo's ulcer drug, had gone off patent and companies pushed to make them available over the counter (OTC). FDA had to be seen to do something to manage the risk. They set up a "talk to your doctor" option to give consumers someone to talk to *before* taking an OTC drug. The OTC label also had to carry a direct number to the manufacturer for any questions *afterwards*.

After DTCA came onstream, the adverts for prescription drugs also sprouted 800 numbers, but these were not direct to the manufacturer. Then in 2007 the package inserts for prescription drugs and company websites began encouraging a reporting of adverse events to FDA's MedWatch scheme.

Direct-to-Company communication from patients is awkward for companies. It can force a company to add a warning to their label, if the company decides their drug has caused an adverse event. Judgments that there is a causal link become more likely if the event is followed to see what happened when treatment stops, or on re-exposure. Manufacturers are obliged to track events reported to them. FDA can't follow events because reports to them are anonymized. Encouraging patients and doctors to report directly to MedWatch sounds responsible but makes the recognition of a drug wreck less likely. People get paid to notice how to game the system in ways doctors and patients are unlikely to spot.

---

71 This material all feature as exhibits which were explored in the deposition of GSK's Dr J Nieman in "Kilker v GSK, Philadelphia," (September 2009).

On May 31, 2001, J. T., an American woman taking GSK's Paxil, emailed a Customer Response Center:

My name is J........ I was diagnosed with panic disorder about four-and-a-half years ago. Since that time I've been taking Paxil, which is truly a miracle drug. I've been panic-free with this drug and have been able to go on with a normal life.

I was married in October of 2000. My husband and I found out we were pregnant at Christmas time. I was so excited. I love children. The only problem is that I carried the baby to six months gestation and then had to have a termination.

The doctors diagnosed my son with Truncus arteriosis. They said he would not lead a normal childhood and would most likely not make it through the open heart surgery that he would need as soon as he was delivered (if he was able to make it to that time.)

To say the least, I was absolutely distraught with this news. I thought this was something that I did, was because I stayed on the Paxil for selfish reasons.

I wanted to know if you could direct me to any information you might have of any woman that has taken Paxil and still had healthy babies.

My husband and I are ready to try again to get pregnant in the next month or two. I am so nervous. I don't want to stop taking my miracle pill. But, then again, if there is a chance that this might hurt or affect the baby I want to know upfront. And I will somehow stop taking it for the time being.

Please contact me as soon as possible. I love everything this drug has done for me. I am so thankful that your company had this available for me. I just want to continue to have a normal life and have the child that I always wanted. Please contact me as soon as possible.

JT

Please don't forget about me. Thank you in advance for your time.

JT had contacted a Customer Response Center for OTC drugs. The Center responded the same day:

> *Thank you for your inquiry. We are attaching a copy of our current product information for Paxil. Please review the section on use during pregnancy. Further questions about your treatment should be directed to the physician, pharmacist or healthcare provider who has the most complete information about your medical condition. Because patient care is individualized, we encourage patients to direct questions about their medical condition and treatment to their physician. We believe that because your physician knows your medical history, he or she is best suited to answer your questions.*
>
> *Our drug information department is available to answer any questions your physician or pharmacist may have about our products. Your healthcare professional can call our drug information department at 1-888...*

Following a company decision in 2001, the label for Paxil no longer mentioned the number of reports of congenital abnormalities associated with Paxil, where previously it had. JT's OB-GYN could not have answered her question.

On June 1, JT wrote again:

> *This response is in regards to an e-mail that I had sent you previously. I was asking to see if you have any or are in the process of any clinical trials for women who are currently on Paxil and pregnant. I wanted to find out information to see how many women were on Paxil during pregnancy and if they were able to successfully have healthy babies.*
>
> *I am in no way insinuating your product did this to my child. I love the product, and I don't think I could have gotten through my panic attacks without the wonderful help of this miracle drug. I just want to start to try and get pregnant again soon. I do not want to put my unborn child through anything that would hurt him/her. Please, if you do not have this information, where is this information held?*

Does anyone do studies like this? Please, any information you may give me would be great. Thanks again for your help.

The 1-888… number mentioned by the Customer Response Center did not connect to GSK. Paxil Ads in medical journals also had a number that did not connect to GSK. The Paxil DTC adverts linked to a call center that was neither a medical information center, nor a Customer Response Center. No matter what number JT called, she could not reach GSK.

Six days after her second email, the Customer Response Center notified GSK's safety department. On June 13 the safety department sent a letter to an address:

…In order to follow up on your report, it is necessary that we have the contact details of your clinical course as it relates to your report. To obtain this we need the name and address of your OB/GYN.

Seeking JT's OB-GYN details is a first step in an ABCD analysis. It allows a company to check on other medications and conditions that might let it off a causality hook.

Companies have a duty to notify FDA within 15 days of a serious event. GSK's Dr Jane Nieman submitted a MedWatch form to FDA on June 13 noting the events listed in the email, and "mother's concurrent medications and medical conditions were not specified." It included her phrase: "I am in no way insinuating Paxil did this to my child."

The letter that had been sent to JT came back on July 5 marked "undeliverable". A later GSK report to FDA notes the unclaimed letter.

On June 13, 2001, a division within GSK monitoring adverse events decided this abnormality was "almost certain" to be linked to Paxil. This was not communicated to JT, her OB-GYN, or FDA. When later questioned under oath, Nieman offered the view that GSK had played it by the book but that as a mother she would have liked to have been told.

"Talk to your doctor" is not much use when you are swept overboard. Companies go to great lengths to conceal the true efficacy of their drugs, sequestering data, having ghosts conjure positive findings out of negative data, leaving trials unpublished. Faced with a drug wreck, they go into overdrive. What's done cannot be undone.

Tort Wars

Facing compelling clinical reports in 1990 that Prozac caused suicide, Eli Lilly deployed selected data from sequestered RCTs and a sophisticated understanding of doctors to transform these reports into anecdotes. What happened is caught in a 1991 memo from Lilly's Leigh Thompson, contrasting the fate of Prozac with the company's painkiller Oraflex which had foundered in 1981:

> *Today at PSC was LRL/Medical's finest hour. Dave Thompson and Gene Stap told me that it suddenly gave them a glimpse of how far medical has come and the vision that they knew (about global databases, super handling of ADE [Adverse Drug Events], proactive excellent relations with FDA, complex analyses and presentations made simple, DEN, GPT etc) but had never really had burned into their brains the elegance and mastery of the complexity!*
>
> *So many of us were not here for the Oraflex, Moxam, etc. crises, that it is very hard to measure the progress over the last few months on so very very many fronts. When you battle the media and politicians, the only thing that counts is the first word. The rebuttals are always on the last page and forgotten. You have to get out front and enlist your allies. The rapid flights to Boston to visit Teicher, the trips to FDA, the consultants coming in, the huge complex database, having so many large trials, the ability to quickly perform elegant analyses, DENs mastery of ADEs, have all come together in a significant effort...*
>
> *I'd like to have some buttons or mementos of other kinds made with a logo along the lines of: "I saved Prozac." Suggestions please for design, memento and words.*[72]

---

72 Exhibit 10 in Deposition of J. Potvin in "Fentress Vs Eli Lilly." See: Healy, *Let Them Eat Prozac.*

As of 1991, things changed so that now it takes several decades from a point of first description before major hazards of an on-patent drug, from compulsive gambling and prostitution on dopamine agonists, to cognitive failures on statins are accepted clinically. While these drugs are being saved, hundreds of thousands of lives are lost or blighted.

In the 1970s, Merrell-Dow faced legal actions from women who had taken Bendectin, a combination of doxylamine, dicylcomine and B6, for morning sickness in pregnancy. The women had given birth to babies with limb deformities. Some actions were settled out of court. Then epidemiological evidence began to come in, which while offering a risk signal did not nail Bendectin. The explanation for this may be that women only begin taking Bendectin as they are coming out of the critical period for organ formation. A fetus can be safe if a mother begins the drug after 8 weeks but not if she starts in week 6. Thalidomide taken later would have produced a weaker signal. Thirty years later, data from SSRIs, strengthened the case that doxylamine, a serotonin reuptake inhibitor, can cause birth defects.

Based on the early epidemiology, Merrell-Dow fought back. The term junk science was coined to refer to anything but conclusive evidence from large-scale epidemiology studies. These are studies that only a drug company can afford to sponsor. This tactic also helped companies repel legal cases claiming breast implants caused connective tissue disorders.

By 1991 Lilly had honed the tactic to include meta-analyses of their clinical trials. Although no investigators had access to the data from these trials, in legal cases from 1994 onwards, Lilly argued that courts were obliged to prefer these analyses to the views of experts based on challenge-dechallenge and rechallenge cases. Even though challenge and dechallenge was the method endorsed by the Federal Judicial Manual, Lilly lawyers argued that clinical cases has to be regarded as anecdotes. Only RCT evidence met the requirement for reliable science. If, in the few cases that get that far, a judge looks like s/he is not inclined to accept this argument, companies always have the option to resolve the case before trial.

Hatch-Waxman Revisited

This new ability to hide hazards made for a legal conundrum when Prozac went off patent in 2001. The 1984 Hatch-Waxman Act required generic companies to adopt the branded label for their drugs. What would happen if someone commits suicide on a generic SSRI?

Stewart Dolin was born on December 27, 1952, the youngest in the family. He grew up in Chicago where his father worked as a luggage salesman, and his mother at Marshall Fields. He did well in school and sports. On Spring break in Florida in 1968, he saw Wendy across a crowded room. They married six years later.

After graduating, Dolin joined a succession of Chicago law firms before setting up his own with colleagues. He then joined Sachnoff Weaver, a well-known Chicago firm. Twenty years later, Sachnoff Weaver merged with Reed Smith, who with 1,500 attorneys in twenty offices were one of the largest law firms in the world. Dolin pushed for the merger, but he keenly felt the lack of an Ivy League background to match the high-flyers they were joining. He and Wendy still took local holidays with school friends, even though he was earning a million dollars a year.

Before the merger, he had two courses of paroxetine for anxiety from his family doctor and friend Martin Sachman. Shortly before the merger, he saw a therapist who noted he saw himself as shy, somewhat unsupported by his family, and pressured by non-stop demands including juggling the needs of two sets of aging parents.

Paroxetine had caused him some difficulties so when anxious in 2007 Sachman gave him Zoloft. This agitated him initially, and later caused weight gain and sexual dysfunction. He stopped it. In May 2010, he had a further nervous spell and Sachman tried Zoloft again. It caused agitation. Sachman switched back to paroxetine on July 10. Over the next few days, he became desperately anxious. His therapist, unaware of the medication changes, was alarmed and called him at work to see if he was okay.

He seemed normal at lunch with a colleague on July 15, talking about future projects. Half an hour later, he walked to a Blue Line train station.

A nurse noticed a restless man on the platform who then dived in front of a northbound train.

Wendy Dolin, convinced her husband's paroxetine killed him, explored legal options. He had been taking generic paroxetine, made by Mylan, rather than Paxil. A year later, in June 2011, the US Supreme Court handed down a verdict in Pliva Inc v Mensing that seemed to put paid to any possibility of Dolin taking a case.

Gladys Mensing was given metoclopramide for gastric issues in 2001. Metoclopramide is related to antipsychotics, which can trigger tardive dyskinesia, a disfiguring neurological condition. Branded as Reglan when first marketed in 1980, its label noted this risk. The warning was strengthened as evidence of the risk accumulated. FDA mandated a Black Box warning in 2009. Mensing claimed the makers of her generic drug had enough information to strengthen the warning and should have done so. The Supreme Court responded that the Hatch Waxman Act meant generic companies had no option but to take over the brand label and Mensing had not sued the brand company.

Dolin's lawyers represented to Judge James Zagel that she was being denied natural justice. She should be allowed to sue GSK. GSK objected. Zagel, a former policeman, prosecutor, and a thriller writer in a Chicago legal tradition, agreed with Dolin.

The trial ran from mid-March to mid-April 2017. The jury were presented with the many ways in which GSK had hid suicidal events in their clinical trials. The jurors also heard how GSK had designated some trials as central and some as local. The central trials were coordinated and run by GSK. Local trials were run by affiliates or academic investigators. When concerns about suicide on SSRIs blew up, FDA asked companies for their trial data. GSK only handed over the central trials and not the local trials with their additional load of suicidal events.

GSK's lawyers blamed Dolin, who they claimed had a severe illness. They stressed he was not on their drug. They said Martin Sachman, his learned intermediary, was adequately warned by the label, supplemented by his clinical experience. This argument was straight from the Learned

Intermediary strategies developed by the leading legal company in that area—Dolin's firm Reed Smith.

GSK also cast FDA in an ambiguous light. The company had sought further approvals for social anxiety disorder, PTSD, and maintenance therapy in depression from FDA. "Don't you think if these medicines caused suicide someone [in FDA] would have spoken up?" Dolin's lawyers responded: "GSK's argument is akin to a car speeding past a cop, the cop doesn't stop the car, and the car crashes into another car and kills someone—the driver who killed someone cannot state it's not his fault because the cop didn't stop him."

The Dolin team hoped the jury would return within 3 hours. They were out for 3 days. The jury had difficulties allocating blame between GSK and FDA. FDA had seen a lot, as GSK said. The clincher appears to have been the fact that FDA had no idea GSK was withholding trials with extra suicides on paroxetine. Despite several hearings on the issue of SSRIs and suicide from 2004 to 2006, for which companies were asked for all their data, the regulator was still not in possession of all the data. The jury laid the responsibility on GSK.

When Hatch Waxman was adopted in 1984, no-one expected a major adverse effect might remain contested a quarter of a century after a drug's launch. GSK appealed and in August 2018, a Seventh Circuit Court reversed the Dolin verdict on a truly extraordinary ground, namely that GSK had tried to put a suicide warning on Paxil in 2006 but FDA had blocked them. A jury decided paroxetine was to blame but the system decided no-one could be held to account. The Supreme Court refused to hear an appeal.

Informing Consent

Ten years after creating Learned Intermediaries, US Courts created Informed Consent, an incompatible legal bedfellow. In 1957 and 1958, cases involving injuries from radiation for breast cancer, radical mastectomy, and electroconvulsive therapy (ECT) gave rise to the idea that treatment without consent is assault. We have a right to "any facts which are necessary to form the basis of an intelligent consent… to a proposed treatment."

In *The Duties of Patients to Physicians* in 1811, Benjamin Rush advocated informing patients of as much as possible so their obedience would be "prompt, strict and universal. He should never oppose his own inclination or judgment to the advice of his physician." This view hinged on an acceptance of medical beneficence, which could stretch to lying to patients in their best interests.

Informed compliance makes sense in acute medical emergencies. It made some sense when the key information a physician could impart was based on his own experience. When there was very little other information 'out there', the idea we could be brought up to speed about the knowledge physicians had spent a lifetime acquiring seemed bizarre.

Lasagna introduced consent forms to drug trials as a means of informing people they were participating in a trial. These forms have now become a means to deny access to trial data as company wording assures us, they will never show our data to anyone other than regulators. This emphasis on privacy sounds good. Hiding the evidence of injuries in trials, and the use of ghostwritten publications to deny that injuries can be linked to treatment, however, has made clinical trials a source of legal jeopardy

Early treatment trials were experiments that supported the rule of the people by the people. We participated in the belief we were extending the range of freedom from illness on behalf of our communities. The rhetoric around company trials suggests this is the mission still but company trials are now assay systems run to get a license. Most trials happen in settings of deprivation, often recruiting people who don't exist. When the data on adverse events is hidden, common purpose is lost. When the experience our doctor might have brought to an encounter is dismissed in favor of junk information, we have ended up in the worst of all possible worlds.

The US Supreme Court threw an ironic light on informed consent in a 2010 case. Zicam, a nasal decongestant was marketed by Matrixx Pharmaceuticals. Company shareholders concerned about reports it could produce anosmia (an inability to smell) and parosmia (a distorted sense of smell)

asked to look at the data. Arguing it only had animal studies and clinical reports of this condition, rather than statistically significant trial results, the Matrixx board decided there was no data to share. The Supreme Court disagreed. Anyone gambling with their money is entitled to make up their own mind about the evidence. We who gamble with our lives are not so entitled.

Twenty years earlier, in 1981, Dr Erling Oksenholt exploited the interface between informed consent and learned intermediaries in an intriguing way. He was sued by a patient who went blind after he gave her Myambutol for tuberculosis. After settling with her for $100,000, he sued Lederle Laboratories for withholding information Myambutol could cause blindness. He won $50,000 in damages, an unspecified amount for future loss of earnings, and $5 million in punitive damages.

The crowd passing by Drug Traffic Accidents gets jolted every so often by mass shootings, or the downing of a plane. None of the doctors who gave medication to the mass shooters or pilots who have crashed, and there have been many on antidepressants, have interrogated companies about withheld data. None have followed in Oksenholt's footsteps.

Lepers

Despite the success of AIDS activists, if we have a disease from cancer to psychosis, we are seen as losers in life's lottery. If something goes wrong on treatment, in addition to a further threat to our survival, there is a threat to our identity. Superficially we who are ill are less stigmatized than ever. In fact, from AIDs to nerves the stigma remains but is contained by the taking of a drug. Many women report others breathe a sigh of relief if she declares her competence by saying she is taking an SSRI, just as they do when hearing that someone with epilepsy is on an anti-convulsant, or someone with AIDS is taking Triple Therapy.

Untreated conditions are alarming. Drug wrecks break the treatment veneer. They unleash a latent stigma, making us lepers that even branded medicines shun. When we start to limp, the community, the herd moves on. At this point, we need someone who listens to lepers.

Our doctor will usually know more about our original condition than we do. She will be a good doctor if she notices pitting in our nails, a slight discoloration of skin, a change of smell or gait, and can hear things we might be reluctant to mention. Her ability to do this is increasingly compromised by service models that mean she may not see us more than once or indeed now may never physically meet us.

When things go wrong on treatment, though, Doc Friday has less expertise than you think. Only you can know if you have cognitive difficulties on a statin. She has no test to confirm it. When put on a bisphosphonate, before fracturing a femur, you were more likely to get a hint of what your drug was doing if a dentist mentioned the bone in your jaw was like marble than from your doctor. When you took a contraceptive, your hairdresser was more likely to notice changes to your hair than your doctor. If you become suicidal on an antidepressant, everything hinges on whether your doctor hears you when you tell her this is different from the suicidal ideation you are used to with depression.

For two decades, an increasing number of doctors have regarded the idea they poison or mutilate us as a touch last millennium. If she doesn't dismiss a link between treatment and our difficulty out of hand, the commonest response is likely to be that this was an accident. The luck of the draw. But unless your event is the first of its kind, this is unlikely to have been an accident any more than the deaths from Elixir of Sulfanilamide in 1937 or the birth defects on Thalidomide in 1956, 1957, 1958, 1959, 1960, 1961 and 1962 or the 100,000 birth defects since. After the first event, someone is no more innocent than James Massengil in 1937, Heinrich Mückter in 1957, Astra staff faced with suicides on Zelmid (the first SSRI) in 1977, or the Sacklers with addiction and overdose deaths in 1997. Someone knew about the risks but opted to keep their mouth shut.

With a new condition, like Anne-Marie's alcoholism (introduction), the internet leaves us as well placed to research what a drug might do as our doctor. We have the motivation that comes from being a castaway needing to master an alien terrain. Having skin in the game often counts for more than expertise. Doc Friday may turn out to be a great companion if we can rescue her from the pot of regulations in which she stews. But neither of us will have much chance if faced with a band of Fridays.

The greatest risk to us stems not from novel hazards we should be warned about but from a failure to monitor hazards like addiction to opioids or sexual dysfunction on antidepressants because they have become invisible. Across medicine, doctors spend an increasing amount of their time treating illnesses they cause. The label on the drug may indicate it can cause a difficulty, and the patient may suggest it is causing this difficulty, but her doctor may be unable to see or hear her.

If the learning of a learned intermediary is as constructed as it appears to be, the learned intermediary doctrine puts the fox in charge of the chicken coop. If professionalism is as dead as it seems to be, our safety is down to us.

15: CRUSOE WE SAY WAS RESCUED

Sara, little seed,
Little, violent, diligent seed. Come let us look at the world
Glittering: this seed will speak,
Max, words! There will be no other words in the world
But those our children speak. What will she make a world
Do you suppose, Max, of which she is made?

George Oppen
Father's Arms

Dangerous currents made escape difficult. Crusoe got away when a mutiny on a passing ship went wrong, leaving the mutineers behind, as "property owners".

Influenced by romances of a bygone golden age, in 1605 Miguel de Cervantes had Don Quixote tilt his lance at windmills. Between 1780 and 1820 and between 1980 and 2000, despite apparent continuities 'medicine' crossed divides from humoralism to medicine and then to health services, leaving golden ages behind.

Medicine hinged on a medical model that tied interventions to discrete bodily dysfunctions rather than general imbalances. As with weapons, measures, and methods of execution, medical techniques developed and interacted with military, urban planning, public health, political, and other systems in a way that humoral medicine had not. Humoralism, however, had embraced our concerns about beauty and identity (cosmesis) along with health and it underpinned a trade in commodities. The medical model defined itself in opposition to this trade but since 1980 it has been outflanked. Its largely male advocates had less of the Right Stuff than they gave themselves credit for.

Health services differ from medicine in a turn to standardization and management that make them de facto drug and device distribution channels, almost eliminating the boundary between health and cosmesis (Wellness). Defining health services this way makes traditional medicine sound romantic but a wish to return there would be quixotic.

While the image of solo medical practice might give some a sense as to why liberalism appealed to many doctors, few of us worried we might have something seriously wrong would now turn to a doctor who didn't have access to a full range of scanners, medications and other techniques. We need a 'system' but our current systems are more likely to serve us up medical conditions to consume rather than minister to us when we bring them diseases. We need to create a new HealthCare and avoid tilting at windmills.

Around 1605, there was a turn from land to trade as a source of wealth exemplified by the transformation of an age-old trade in *materia medica* into a proprietary medicines' industry. The rent-seeking condemned by religion, previously linked to land and money (usury), extended to goods. Driven by greed and trading on our fears, later charging the greatest rents any commercial enterprise had ever seen, proprietary medicine boomed on the back of a marketing and advertising made possible by a new media. Religion was turned inside out; self-interest was enshrined, and we had a new set of sacraments.

This trading activity and rent-seeking colored both the capitalism and medical model that came next. The medical model appeared before the word capitalism. The turn to technique that gave rise to the medical model, also gave rise to a capitalism that was as distinct from a prior commerce

that traded on our vices, as medical model medicine was from the proprietary medicines industry. There was still exploitation but a new way to
make money through an application of technology made it possible to
spread affluence, in a way that simple trading could never have done, just as
medical techniques extended life expectancy. There was enough for socialists to figure it made more sense to have a seat at the table than try to tear
the system down.

"Estate's a pond, trade's a spring, technique's a river." The industrial
and medical techniques that gave us things that worked were and are
capitalizable. Both emerged within a business model built on trade and
contracts. Novel goods were the substrate for one, we were the substrate
for the other. This difference underpinned a divide between medicine and
economics until health became the biggest industry on earth.

More recently capitalism, in the sense of a developing set of technologies financed by individuals or governments, has given way to a neo-liberalism that parallels the neo-medicalism that has given us health services.
Neo-medicalism turns the medical model inside out. Most prescription
drugs are now taken by people who have nothing wrong with them, with
ever fewer drugs to remedy diseases that need remedying. Something
similar has happened to capitalism.

The medical model and capitalism have drawbacks, but we should not
blame all our difficulties on them. The rent-seeking and exploitation of our
fears that predated both capitalism and the medical model meshed with
the additional failings of both capitalism and medicine. In the mix, we now
also have financialization and pharmaceuticalization.

Shortly after World War II, a new managerial class grew in a space in
US manufacturing industry between entrepreneurial owners and shopfloor
workers. Supported by the military, these managers favored automation,
as it would reduce worker numbers and deskill the remainder, thereby
removing a competing source of power, an 'enemy within'. In addition,
automation is essentially a bureaucratic process, in which all steps in a
procedure are laid out. It gave managers, the new masters of procedure, a
sense they knew more about how to do the job than those on the shopfloor.

Entrepreneurs previously didn't claim to know more about how to handle complex machines than their machinists, any more than the religious who notionally owned Catholic hospitals would have claimed to know more about clinical issues than nurses or doctors. The managerial cuckoos landing in health service nests in the 1980s, replaced administrators who looked after payroll and estates. Few doctors paid much heed in the 1950s when the expertise of machinists was downplayed. Now doctors are in the procedural firing line.

What is happening now is also capitalizable, creating a confusing continuity. Is the continuity substantive or apparent? An application of technique through to 1980 seemed to increase wealth and health. Is the new dystopian pharmaceuticalization that has drugs chasing drugs even as life expectancies fall, and a financialization that has money chasing money as poverty rises, an inevitable consequence of medicine and capitalism?

Through a Glass Darkly

Crusoe's tale echoes with archetypes from the Bible to Plato. Crusoe glimpses a reality beyond the everyday through a glass darkly, while reading the Bible. Plato had us prisoners in a cave, with a fire at the entrance, casting shadows on the wall. He disparaged this form of knowing as less than the knowledge we were capable of when grasping the 5 geometrical shapes and prime numbers. Holding true in any universe, these seemed to point to a realm of pure knowledge beyond corruption by our passions. For two millennia, pure knowledge, which included mathematics, logic and what could be said about a prime mover, trumped all other knowledge, except that of Biblical Revelation.

The allure of pure reason lay in its seeming objectivity. Its fruits held true over time and from whatever angle. The sciences that had a mathematical input aspired to the same objectivity and the aphorism that if it couldn't be quantified it wasn't science packed a punch. Both science and Plato's pure knowledge appeared to rescue us from a chaos into which Heraclitus had thrown us when he remarked that we can never step into the same river twice. We now know we are no more unchanging than the river. No constant spirit hovers in our changing machinery. We are as singular as the events that befall us, but with a compelling common need—to grasp an Us.

'Objectivity' underpins the allure of techniques like RCTs, which seem to take us beyond the flickering appearances of individuals, and the momentary variations within each of us, to truths which if not eternal are ones the Drugs' Magisterium are prepared to stand behind.

But once we found that working with the shadows on the wall, we could build models that helped us navigate our way in the world, to the consternation of philosophers we hitched our wagon to the star of instrumental rather than pure knowledge. In 1847 in *The Poverty of Philosophy* Marx threw down a gauntlet to philosophers: "The windmill gives us society with the feudal lord; the steam mill, society with the industrial capitalist." Society, he argued, develops according to a logic that has little to do with pure knowledge. We need to control this logic, rather than interpret it.

Today he might have mentioned contraceptives or Viagra, techniques that change us and the relations between us. Like other techniques, these can alienate. Are we more authentic if we manage ourselves naturally rather than artificially? How much depends on the extent to which our awareness of what we are doing has been compromised by the marketing of drugs like the bisphosphonates? What happens if a marketing that promises enhancement, and control over our destinies is as fraudulent as the marketing of Samuel Lees' Bilious Pills or similar remedies Marx likely used?

Beyond a potential alienation arising from doing things artificially rather than naturally and the further alienation inflicted on us when we are misled, in giving rise to drug wrecks, drugs produce a full-blooded alienation. They maroon us.

A century after Marx, Albert Camus said that suicide, deciding whether to live or die, was the central philosophical question. The 200 or more drugs that cause suicide smash right into this central question. As do drugs that inhibit sex. What would Marx, Freud or Camus have made of the fact that around 20% of us daily take drugs likely to cause suicide or inhibit sex? Philosophers don't engage with these issues. No-one does.

Drug castaways can't avoid these questions, which point to the limitations of our physical techniques and the power of propaganda to prompt the herd to move on leaving the injured behind. In 1880 facing health hazards in cities created by industrialization and factories, we organized, stood together, and made a difference. Standing together now in the face of drug wrecks is nearly impossible.

Drug wreck knowledge derives its validity from the fact that we are made of flesh and blood so that if we bump into things in the cave, we feel pain, we bleed, and end up knowing something. We know something more if someone else bumps into the same object. If we co-operate, we can build maps of where the bumps are. The objectivity of this knowledge lies not in mathematics but in collaboration. If others can reproduce what we have found, and if the finding keeps us alive or gets us places, while our understanding of what we have bumped into may shift, this way objectivity lies.

Drug wrecks offer the clearest point in the modern world where an exercise of judgment rather than a further application of technique is called for. Judgments that are incompatible with the neo-medical, neo-liberal, ethos of our times. Those injured by drugs, or caring for those injured, face a Lutheran "Here I stand, I can do no other," moment.

Getting a handle on the interior of our cave enables us to manipulate our surroundings to our advantage. The techniques and maps we have developed from bumping into things have advanced humanity more than the great men we celebrate. If we want to cure Alzheimer's, solve poverty, even survive, we must continue exploring our cave and developing techniques. To do otherwise would be to wander around blindfold, which is neither efficient nor safe in a cave full of others.

Bumping into each other also gives rise to techniques, from randomization to operationalism. These techniques can kill spontaneity, facilitate homogenization, and create obstacles we can also bump into, but their application is inevitable in an increasingly crowded cave.

Shipwreck charts the emergence of both sets of techniques and since 1962 the combination of both in a medicine. These techniques, embodied in RCTs, consign the injuries we get from bumping into drugs to the realm of old wives' tales. To push for a recognition of drug wrecks is to frustrate health systems. Calling as they do for diagnoses and verdicts, drug wrecks frustrate both instrumental thinking and the dreams of pure reason. Can creatures of flesh and blood whose judgments are made under uncertainty ever be believable, much less definitive, about these wrecks in which they have so much invested? Can we control our situation, rather than just interpret it?

ECONOMICS IS FROM MARS, MEDICINE FROM VENUS

There is that one word
Which one must
Define for oneself, the word
Us

George Oppen
Semantic

Marx's quote about steam mills launched a century of debates that split us into Left and Right. But even though anesthetic techniques were invented as he wrote and public health was a revolutionary force in France, and Marx spent lots of time with doctors and none in factories, neither the medical techniques then developing in Paris, Berlin, and Boston, nor the thriving trade in proprietary medicines came on his radar.

Drugs, materia medica, have been around for longer than coinage. Tobacco, alcohol, tea, coffee, ayahuasca, spices and other drugs drove a seventeenth century increase in trade, transformed our later ideas about freedom of trade, probably colored our religious ideas for millennia, and certainly many of our ideas about public morality, competing with money for the title of the root of all evil. Few things in the last two centuries aside from infective agents can have killed or disabled more people than tobacco.

Disease impacts us more than poverty. While a Dives might dislike a Lazarus foraging for crumbs from his table, he wouldn't stay sitting if Lazarus had the plague or leprosy. The Black Death kept Europe in its place and feudal for a millennium. Smallpox then eradicated the Aztecs and American tribes, while measles defeated the Incas, making Europe wealthy.

The mapping of our world and bodies from 1605 coincided with the first mapping of gross domestic and gross health products, shaping ideas about how social bodies might function. The idea of human capital emerged at the same time as financial capital, leading to public health, a marriage between economics and medicine. Some like William Petty and Josephine Baker saw wealth lying in people; the French government saw the need to match the German population. The upshot was a dramatic growth in human capital so that forty years before financialization became an international crisis, the greatest threat to our way of life, aside from nuclear weapons, was thought to be an annual population growth projected to leave us standing side by side on the planet by 2020.

Medical and economic developments have run side by side from Petty's political medicine, through the French Revolution, the revolutions of 1848, the discovery of our immune systems and psyches in the 1880s that made us individuals in a new way, the central planning that underpinned 1920s medicine before it appeared in 1930s politics, 1970s neo-medicalism and neo-liberalism, 1980s medical and political risk prevention, and 1990s pharmaceuticalization and financialization. The 2020 pandemic is a great example of disaster capitalism. The common factor lies in a development of techniques. These have driven medicine and economics forward displacing previous ways of doing things and shaping insights on our dislocation from Marx's class struggle, to Marcuse's one-dimensionality, Foucault's biopower and *Shipwreck*.

Despite this the medical and economic worlds remained almost entirely separate until 1990 when health and care services emerged as the biggest industry in most Western countries. These services now employ up to 20% of the population. There is a real prospect US health spend might bankrupt America unless, in a replay of 1930s totalitarian empire building, US services are allowed to take over health services elsewhere.

The Covid pandemic looks set to fuse the economic and medical worlds more completely. It has increased the rate of commodification of health and educational services. Global vaccination programs are now spoken of in terms of universal health coverage. Debates about policies on masks, lockdowns and vaccines play into a much wider set of values and make the Crowd seem as unmanageable as revolutionary Parisian crowds. Further pandemics or disasters linked to climate change will likely increase this social fever.

When mapping the dimensions of an emerging capitalism in 1867, Marx conflated the emphasis on activity found in commercial enterprises like the proprietary medicines industry, with the capitalizability of new techniques. He focused on the role these techniques might play in alienating us from our labor and how this, rather than the World Wars and climate change inherent in technique's capitalizability, might trigger change.

Had he focused on medicine, a distinction between activity and technique might have been more readily drawn. Viewed through a medical lens, the accidental effects of technique seem a more obvious driver of history than class interest. The role thalidomide and the adoption of RCTs have had in shaping health services, and how we handle drug wrecks, brings this point home.

Some aspects of the AIDS crisis, such as the struggle for access to Triple Therapy in the Global South, as well as access to healthcare in the United States, and the effects of Covid, can be mapped onto class politics. But we are all now more deeply alienated than this. At a time when the Catholic Church, formerly the chief purveyor of sacraments, acknowledges that the Eucharist can harm, so that it now comes gluten free, branded drugs have become a global religion, offering salvation through sacraments that cannot harm.

(Religion is an ambiguous word here. Religions at their best have supported exploration and debate. The idea of a religion of technology just might work in this sense. It doesn't work well when applied to the devotion to operationalism that now keeps the tribe, the herd, moving in one direction. This however is a function religious badges once fulfilled. The religious nature, in this sense, of what we now have can be seen in the struggles vaccines trigger.).

In the face of Health Services mobilized around pharmaceuticals, a rallying cry, "Patients of the planet unite, you have nothing to lose but your pills," will not work. From the start, polypharmacy was an obvious risk factor for increased Covid mortality. The data now bear this out. But at a time when leading medical journals would publish even a Denis the Menace cartoon that had the word Covid attached, none would touch a proposal to collect data on the interactions between Covid and polypharmacy[73]. The rationale for not publishing offered was, "We publish nothing but Covid articles these days," even though no journal has published anything on polypharmacy and Covid.

Marx thought a newly forming working class would stick together. This made sense before the seductions of consumer goods clouded the picture. Class solidarity melted away once those goods held out the promise of saving lives, particularly the lives of our children. Drugs and drug wrecks expose a more primitive divide between people than class, race, gender, or nation. A divide between the fortunate and the unfortunate.

A Nuclear Moment

Efficient techniques are adopted as certainly as water flows downhill. The perception that medicines are efficient techniques is caught in a 'we are a quick fix culture' response to questions about why we don't exercise more, control our appetites more, or endure more pain rather than turn to pills.

---

73 "Medications compromising Covid Infections," see: rxisk.org/medications-compromising-covid-infections/ and "Covid and the Market in Research" see: rxisk. org/covid-and-the-market-in-research/

Part of our current predicament hinges on new abilities to create a perception of medical effectiveness. Since 1980, there have been few life-saving medicines. A few drugs like Viagra offer functional benefits we didn't have before but even these are over-hyped. The perception that medicines work is increasingly based on their effects on numbers rather than tangible benefits and on a freedom not seen since the 1906 Food and Drugs Act to portray drugs that don't work as miraculously effective.

The minimally efficient drugs developed since 1980 however are adopted almost as certainly as water flows downhill unless a bump gets in the way. The disappearance of drug wrecks, the bumps, has played a key role in making medicines a modal form of death, an increasing source of blight for many, and perhaps the leading cause of recent falls in life expectancy. We who are drug wrecked are ever more likely to perish than be reprieved.

Chlorpromazine was discovered in 1952. Despite transforming patients never thought likely to leave the asylums, by 1959 it was linked to tardive dyskinesia, a disfiguring neurological condition, with a distinctive feature inhibiting the recognition of a link to treatment—it often appeared only after treatment had stopped. The recognition of tardive dyskinesia didn't come from the patients whose conditions meant they were ignored. It came from doctors, who forced companies and regulators to warn about it.

Compare this with finasteride (Propecia) used to reverse hair loss in young men, isotretinoin (Accutane) for acne or SSRI antidepressants used by both sexes and all ages. These can all cause a permanent loss of sexual function with a distinctive feature—it often appears only after treatment stops. Tens of thousands of people, well-placed to get media attention, are affected. But thirty years after the first reports of enduring post-treatment sexual dysfunction, they meet disbelief. The media are reluctant to cover an issue, whose solution would prevent suicides and relationship breakdowns, would merit a Nobel Prize, and would underpin novel treatments. Doctors are nowhere to be seen.

The best-selling fluoroquinolone antibiotics, children of Panalba (chapter 6), when introduced in the 1980s were expected to be second line antibiotics. They were almost immediately noted to cause mental illness, musculo-skeletal conditions, including Achilles tendon ruptures, and chronic pain syndromes fueling opioid use. Regulators only warned about the mental health issues in 2018 when long-set prescribing patterns meant warnings had little effect.

The commonest treatments for gut acid, the proton pump inhibitors (PPIs) cause an anxiety that perpetuates PPI use but, rather than recognize this, doctors add psychotropic drugs to the mix. The most profitable drugs for asthma, the leukotriene antagonists, are relatively ineffective but hugely prescribed despite causing personality changes, psychotic reactions, and aggression, especially in children. These hazards took 40 years to be recognized.

It took two decades for the promiscuity, sexual deviance, compulsive gambling, and other risk seeking behaviors caused by dopamine agonists to be recognized in warnings, aided by the fact that members of the judiciary were affected. Whatever about risking complications like these in the treatment of a disorder like Parkinson's, these drugs are promoted for restless legs syndrome, for which there are more effective, safer, and cheaper older options.

Delays in recognition are growing in number and duration, driven by a medical literature that has been transformed into fools' gold and by the one-dimensional nature of technique.

Life expectancy across the Western World in 2020 is less than it was in 2015. For the seriously mentally ill, life expectancy is no better than it was in 1890. This fall is taking place even though cardiovascular deaths, our biggest killer, have been falling for decades as more recently have cancer deaths, our second biggest killer.

Most cancer and cardiac deaths are coded under cancer and cardiac headings rather than drug-induced, which many are, yet still the data on deaths in hospital settings show treatment to be the third leading cause of death. Drugs must be an even commoner cause of death outside hospitals where the conditions treated are less severe and less likely to kill. But drug wrecks are not as yet in the frame as the source of the drop in life expectancy.

Talk of a precautionary principle gained ground in medical circles in the 1980s. This sounds Luddite. If we insisted on only doing things that are safe, would we ever do anything? The precautionary principle gave way to concerns about overtreatment. This invokes the specter of rationing. If treatments work, we will always resist anyone who tries to take them away from us.

The radical solution is to talk about the harms of drugs, but even if dressed up in terms of safety, such talk takes most of us beyond our comfort zone. Other than in the abstract, few can contemplate the idea that medicine is about bringing good out of the use of a poison.

There is another option. Around 1962 most of us were on 1 drug at a time and then only for limited periods. By 1990 many of us were on enough drugs chronically for the idea to take hold that being on more than 5 medicines might cause complications. Since 2010 there has been mounting evidence that reducing medicines from 10 or more to 5 or less increases life expectancy, reduces hospitalizations and can dramatically improve quality of life.

This is medicine's nuclear moment. Military technique improved remorselessly through history, dramatically so from 1800 onwards, because the possessors of the most effective techniques won wars. But with the nuclear bomb, it became clear that if it couldn't be used extreme efficacy might no longer be effective.

Now 40% of us over 45 are on 3 or more drugs every day, and 40% of over 65s are on 5 drugs. Because some are on no drugs, the norm for over 65s is to be on 7 drugs. If our doctor keeps to guidelines, our medication burden will increase year on year, even though being on 5 or more drugs is just not as effective as being on less. We have reached a limit.

We who take medicines, and those who give them to us, can have our cake and eat some of it. This is not about rationing or taking medicines away. Ensuring optimal efficacy forces us to introduce the values of the person being treated into a sustainable treatment. What do you want to gain from treatment and what do you want to avoid?

School shootings in America bring the ambiguities of one-dimensional efficacy into view in another way. These shootings led to calls to have a good guy with a gun posted in schools. Those horrified by this idea are liable to be stumped by a follow-up question as to whether they would then remove the armed guards from outside the White House? If guns work outside the White House, why not outside a school? Efficacy always has a context, and we sense that letting it leak outside specific contexts or develop beyond certain points is liable to be counterproductive.

The Covid pandemic has exposed the consequences of a one-dimensional, no-spare-capacity, just-in-time efficacy culture in health. Health care can never be engineered like a bridge, which even if built before any automobiles appeared can still safely hold a string of juggernauts. But it shouldn't be like a rope bridge with most of its slats missing.

One-dimensionality

The dynamics of efficacy map onto the entrapment by consumption that Herbert Marcuse framed in terms of a one-dimensionality, from which he could see no exit other than a turn to philosophy.

From the Greeks to the Enlightenment, the narrative underpinning Western thought has been of a struggle between reason and magic with science being a prime exhibit for an inevitable triumph of reason. While Marx, Freud and Marcuse saw the commodities of capitalism as fetish items, techniques and algorithms embody an intelligible component that makes them capitalizable.

Health services offer compelling examples of one-dimensional fetishes, best symbolized by sacramental drug brands, these hyper-real items, which can only do good and from which harms cannot arise. In creating conditions for which drugs seem the answer, figures like those for cholesterol, blood pressure or bone density are a driver of one-dimensionality that is difficult to argue against. The algorithmic if X then Y appears to replace the idiosyncratic views of patients and doctors with 'objective' solutions. When risk benefit jargon comes into the frame, everyone assumes both benefits and harms have been weighed by regulators who find a positive balance, at least on a population basis, sufficient to prevent warnings being put on treatments. No such calculations can be undertaken but the perception they have been trumps our experiences of real harms.

This is a hazard of all technique, not just medical technique. In *God and Golem*, published in the same year as *One Dimensional Man*, Norbert Wiener pleaded with us to recognize that algorithms can work for closed systems (where we know all the moving parts), but open systems, such as a human life, require choices and responsibility.

With the adoption of an effectiveness criterion in the 1962 FDA Act, even while accepting that medicines are inherently dangerous, we relegated drug wrecks to the realm of the accidental or incidental. We compounded the problem when we interposed prescription only arrangements, guidelines, and regulators between us and our fate. These moves were a tragedy in the Shakespearean sense of bringing our fate on ourselves. The only consolation is that any other course of action or non-action would likely also have thrown up difficulties.

Before climates began to change, technical developments faced no economic pushback. Growing personal wealth was not an issue other than in a spiritual 'money can't buy me love' sense. But our embodiment inescapably subjects our collective health to a pushback from the world. And we can't accumulate or pass on health as we do wealth.

Grappling with drug wrecks and how to deploy medicines in a world in which efficacy has limits offers a route to restoring complexity and discretion. It is operationalism, rather than technology per se, that stands in the way. This is what straps us to technologies and techniques rather than enables *Us* to benefit from technical developments.

A coherent answer can only arise from the bottom up; it cannot be imposed from the top down. The HealthCare we need hinges on enough of us realizing our actions make us, in contrast to health services which pivot on our adherence to guidelines (operations) set by others. Algorithms can be used to support a deprescribing process but attempting to magic good out of the use of a poison cannot be algorithmicized. It is a personal moment that requires a diagnosis and choice.

Philosophers and medical scholastics in ivory towers debating the equivalent of how many angels might fit on the head of a pin, how many vaccines infants can tolerate, or efficacious drugs we should take, cannot help us. Far removed from the cave in which we stumble around, get injured by drugs, build maps, and make judgment calls about our next step, they tell us that our knowledge is not real knowledge.

If things go wrong on a drug, or we need to decide between treatments, making a judgment call, a diagnosis, is critical. But judgments, verdicts, are what modern technique sidelines in the name of objectivity. Our judgment may be influenced by prior events, current difficulties, or be thrown off course by other currents, and this is where another's input can provide perspective and balance. But the bottom line is a different kind of learning happens when we make a call and take a risk. At points like this, we can mobilize in astonishing ways and be driven by a motivation worth more than expertise.

This is not a novel theory of knowledge. Legal systems wouldn't work if our hunches about how the evidence stacks up aren't mostly right. Deciding clinically about what a drug has done is similarly judicial rather than technical.

In medicine now, however, but especially around drug wrecks, knowledge gets as bent as light does near a black hole. Focusing on the merits of pure versus instrumental reason, whether we are minds or bodies, obscures the fact that operationalism increasingly determines what passes for truth, mediated through social techniques and social media (Google and Facebook) that keep the herd together. Keeping together is key but not as a herd. We apparently have more Liberty and Equality than at any time since the French Revolution. But Solidarity is in ever scarcer supply.

Drug wrecks, even more than nuclear weapons, bring out the limitations of technique and point to a world beyond a purely technical one. A personal rather than an impersonal world. Will technology be our religion? Or can we find something else?

ALGORITHMS ARE FROM MARS, MAGIC FROM VENUS

Looking through an economic lens, the boundaries between individuals and groups have shifted over three centuries. Up to 1700 we saw the invisible hand of Providence guiding discoverers, inventors, artists, and heroes to breakthroughs. After 1700, we recognized 'individual' genius in patents, copyrights, and property owning, while some held out for the importance of 'us'.

Re-viewing our history through a medical lens highlights other options such as the interplay between the personal and impersonal. The personal is not the same as the individual. There is much that is impersonal in everyone, from our genetic make-up to our personas (masks), which are largely given to us by society. It may be only when we get sick, and the masks and routines that slot us into the herd fall away, that the personal flickers into view with its need for other persons, for a healing that impersonal health services cannot comprehend, along with the judgment calls critical to healing.

For nearly two centuries, single-handed family doctors delivered most healthcare. Despite the concerns of religious folk, the image of the good doctor was of someone present for us at personal moments. The pharmacological revolutions of the 1950s brought a sense that cures might count for more than care. The growth in scale of health services has aggravated this but even in hospitals until recently doctors were celebrated if they retained a human touch. If they didn't, nursing staff compensated for them.

Nothing Personal Just Systems

"The windmill gives us society with the feudal lord; the steam mill society with the industrial capitalist; the operational-mill society with managers." In the last three decades, we have moved decisively into a world of medical systems. Systems treat us, where once people did. Exhortations to person-centered care in health service management manuals increase in inverse proportion to the extent to which meaningful personal engagement is lost.

Health services have become a hostile Kafkaesque environment for many working in them. To adapt the words of another Czech, Vaclav Havel, from 1978:

> *A specter is haunting [Health], the specter of dissent… You do not become a 'dissident' just because you decide one day to take up this most unusual career. You are thrown into it by your personal sense of responsibility, combined with a complex set of external circumstances. You are cast out of the existing structures and placed in a position of conflict with them. It begins as an attempt to do your work well and ends with being branded an enemy of society. … The dissident does not operate in the realm of genuine power. He is not seeking power. He has no desire for office and does not gather votes. He does not attempt to charm the public. He offers nothing and promises nothing. He can offer, if anything, only his own skin—and he offers it solely because he has no other way of affirming the truth he stands for.[74]*

The emphasis on effectiveness that now dominates medical goals is central to this loss of meaning. Effectiveness drives us toward partialism and fragmentation of services. Under this influence, both the notionally private US and public UK systems are falling apart as the mission gets ever more fine-grained, with ever more interfaces, ever less continuity of relationships, and managements ever more likely to blame the person at the point on the assembly-line where things come unstuck. Our pets now get more continuity of person-centered care when brought to a vet than we get in health services.

When managers insist psychiatrists use rating scales, assuming these checklists are more scientific than a free-floating interview, the embrace of technique has gone mad. Scores on rating scales, just like scores on blood tests, are the basis for the algorithms that mandate prescriptions, if X give Y. They also provide a basis for replacing doctors with specialist nurses or physician associates, for procedures from prescribing to colonoscopies.

---

74 Havel V.,"Power of the powerless", *In Living in Truth*, (Faber Books, London 1978), 83.

Electronic Medical Records (EMRs) now dictate questions to be asked in clinical interviews, so that rather than a repeat visit to a doctor being a moment where growing trust leads to key information, it becomes stultifying for us and whoever we see. The rise of digital consults means we may now be prescribed treatment based on checklist scores by prescribers in a different part of the world, who have never met us and will never follow us up.

Even before Covid, doctors had become supervisors of counters manned by nurses or physician associates. Paramedical staff are keen to replace physicians, but some voyage soon will dump robots on our shores to work our plantations, drive our vehicles, clean our houses, handle our insurance claims, and deliver health services.

The development of computers raised questions about professionalism. Early predictions saw much of law and architecture being swept aside. Claims for professional status, it was argued, hinged on specialist knowledge. Computers with a capacity to crunch vast amounts of data would break the monopoly the few have on this kind of knowledge and make it available to the many. Fintech has been the latest to storm the professional barricades. Indeed, *Shipwreck* might mark the last time readers can be sure that a book like this will have been written by a creature of flesh and blood rather than a machine.

Doctors, to date, have seen Artificial Intelligence (AI) as no more than an extension of smartphone apps, which seem to increase medical business. This insouciance holds even though surgery by robots, developed in the 1990s by the US military for battlefield situations, and then through a commercial spin off, Intuitive Surgical, has rapidly taken over fields such as prostate surgery. In 2011 a surgeon tele-operated on a patient over 3000 miles away. This development was aimed at enabling warfare and space exploration capabilities.

With a new generation of robots that can learn, physicians will face new challenges. Current systems mandate adherence to the algorithms embodied in guidelines, even though these guidelines lead doctors to kill and injure. What doctors at present learn from patients dying is not that drugs can harm, but that non-adherence to a guideline leads to job loss. If a future system, with a goal of keeping people alive, introduces robots who can not only crunch data but learn, accepting that some patients will be killed in the early stages, the robot will likely keep more people alive and well than doctors at present. It will do so by going off guideline, deprescribing, and listening for drug wrecks.

If the system doesn't decide drug-induced disability is good for business, the robot won't succumb to the bias that makes physicians unable to see the harms they cause, or the behavior that stems from fear of losing a job. At present, physicians do not see the suicidality or withdrawal antidepressants cause in their patients. They dismiss an 80-year-old woman's complaint of fatigue as age-related when it is more likely to stem from her blood pressure being too low from medication, the effects of statins she should never have been on, or the horrors of osteoporosis drugs.

Just as with Google cars, the doctor won't decide whether she or the robot drives or whether she or the robot sees the next patient. It may be the insurance industry or even the EMR.

"Estate's a pond, trade's a spring, technique's a river, AI's the ocean." If AI brings the capitalizability of technique to an end, then what?

Nothing Personal Just Regulations

In a 2016 political earthquake Britain voted to leave the European Union. Exit polls showed the main concern of those who voted Leave was sovereignty. Given Britain had bombed Iraq, Libya, and Syria in the prior decade, sovereignty to do what you might ask?

The seeds for the break-up were sown on January 1, 1973, the day Britain joined, and the Chocolate Wars began. Other European countries argued British "chocolate" contained vegetable fats rather than just cocoa and couldn't be called chocolate. A Thirty-Years War followed that contributed to English perceptions that Europe meant rule by bureaucrats, while European choclatistas saw nation based artisanal enterprises threatened by multinationals bent on replacing wholefoods with processed foods.

Behind this War lay the role of regulation in modern life. Regulators license a drug if it meets criteria in the same way as they apply criteria to butter or chocolate. Meet the criteria and you can claim your product is butter, chocolate, an analgesic or hypoglycemic. Your product might kill people, be an inferior butter or drug but it's not the role of the regulator to keep people alive (other than by banning egregiously false claims), nor to mediate between artisanal and multinational sectors of the market. They apply criteria. When Chinese, American, or European trading blocs meet, the issues to be negotiated are about achieving regulatory rather than ideological alignment. The criteria applied to feta cheese, diesel emissions and drugs determine the political room to move.

Where in the 1860s both liberals and communists saw the State withering away, by 1970 regulatory systems were nuclear bomb proof. Having no regulations for food and drugs is no more an option than removing road signage and driving codes. Companies have preferential access to the regulatory apparatus through appeals and other processes. Regulators are also encouraged to partner industry and consider the impact of regulations on jobs. With drugs, however, industry primarily win by withholding the raw data. They also win by being able, without pushback from doctors, to game the system by working on possible meanings of organic, artisanal, chemical imbalance or mood-stabilizer.

In the 1980s, Pharma was among the first industries to push for a global harmonization of regulations. This underpinned a globalization of the industry. This necessary feature of modernity would notionally be balanced in health by physicians acting as a counterweight to industry and as advocates for consumers.

Facing a plurality of interests, regulatory criteria must aim at a lowest common denominator rather than nuance. Although these criteria were not supposed to interfere with the practice of medicine, they have displaced judgment at junctures key to healthcare. Can this be rolled back? The forces that will resist a change, easily characterized as a descent into unreason, are now deeply entrenched. As in a movie plot, where faced with an approaching asteroid, one-time campaigners against the nuclear bomb are thrilled to have one, so it's not difficult to see the appeal a once scorned wrecking ball of a plutocrat or dictator complaining about the Deep State might have.

In England's Civil War in the 1640s, Thomas Hobbes argued that without rule from the top-down, life would be nasty, brutish, and short. The Enlightenment later gave us rule by reason. We now have a rules-based order on which liberal democracy supposedly depends. Medicine once offered a potent symbol of the power that comes from hanging together— white coats closing ranks. The new rules favor companies hanging together. In the new dispensation, the rest of us are rule-takers (vassals). The idea of discretion doesn't compute especially in contracted out services.

It once seemed that the regulated power that emerged with the French Revolution could always be undone. There are few better illustrations of this than the interplay between Ireland, then Europe's most destitute country, and England, the global superpower. After Ireland was forcibly absorbed by Britain in 1800, Daniel O'Connell, realizing that power in this new world was constrained by laws, and boasting he could drive a horse and carriage through any English law, campaigned to get people to hang together peaceably. He brought out a weakness inherent in England's apparent strength. This led to Catholic emancipation in Ireland (not yet England). It also led to a series of Irish inventions including the boycott and the hunger strike that against the odds delivered freedom to the Irish to oppress themselves—and even hand over sovereignty to Europe.

The 1962 FDA regulations strikingly illustrate how laws and processes now shape our world and lead us to concede power to others. Facing up to Big Pharma in 1984, Alfred Engelberg and Bill Haddad used the weapons of the enemy just as O'Connell had. Since then, industry has transformed even the regulatory apparatus into a learned intermediary between us and it, facilitating their claims to be rule-abiding and ethical. The more we drift toward Google cars and away from Horses and Carriages, the more difficult it will be to pierce this system.

Regulatory capture initially referred to industry's ability to have its people occupy key positions in the apparatus. A subtler phenomenon became apparent after passage of the 1875 Food and Drugs Act in Britain when companies realized the potential of regulations to squeeze out competition. But our current difficulties stem from something more subtle. They hinge on the capture of the mental sets of physicians and other key stakeholders. We would face the same difficulties, whether there was a revolving door between the bureaucracy and industry or not.

In terms of drug wrecks, the key factors have been a belief in RCTs and losing access to data from the RCTs in which we have participated. This data should be as inalienable as our vote. If we take our data back so that our consent must be sought for its use, we take back not just data but power.

Electronic Medical Records also generate data from our encounters with health services. Starting from IMS' transformation of prescriptions our doctors wrote in the 1950s into data that could be mined, an industry has grown up that transforms every entry any healthcare worker makes on our EMR into data that can be mined. We are told it is in our interests to allow this mining. The claim that our data is deidentified and this business poses no threat to us is false. These mines will collapse, and when they do it will be us not the mine owners who are injured. Our injuries will be passed off as accidents. But are they inherent to or incidental to the process?

Nothing Personal Just Business

The phrase "nothing personal just business" emerged in the 1930s. Dubbed the hitman's dilemma, it was adopted as emblematic of business. The inverse of the customer always comes first. There is no better illustration of this than Otto Ambros sitting down with Jewish doctors to look at the business opportunities thrown up by thalidomide.

The pharmaceutical industry sells itself as doing well by doing good. Many who work in it believe that while companies play the system in whatever way they can (to do otherwise risks going out of business), their companies contribute to national productivity by saving lives and reducing disability. They contribute to research productivity by providing research tools to help us understand biological systems, and to health productivity as evidenced until recently by increasing life expectancy. Most of what we know about company abuses have come from industry whistle-blowers, not from physicians.

The shifting tectonic plates of falling life expectancy and robots able to learn to save lives, however, will soon bump into the plate from which the pharmaceutical industry now operates a de facto rent extraction 'If you don't pay us what we want, we will stop doing research and you will die' business model.

Industry has an Achilles' heel. Despite its evisceration of WHO for the temerity in producing an Essential Drugs List in 1977, it has produced nothing since that keeps us alive saving Triple Therapy for AIDS, Gleevec for leukemia and treatments for Hepatitis C. There have been no improvements on the psychotropic, antihypertensive, hypoglycemic, and other drugs available in the 1960s, but dismissed by industry in 1977. The essential drugs list now includes statins, bisphosphonates, and fluoxetine for children.

Pharmaceutical profits, now the greatest of any industry, would be fine if we got returns commensurate with our money. Patents are often blamed for our failure to benefit from research but the monopoly over medical minds has little to do with patents. Company power stems from marketing techniques, the sequestration of trial data, and the fact they sell to the most naïve consumers on earth rather than from patents.

Patents are blamed for high prices. Companies holding patents can charge what they like but their ability to do so stems from a lack of access to data. This enables them to trade on the fact that if someone withholds a treatment from us, we are liable to be irate. Our doctors also think it's good for their business to lobby for access to anything that costs a lot. So long as the object of desire is not seen as a source of infection, this pimping can work.

The AIDS crisis showed how ruthless industry can be. With new drugs now 10 times what Triple Therapy for AIDS initially cost, what was a Third World difficulty is now an issue for everyone. At present, advised by NGOs, and others untainted by links to industry, Western governments question the cost, not the safety, of these new drugs. This puts them on the wrong side of the people for whom they think they are advocating.

There are options other than product patents such as process patents and prizes. We could offer industry the billions they now get but only in return for drugs that save lives in the manner we specify. We could also help companies maximize their profits by asking them to withdraw from marketing. Drugs that save lives or clearly enhance function need little marketing. Health services, whom one might have thought shouldn't want drugs that don't work, as they operate at present, won't support this move. Shrinking the iceberg of 'unmet need' would leave a lot of managers drifting on ice floes in open waters.

Through this book, technologies have been collapsed into the category of techniques. All techniques function on the generic principle of if X then Y. The chemicals in a medicine would more usually be called technologies; the information about drugs involves techniques. At the start of the pharmaceutical era, the technologies were more important than any techniques, as is the case at the start of any technical era. The balance began to shift soon after, and the techniques surrounding drugs are now so good that doctors routinely prescribe previously junked drugs or derivatives of a parent compound passed off as a new marvel.

But in addition to robots who learn, pharma will soon face a new technology—CRISPR. These new gene editing technologies, first developed by bacteria and viruses, will soon be commonplace, offering possibilities to remove genetic disorders, treat antibiotic resistant infections, enhance immunity, personalize medicines and make vaccines in pandemics.

CRISPR will challenge Pharma. But it will be born into a world dominated by sophisticated marketing techniques, a regulatory apparatus comfortable with the concealment of key data and a medical profession difficult to see as a more reliable bulwark between us and corporate power than German medicine was in the 1940s.

Companies, regulators, and physicians now force us to view drug wrecks as accidents in the sense of random Acts of God; events that are incidental to the logic of the therapeutic act. Except they are not rare or incidental. Just as erotic attraction is more promiscuous than any effort to confine it within the framework of marriage, so drugs cannot be confined. Their other effects are more common than their officially sanctioned effects. With Gene Wrecks, we risk finding that Hell has yet another Circle.

Short of finding a desert island, we cannot do without technique. Every technique, however, will compound our dilemmas unless the values of science and Care trump a commitment to algorithms. We need a sustainable HealthCare, not more and more health services.

Who then is to keep us safe on the Big Dipper we are now riding where the drops seem to be getting ever steeper? Doctors are probably still most people's answer.

HealthCarers?

When the medical model emerged around 1800, the religious who had previously cared for the sick and dying were concerned that the brash newcomers, eager to remove religion from health, would lose sight of the most personal and magical of functions—the need to heal.

Before the French Revolution, doctors had been learned gentlemen. After 1800, responding to a development of medical technique, they became liberal professionals. Fifty years later the first shoots of academic medicine appeared in Germany. With Bismarck's co-option of medicine for the establishment, academic doctors gradually became medical bishops and cardinals, ceasing to be the radical bearers of a new faith they had been in 1789 and 1848.

We resist the artificiality of the medical technique that developed after 1800. The romantic streak in all of us would prefer healing to be natural, a restoration of harmony. Any mention that medicine involves poisoning and mutilation draws a hostile response from all sides. We hope that something like a personalized medicine, perhaps linked to human genome research, will allow medicine to return to or advance to its natural roots. But we are always likely to need to insert plates or produce compensatory disturbances in bodily systems to counter abnormalities, even after we fully understand biology. Remedying the troubles toxins and drugs cause will always require a hard-headed belief in science and support for technical developments.

The curative techniques the medical model fostered were applied within a universe of medical care that viewed disease, whether linked to genes, germs, injuries, toxins, or drugs as limiting lives. Good medical and nursing care recognized these limitations and embraced technologies from prostheses to medications as part of the effort to adapt.

Drug and device marketing in contrast portrays people with diabetes, depression, even dementia, as restorable to an Edenic state. These romantic fictions block a recognition of the limitations of our current treatments, the difficulties they bring in their wake, and the need to keep seeking and adapting. Key to care is the act of assisting someone to live the life they want to live and take the risks they want to take. It is a failure of care if a person in treatment becomes invisible, is neglected, or is viewed as a consumer.

The usual translation of the Hippocratic Oath as *First Do no Harm* is incompatible with this medicine. If applied there would be no anesthesia. Lasagna rewrote the Hippocratic Oath, stressing that the duty to save lives meant that First Do no Harm cannot mean *First Take no Risks*. In context, the original Greek is better translated as *Don't make Things Worse*.

Key to not making things worse is engaging with a person. Traditional medical diagnoses involved engagement. Diagnosis by numbers in contrast is a superficial encounter, aimed at reducing risks to a health service. This is driving our central loss, a loss of trust. Ironically, this seems to lead us, particularly in America, to seek ever more tests in an effort to establish a beachhead in the system.

Restoring care, trust, and morale requires a reversal of the partialism driven by treatment by algorithm. For a century, generalists have been pilloried as bringing up the medical rearguard. Given there is more cholesterol in our brains than blood and more serotonin in our gut than brains, however, working out what exposure to statins, antidepressants, or the chemicals around us could cause requires knowing the whole body, not just a bit of it.

Pulling back to 'medicine' should not be rebranded as pulling back to clinical science. Healthcare needs to be Relationship Based before being Evidence Based. Wisdom is at the heart of what a healer rather than a technician brings. The wisdom needed to get a benefit from poisons and mutilations. The wisdom to know when not to screen, so patients don't get sucked under by the rip currents from tests. The humanity to know when to chat to someone off the record without billing. A wisdom to recognize that efficacy has limits and care may mean helping someone to realize what they most value. Wisdom seems a more appropriate word than expertise, which leans in the direction of a one-dimensional technical proficiency. Most doctors, however, buy into the image of expertise, and trusting their own good intentions, cannot see unmet medical need as anything other than Christmas.

Physicians, who can overcome the bias that prevents them seeing drug wrecks, may be better placed than a robot to tease out distinctions between depressive and drug-induced suicidality, for instance. A doctor who listens seems more likely than a robot to be able to mobilize several hundred free research assistants, making the job more fun than a technician's and less lonely than an expert's.

Getting this right requires continuity of care. If being on 5 or more drugs is a hazard, then consulting 3 or more partialists is too. We need to de-partialize as well as de-prescribe. But there is no point replacing partialists with generalists, if at every visit we see a different person.

HealthCare is about healing, which is more than saving lives or managing us. Drug wrecks cause fear, bewilderment, and seething anger. Someone needs to engage with this. Needs to be able to undo a numbness and help us feel again, rather than numb us further with drugs. The word recovery, popular within mental health, refers to a restoration of person-hood rather than the cure of an illness. It is another word for healing. It comes from the bottom up rather than the top down and takes place in relationships.

This healing act needs to be embedded in a system. A re-energized Family Medicine in either a National Health System or a Multinational

Medical Company (MMC) with managers committed to HealthCare rather than health service goals might do it. The economic offer would be to enhance productivity by treating medical disorders (not risks) such that the service paid for itself, even if some grey areas were included. It would also offer advice on what interventions to leave to a cosmetic market or politics. Family Medicine, however, is rapidly being Walmartized, and the option of making it Great Again will not exist for long. Britain's NHS has ceased to exist, other than as a brand. An MMC is a fanciful notion.

Seeing neo-medicalism at close quarters, doctors should be better placed than anyone to understand and grapple with neo-liberalism, but the emerging medical generation complains they have no home within current health systems, and don't appear to understand why not. They shrink from drug wrecks, the one thing that would call on all their training but would also call for courage. They need to decide whether to hang on to the prescription-only privileges that have transformed so many of their predecessors into model (shrunken replicas of the real thing) doctors.

As things stand, prescription only arrangements primarily help companies. Many over the counter serotonin reuptake inhibiting antihistamines can agitate takers and cause suicide or aggression. Uninhibited by our doctors telling us we must continue them, however, we stop these 'SSRIs' if we don't feel right. By checking our natural instincts, doctors regularly make drugs more dangerous for us and more profitable for companies and are blind to their role in this dynamic. Do they dare abandon prescription privileges on the basis that if they really have something to offer, people will not go elsewhere? Or do they have the courage or organization to use their current control of prescribing to get access to RCT data?

In being willing to prescribe drugs for which the data is not available, doctors have let us and themselves down. In portraying themselves as scientists they have been living a lie. In advocating for more services, they compound our dilemmas. In forcing cures on us, they get in the way of healing. Will their new status as vassals (rule-takers) in health services lead them to revolt? The betting must be that some doctors will survive as managers but medicine as a profession will fail to rise to the challenge posed by our falling life expectancies. Doctors will drift and, taken by the currents out to sea, will perish.

DECERNIMUS ERGO SUMMUS

In 1848 Marx, struggling with a transition to liberalism, could turn to philosophers like Fichte and Hegel to provide a framework against which the events of the day could be set. There are few philosophers with anything worth saying about our health dilemmas now other than some feminist philosophers.

In 1968 Foucault, struggling with a transition to neoliberalism, turned to the history of medicine. Historians poured into the breach he opened up. But even though drugs like Valium, Viagra and Vioxx now book-end history in the way Wars once did, historians claim it is no longer possible to write history in a biomedical era.

Drug wrecks should offer social scientists a window on how knowledge is forged today, but social scientists seem not just to have been side-lined by RCTs but colonized by them with the 2015 and 2019 Nobel Prizes in Economics awarded for work on RCTs.

We face a behemoth. The interlocking pharmaceutical and health service industries form a complex like the automobile, oil, plastics, and urban development complex. Up to 20% of our jobs now depend on health services/pharma. Where there was once a divide between business and medicine, health services are now the paradigmatic business.

From 1880, socialism and consumerism helped the economy grow. A socialist option applied to health, deprescribing and departialising, would also transform the economy. Aligning with things that work makes sense. There is no sense in aligning with a Fake literature, the greatest earthly concentration of which centers on our medicines.

Drugs however are now a quintessential consumer item. From 1848 to 1962 the center of gravity in capitalism, socialism, and medicine lay in production rather than consumption. In saving lives and reducing disability, the traditional medical act was productive. We will always need drugs that in saving lives and remedying disabilities increase human and social capital. Pharmaceuticalization does not do this. The flow of drugs we need has become a trickle and the relationships that produced health, sometimes using drugs, are not what they once were. All too often they fuel a health destroying consumption.

Before 2010 social media looked like enhancing key relationships and empowering a new health productivity. Now colonized by industry, they have become vehicles for consumption, with health the most commonly accessed domain on the web after pornography.

Drug wrecks offer another site for production. Finding out what underpins a condition like Post-SSRI Sexual Dysfunction (PSSD) would dramatically enhance our ability to produce novel drugs whose effects endure long after short courses of treatment.

It would likely also transform our understanding of ourselves. PSSD appears to be located on our sensory border, the interface between ourselves and the world. We mistakenly think of our brains as the interface. We know little more about this mysterious border than we did a century ago. Exploring it has the potential to re-orient our sense of what it means to be human as much as the exploration of the heart and the brain by Harvey and Willis once did.

While discoveries triggered by drug wrecks, the stones the builders have rejected, offer one of the best chances not just to find new drugs but to build a new dwelling place, these will be born into a world enmeshed in processes that tolerate a Fake literature. Parties of both Left and Right have tolerated this for decades. Do we need Green or other parties, likely with a strong feminist input, not enmeshed in the Faustian bargain with technology that has brought us to this point?

We Get on the Train

Those of us with aplastic anemia on an antibiotic, a DVT on a contraceptive, or a fractured femur on a bisphosphonate are no more singled out than troops sent over the top in the Battle of the Somme. We should never have been put in this position. Just as socialists and feminists, however, were surprised that women and workers didn't unite to stop the carnage of War, many of us now disabled by treatment go on supporting the consumption of fake medicines. We get on the train hoping that keeping to the rules will deliver us, that someone somewhere will recognize a mistake has been made, an 'accident' has happened, before it is too late. We perish because the System can depend on us to hand over responsibility to it.

In the face of calamities, efforts to get us to realize that black or white, female or male, rich or poor, we are the same under the skin, are only partially successful. We seem less likely to overcome an even more primitive division into the fortunate and unfortunate. This is what AIDS activists achieved, and we who are marooned by drug wrecks need.

AIDS activism demonstrated that the appearance of establishment expertise can hinge on keeping us isolated. The death threat that was AIDS forged communities and kindled a motivation that fractured the wall of expertise. Many drug wreck castaways have as much motivation as anyone with AIDS. But can they become a community? At present, Pharma is supremely good at co-opting the families of those who have died on its drugs into patient advocacy groups to lobby for more of the same drugs.

Emigration isn't an option. Guerrilla resistance is all that remains. Being a guerilla doesn't take Nobel Prize winning brains. The insight on what drugs do that led Arvid Carlsson to create the SSRIs was identical to Anne-Marie's insight that her SSRI was making her alcoholic. The activists behind the AIDs movement like Anne-Marie schooled themselves in things they previously knew nothing about when circumstances called for it. But it will take guts. Do we sign off with a 'we who are drug-wrecked, salute you' or do we fight?

Companies have created a situation where they want us to boycott them. They do not want us to speak to them or have anything to do with them other than take their pills. This calls for a Reverse Boycott, an extreme reporting of drug wrecks with our names attached. Extreme reporting of drug wrecks is a better way to discover new drugs than current company methods. It might also shed more light on who we are, the biological differences between us. In so doing, it might open up new perspectives on our religious or political impulses or tendencies to buck or adhere to Systems, which may be the same thing.

The sacraments and indulgences on offer from our health services face us with a challenge similar to the one Martin Luther faced in 1517. He was up against the powers that controlled access to salvation who were selling indulgences as a way to better and perhaps extended life. The argument was Fake, but dissent was perilous, unsupported by anything other than "Here I stand I can do no other." Standing up to be counted fractured a world order.

Two centuries later, the Enlightenment aimed at a new world order grounded in everyone deciding for themselves rather than handing over responsibility to a System. This was a political challenge to a hierarchy, a patriarchy, that previously reserved discretion to itself.

Two centuries later again, in an effort to strengthen the *Volk*, German doctors began to eliminate the mentally ill and mentally handicapped (before they eliminated anyone else). While some of us, at the time, saw the need to visit our children or other family members in hospital in order to keep them alive, many of us wrote letters thanking the physicians, some of whom were conscientious churchgoers like Hans Asperger, for these merciful releases.

After the fact, and from the comfort of armchairs, those of us not faced with these dilemmas can react with horror. We assume nothing like this could happen again, but ultrasound scans now face women with the logic of the test—take a bisphosphonate, or a statin, eliminate a fetus. The ability to edit our genomes or those of our children will soon pressure us further. Having a hierarchy (management) reserve discretion to itself and decide for us, as it increasingly does, offers comforts. Crusoe, we say, was rescued.

Judgment Day

When Crusoe returned to the island, he was pleased to find that making the mutineers property owners transformed them into responsible citizens. Defoe took a stab in the dark endorsing property owning as a solution to this world's ills, two centuries before Weber drew attention to the consequences of the systems needed to make property owning democracy work. It was two hundred and twenty years before modernity proper took shape, and two hundred and forty years before a French drug in German hands became an exemplar of the banality of evil.

Since Defoe, Turgot, Smith, Marx, Friedman, Foucault and others have offered trade, production, monetary technique and biopower as the source of progress and wealth.

Capitalization now faces a push-back from Gaia, Providence's latest incarnation. Even before our oceans rise, they are filling with plastic, while insect populations are dropping like flies, portents that technique can generate both wealth and destruction. We have landed on an island ringed by dangerous rent-seeking currents on the one side and impersonal policy on the other. Is there a way off?

Full AI, Full Technique, will be a point of peril beyond anything encountered previously. Before we reach that point, the tentacles of social media companies increasingly touch everything we do. Their systems, which build associations as Locke proposed, and Pavlov developed, reinforced with rewards as Bain suggested, and Skinner developed, enable them to predict and shape ever more of our behavior. But they do not diagnose or come to a verdict. They operate one-dimensionally, with the thermostat set to maximize revenue (seek rent) or to provide surveillance (iron cage) beyond managements wildest dreams.

While social media can surveil us, shape our behavior and create dis-ease, our diseases and drug wrecks force diagnosis on us because, as Pinel realized, no amount of nudging by the right associations cures diseases or drug wrecks. In forcing judgment calls on us, our diseases and drug wrecks might restore our humanity.

We clearly benefit from techniques. No-one would want to return to 1789, or even 1962. But, as with anesthesia, any technique involves doing evil in order to do good. Evil in this sense means an absence of good. This evil is an indifference in lieu of care, rather than a demonic or personal evil. If our use of technique is going to enhance rather than diminish us, if we are to bring good out of evil, we need to keep our responsibilities to others in mind.

For HealthCare to be more economic than health services, it must be more than an artisanal version of the services delivered by a health industry. Anything else will be a frivolity for the wealthy rather than something to take seriously.

What might Care do that services don't? Care sees people and our role in making each other. Hinging on an algorithmic loop, in contrast, services hypnotize rather than awaken. This is seen most clearly with drug wrecks, where the thermostat over-rides protests, often adding more of the drug that has caused the problem. Handling drug wrecks requires the kind of judgments made in relationships.

Caring disrupts trances. It happens when we take responsibility for acts in which we make each other and make communities. Drug wrecks challenge our ability to Care. They also point to something else. Unlike Luther's *Credo ergo Sum* and Descartes' *Cogito ergo Sum*, Care cannot be an individual thing. When we bump into things in the Cave we learn by co-operating. Learning hinges on a *Decernimus ergo Summus*—it is in making judgment calls together that We become something other than individuals and something other than a herd that can be stampeded. We face a *Here we stand, we can do no other* moment.

This idea is echoed in the African, "It takes a village to raise a child"and the Zulu, "*Umuntu ngumuntu ngabantu*—a person is a person through other persons."

Relationships are critical to Care. The 1980s morphing of patients into consumers marked a transition from care to services. Becoming consumers suggested we gained rights not to be infantilized. It also marked the start of a progressive atomization that disrupts both care-giving and care-receiving. No-one can be completely self-reliant. We need to recover an ability to accept our dependence on one another.

The wider political expression of this is democratic in the sense of citizens assemblies and co-operatives rather than a property-owning democracy and corporations. Any move that takes us beyond capitalizing intelligibility to celebrating judgment.

William Petty and Josephine Baker hinted at a Pandora hypothesis—that people are the ultimate source of capital. But not in the sense of consumers. The castaways from AIDS navigating the rip tides to their right and left, in setting a course based on the value of people and their right to live the lives they choose to live, flagged up an escape route for all of us.

Robots seem likely to work the land, produce goods, and service us soon. If so, we will need to adjust the rules of our common home (oikos nomos) to distribute our resources to those who literally produce people (payment for labor), turn infants into people who can decide for themselves, make it possible for us to continue being decisive later in life, and treat disease to avoid premature death and disability. Invisible hands have unquestionably played a part in wealth creation up to this but may have less role in future. Even if they have a role, have they created as much wealth or held societies together as much as the decisions made by invisible hearts?

If producing people is the key to whatever wealth might mean once we have Full AI, then treating must be able to recognize when treatments impair us. Albe Watkins and Louis Lasagna were unusual in being male and willing to make drug wreck calls. When it comes to defending children, partners, or parents, women are more likely to take up the warrior role. Companies recognize this and their marketing hinges on appeals to women to 'care' for children, partners, and parents.

Handling drug wrecks is harder now than it was for Watkins or Lasagna. There is neither an evidence base nor clinical expertise to call on. A growing censorship in the midst of apparent freedom, deeply internalized by health service staff to a point where the censorship becomes almost invisible, may make it close to impossible for anyone in health to support anyone our 'services' injure. Yet this support is more necessary than ever. Short of giving birth to a child, this is fast becoming one of the points of maximal social capital generation. If some of us can find a way to reassert the value of collective judgment in the face of threats of excommunication,

AI might yet support our efforts to keep decency alive. Or put another way, it might thwart the aggression that has driven the evolution of all animal life.

Microbeads of plastic can now be found in pristine Arctic waters, and chemicals in breast milk. These are symbols of our dilemmas. We cannot return to a pristine natural state. We were never not alienated. No revolution will ever produce a state of permanent authenticity. We will always be caught between life and death, with a need to find, if not something to live for great enough to die for, something beyond a brand.

After 1848, our families, tribes, or clans, which had provided the networks in which these needs were met, gave way to class and nation. If humanity is not now the group that attracts our allegiance, two World Wars suggest many of us face extermination and the humanity of all will be diminished.

Exodus

George Oppen described himself "as [one of the] descendants of later immigrants… who found refuge in the tenements of these shores from political and financial shipwreck." Despite being well-placed, 34 years old, and with a military deferment, when the U.S. entered the War, he volunteered to fight. He was in the Ardennes and the Battle of the Bulge, and "stood in emplacements, in mess tents, in hospitals and sheds, and hid in the gullies on blasted roads in a ruined country beside many men more capable than I—Muykut and a sergeant named Healy…" He got a Purple Heart for bravery. His unit liberated the concentration camp at Landsberg am Lech.

After the War was over, unlike Art that could sell for millions, poetry seemed to many like fiddling while Rome burned. There was even less interest in anyone trying to produce a 'good' poem. This pushed him to strip his poetry back to specific rather than abstract words aimed at revealing the world as a scientist would. Aimed at making the reader feel again.

Drug wrecks need the very best descriptions. Good descriptions are highly specific and trigger in others a moment of recognition.

In Landsberg, Auschwitz, Birkenau and other camps, the interned fiddled. They also composed music, which is slowly being rediscovered. While this was happening, a French drug may have first been given. Fourteen years later, given as a hypnotic, it caused previously unimaginable injuries.

The children who survived these injuries, armless and legless, had to solve novel difficulties. Had to learn to negotiate relationships and politics. They had been born to Jewish, Christian and atheist parents some of whom deserted them at birth. Others fighting for justice for their children born with the stigmata of thalidomide flickered briefly in the media.

By the 1990s, the thalidomiders began to join together to get at the truth of what had happened. They are the most extraordinary people. To be in their company is to become aware that having arms or legs in the right place is incidental to what it means to be human. Working together they have opened up human possibilities beyond ordinary comprehension.

After the War, for Oppen there was no turning to Providence or Progress. The world was impenetrable. He stuck with describing events and the people they break or make.

When she was a child I read Exodus
to my daughter
'The Children of Israel…'
Pillar of fire
Pillar of cloud

We stared at the end
into each other's eyes
Where
She said hushed
Were the adults

George Oppen
Exodus

Dedication

Nicholas Dobrik, Mikey Argy, Guy Tweedy and Geoff Adams-Spinks, who have a rare link that ties them together.

Leonie Fennell, Linda Hurcombe, Colleen Bell, Kim Witczak, Heather McCarthy, Dorrit Cato Christensen, Kristina Kaiser, Wendy Dolin, Tim Tobin, Terence Young, Julie and Peter Wood, Ian and Tania Morgan, Neil and Alison Cutland, Brian and Maureen Davy, John Stone, Ariane Denoyel and others who have a common link that ties them together.

Anne-Marie Kelly, Annie Bevan, Johanna Ryan, Katinka Newman, Sally MacGregor, Shane Cooke, Bob Fiddaman, Karen Pritchard and Jack Roberts, Justin Oxley, Frank van Meerendonk, and Lara Merli with yet another link.

The many with PSSD, PGAD, PFS, and PRSD whose suffering is intense, leading some, like David Stofkooper, to take their own lives. Despite this, some have done extraordinary things to help others and all of us. Anonymity is forced on almost all of them by us. Their worse than death fate has changed most of what I think about our bodies.

For some, like James Holmes and David Rule, who have to live with other horrors.

For the tens of thousands of people who have filed drug wreck reports with RxISK in the last decade.

For Billiam James who helped launch Samizdat and for Patrick Hahn, Paul Scott and Jim Gottstein who now sail on her and those who might still board.

For the hundreds of friends and colleagues who have shaped every nook and crevice of this manuscript, whom I hope will add to what is here, even if in disagreement.

Index

A

H

I

About the Author

David Healy is a psychiatrist, psychopharmacologist, scientist, and author. He is now based at the Department of Family Medicine, in Canada's McMaster University. He is a co-founder of RxISK.org, an adverse event reporting website, and the co-founder of Samizdat Health Writer's Co-operative Inc. Healy's research covers treatment-induced problems, and the history of physical treatments in medicine. He has written more than 200 peer-reviewed articles, 200 other articles, and 24 books, including *The Antidepressant Era*, *Let Them Eat Prozac*, and *Pharmageddon*. He is also the co-author of *Children of the Cure*.

www.ingramcontent.com/pod-product-compliance
Lightning Source LLC
Chambersburg PA
CBHW020857060726
47591CB00004B/989